Hatfield's Herbal

The Curious Stories of Britain's Wild Plants

GABRIELLE HATFIELD

PENGUIN BOOKS

*To my husband John, with love and gratitude for all he has
given me – including his name for the title of this book*

PENGUIN BOOKS

Published by the Penguin Group
Penguin Books Ltd, 80 Strand, London WC2R ORL, England
Penguin Group (USA) Inc., 375 Hudson Street, New York, New York 10014, USA
Penguin Group (Canada), 90 Eglinton Avenue East, Suite 700, Toronto, Ontario,
Canada M4P 2Y3 (a division of Pearson Penguin Canada Inc.)
Penguin Ireland, 25 St Stephen's Green, Dublin 2, Ireland
(a division of Penguin Books Ltd)
Penguin Group (Australia), 250 Camberwell Road, Camberwell,
Victoria 3124, Australia (a division of Pearson Australia Group Pty Ltd)
Penguin Books India Pvt Ltd, 11 Community Centre,
Panchsheel Park, New Delhi – 110 017, India
Penguin Group (NZ), 67 Apollo Drive, Rosedale, North Shore 0632,
New Zealand (a division of Pearson New Zealand Ltd)
Penguin Books (South Africa) (Pty) Ltd, 24 Sturdee Avenue,
Rosebank, Johannesburg 2196, South Africa

Penguin Books Ltd, Registered Offices: 80 Strand, London WC2R ORL, England

www.penguin.com

First published 2007
Published in paperback 2009
1

Set in The Antiqua
Typeset by Palimpsest Book Production Limited, Grangemouth, Stirlingshire
Printed in England by Clays Ltd, St Ives plc

ISBN: 978-0-141-02514-8

www.greenpenguin.co.uk

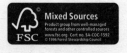

Some writers make their readers feel
Provided with a good square meal,
While others – such a task is mine –
Supply the walnuts and the wine.
A sip of truth – the merest smack,
A pinch of salt, a nut to crack.

Some writers take you by the hand,
And lead you far through Fancy's land,
Through cultured gardens where the soil
Is redolent of care and toil.
My path less formal you will find;
My labour is of humbler kind.
A few wild flowers – by some called weeds –
I pluck from Nature's tangled meads.

Charles E. Benham, *Jottings*

Contents

The illustrator

Frederick Edward Hulme, F.L.S., F.S.A. (1841–1909), came from an artistic family. His father was the landscape painter Frederick William Hulme and his grandmother had been a porcelain painter. He was a keen amateur botanist and in 1869 was made a Fellow of the Linnaean Society. He taught drawing at Marlborough College and later became Professor of Freehand and Geometrical Drawing at King's College London, a post that (very suitably for him) covered both the arts and science faculties. The illustrations used in this book come from his best-known work *Familiar Wild Flowers* (Cassell, Peter & Galpin & Co.), which originally appeared serially, in nine volumes, and was completed just before his death at Kew in 1909.

Introduction

The birds are singing and the wind is blowing in your hair as you push aside the clinging bramble shoots and step carefully over the nettles. Bending under the low branches of a sloe tree, you are into the woods. The young leaves of the silver birch are unfolding and under your hand its pale bark is cool and smooth, peeling in places to show its pink lining. There are ferns clumped around its base, and a single primrose plant, its downy buds just showing lemon cream ...

All these plants are reassuringly familiar, as they must have been for countless generations, and it is all too easy to take familiar things for granted. Stop a moment and look at them again. Chewing those bramble leaves can cure a toothache. Did you know that you don't necessarily need a dock leaf to cure a nettle sting? The juice of the nettle itself can do the trick. Sloe berries are good for an upset gut. Birch wine can help rheumatism and ferns can kill intestinal worms. The primrose yields a cosmetic as well as an ointment for burns. Such ordinary plants – and yet we are in danger of forgetting how powerful so many of them are.

The elder tree can provide us not only with remedies but also with cosmetics, dyes, fencing, insect deterrents and painkillers, not to mention the popguns that children have made for centuries from its tough, hollow stems. So many plants that we regard today simply as nuisances in gardens or agricultural land were once used and respected. The very term of 'weed' is used in a derogatory sense today, but in Anglo-Saxon times *weòd* was the name given to any small plant. The lowly plantain that many of us regard simply as an inconvenience in our lawns can help in healing cuts and soothe insect bites. The list could go on and on; we have found human uses for so many of our native wild plants, but as we have become more and more urbanized, much of this knowledge is being lost.

THE ORIGINS OF HERBAL MEDICINE

When humans first colonized Britain, the surrounding landscape had to provide all their needs since they lived mainly on wild plants, with meat as an occasional variation. Gradually they would have learned, by trial and error, which plants and seeds and berries were good to eat and which were poisonous. The last meal that was eaten by Tollund Man, preserved in a Norwegian bog about two thousand years ago, included fat hen and heartsease. As the forests were cleared and the hunter-gatherer lifestyle gave way to farming, domesticated animals and plants began to supply food, but there would still have been considerable reliance on foodstuffs gathered in the wild to supplement these first crops.

The origin of herbal medicine is unclear, but is highly likely to have been a by-product of the use of plants in other ways. People would notice that a particular leaf used to bind a wound seemed to help it to heal or that a particular berry when chewed eased a headache. First aid was just one of many ways in which wild plants served early man. They provided bedding, fuel, housing, roofing and weapons as well.

As other materials replaced plants for many of these functions, plants still formed the basis of medical remedies until relatively modern times. It has been claimed that the Anglo-Saxons had a greater knowledge of their native plants than any other race, but the written evidence of such knowledge is, literally, fragmentary and consists of frequently incomplete manuscripts.

Meanwhile continental Europe, and in particular Italy, became the seat of medical learning. In the first century AD, Dioscorides, a Greek physician, produced *De Materia Medica*, the first European herbal. His work and that of his Roman counterpart Pliny the Elder was translated into innumerable languages and became the basis of all the later European herbals.

These herbals became increasingly fossilized and inaccurate as they were copied and re-copied through the succeeding centuries. Their illustrations, although of great beauty, were often too stylized for the identities of the plants depicted to be certain, so increasingly the herbals became filled with approximations of plants that the artists had never actually seen. In Britain as on the Continent generally, monks devoted their entire lives to producing the wonderfully illuminated early herbals. Usually their copying from the early classical authorities seems to have been unquestioning, but in the twelfth century an enterprising monk in Bury St Edmunds replaced at least one of the illustrations in the manuscript he was copying. He included instead a plant with which he was more familiar. All these beautiful manuscripts were, of course, accessible only to the few who could read Latin.

Even the earliest printed herbals, which began appearing in the fifteenth century, represent a distillation of the knowledge of mainly classical authorities. Since they were also written in Latin and incomprehensible even to many literate laymen, this immediately set apart the learned practitioners of official medicine from the majority of their patients. The gulf between doctors and the illiterate majority was even wider, but ordinary people continued to use plants for first aid, just as they and their forbears always had. Moreover, they used local plants that were freely available to them, whereas the authors of the printed herbals for the most part still described Mediterranean plants that had been recommended by the Greeks and Romans.

The classical authorities held such a dominant position in medical writing that John Gerard's herbal of 1597, even though it was based on classical texts and largely lifted from an earlier English translation of Rembert Dodoens' *Pemptades*, was revolutionary because it included some plants that actually grew in Britain and which he had seen for himself. Gerard's herbal was novel in another way too: it was written not in Latin but in English and was therefore available to anyone who could read and had access to a copy. However, Gerard, as a member of the Company of Barber Surgeons, was still firmly aligned with the medical profession and had scant regard for any non-professional practice. He does make some condescending references to the practices of the 'common people', and from these we can glean useful information about the popular folk medicine of his day.

The rebel Nicolas Culpeper broke the mould of the English herbals with *The English Physitian*. He had some medical training, having been apprenticed to an apothecary for a while after studying at Cambridge, but he had no time for members of the medical profession (nor they for him). Not only did he write in English but he also included in his book 'such things only as grow in England, they being most fit for English Bodies'. His book became a bestseller. He championed the ordinary people and tried to make his work accessible to them. Even Culpeper's book drew heavily on the classical authorities when he described medicinal applications of the plants. His own firm beliefs in astrology and in the doctrine of signatures further obscured his knowledge of British plant use. However, as with Gerard, we are indebted to Culpeper for recording some folk practices of medicine.

Another of the writers whose work is extensively quoted in this book is John Pechey. He was a more orthodox medical practitioner and a member of London's Royal College of Physicians. He wrote *The Compleat Herbal of Physical Plants* at the end of the seventeenth century in English and clearly intended it for a literate, but non-medical, audience. In his preface, he writes that he hopes his book will be 'serviceable to Families in the Country, that are far distant from Physicians'.

His contemporary William Salmon, although describing himself as 'a Professor of Physick', was a more eccentric character and not a member of the medical faculty. However, his book *The English Physician* draws largely on the same, ancient classical sources used by physicians of the time. In flamboyant style, he declares on the frontispiece that this is 'A Work of exceeding Use to all sorts of men, of what Quality or Profession soever. The like not hitherto extant.'

Generally, it remains true to say that folk practice of medicine in Britain remained largely an oral tradition, handed down by word of mouth through the generations. Today's folk medicine represents the broken fragments of this body of knowledge, mingled by now with input from printed sources.

This herbal attempts to refocus attention on our own native wild plants and to describe the varying ways in which they have been used by ordinary people as well as by health professionals. It is unashamedly a book about British uses of British plants and does not decry the use of worldwide flora, but champions, and encourages further study of, our own largely neglected one.

THE DIFFERENCES BETWEEN FOLK AND OFFICIAL MEDICINE

Although it is impossible to separate out completely the folk tradition of healing from the learned one, the two traditions do seem distinct as far as

Britain is concerned. One obvious way in which folk medicine differs from official medicine is that the former almost entirely uses native plants – those which, as far as we can tell, occur in Britain naturally and have not been brought here by man. Official medicine has drawn on a much wider flora, using many Mediterranean plants described by classical authors and herbs and spices from the Arabic tradition. Another distinction is that folk medicine is primarily an oral tradition, passed on through generations and rarely written down because its practitioners had neither the time nor the skill to do so.

The country names that people gave to the plants around them are as varied as the communities that gave rise to them. East Anglia's 'paigles' are Somerset's 'totsies' and Hertfordshire's 'cowslips'; Scotland's 'bluebell' is England's 'harebell'. The possibilities for confusion are endless. The plurality of common names makes it difficult to be sure, in modern taxonomic terms, exactly which plant species is being described. However, this is not a problem that is confined to folk medicine. The early, printed herbals were largely descriptions of Mediterranean plants that had been used by the Ancients; the authors 'best-guessed' which plant was meant by the Ancients, and sometimes even substituted a local plant. Meanwhile the country people, without access to the written word, continued to use their local native plants and to refer to them by local names. Written records of this unofficial practice were scarce, but occasionally authors of printed books and later of local 'floras' (that listed the plants occurring in a particular area) referred to folk practices. Sometimes ballads and poetry refer to them. The 'kitchen books', notebooks of culinary and medicinal recipes kept by many members of the gentry from the seventeenth century onwards, sometimes provide glimpses of folk practice; here and there is a remedy described to the writer by a servant, a gardener or a local tradesman. But for the most part these collections of medical recipes represent the official medicine of their day.

'Simples', single species of plants used as remedies, are more common in folk medicine. In official medicine, polypharmacy was common – some eighteenth-century herbal preparations contain literally hundreds of ingredients. Venice treacle, a commonly used preparation, is listed in the eighteenth-century pharmacopoeia as containing more than seventy ingredients, and Venice treacle was itself often combined with other medicines. Even where official and folk medicine used the same plant for a given condition, in the former it was often combined with numerous other ingredients to make it more impressive, more costly, more exotic and distinct from what the 'common people' used. In a seventeenth-century manuscript entitled *The Winnowing of White Witchcraft*, a doctor decries the ignorance of the common people. He disparages their willingness to submit themselves to their own practitioners, or 'white witches' as he calls them, who use 'few salves and medicines for manifold maladies'.

Another belief has been much quoted as a symptom of the ignorance of country people – even though it was invented by an official practitioner. The 'doctrine of signatures' was propounded in the sixteenth century by a Swiss doctor, Theophrastus Bombastus von Hohenheim (better known as Paracelsus). It suggests that each plant bears a physical sign, left by its Creator, to indicate for which human illness it should be used. However, the belief was probably based on a much simpler concept: the lesser celandine was good for piles not because it had swollen bulbils (which resembled piles) but the bulbils did provide a useful reminder of the plant's use.

THE SPLIT BETWEEN OFFICIAL AND FOLK MEDICINE

The eighteenth century became a watershed in medicine: official medical practitioners wanted to distance themselves from the earlier, unscientific practice of medicine. They also wished to appear to have something different and exclusive to offer that was far removed from the 'simples' of the common people. Increasingly, exotic plant and animal ingredients appeared in their pharmacopoeias, a trend already criticized by Gerard at the end of the sixteenth century: 'Yet it may be more truly said of phantasticall Physitions, who when they have found an approved medicine and perfect remedy neere home against any disease: yet not content therewith, they will seek a new further off, and by that means many times hurt more than they helpe.'

The almost exclusive use of Latin in prescriptions and books widened the gulf between the learned and the unlearned. The use of minerals was seen as 'scientific' and they were increasingly used in official practice. Blood-letting, purging and administration of mercury were all aspects of official medicine which the poor may have done well to avoid. Even those wealthy enough to afford physicians sometimes resorted to simple home remedies, as an eighteenth-century letter describes: 'When the medicine of Dr Cullen failed, I shall give him garlic in brandy ... I shall engage it will free him of worms and it is attended with no inconvenience, but his breath will perfume the air.'

Simple plant remedies were used less and less in official medicine and, by the nineteenth century when 'active ingredients' began to be isolated in the laboratory, the divorce between herbal medicine and orthodoxy was almost complete.

THE GROWTH OF HERBALISM

It was through herbalists that written plant traditions survived, in so far as they did at all. Throughout the sixteenth century, Parliament passed a series of acts aimed at making peace between the rival physicians, barber surgeons and apothecaries. In effect though, the legislation ensured that the College of Physicians had a near monopoly of medical practice and power also over the apothecaries and barber surgeons. One unforeseen result was that it left a huge proportion of the population without any medical care at all because they were too poor to afford physicians' fees. Parliament therefore passed yet another act, allowing any of His Majesty King Henry VIII's subjects who had knowledge of herbs to practise herbal medicine for a wide range of ailments. This act was the single most important factor in ensuring the survival of herbalism.

Rivalry between official practitioners and unofficial herbalists in Britain continued unabated. Meanwhile settlers in North America had discovered a wealth of herbs used by Native Americans and the medical practice that began to develop in North America incorporated many of these herbs, as well as the domestic medicines brought from Britain and elsewhere by the settlers.

In the eighteenth century, Samuel Thomson (1769–1843), a farmer's son from New Hampshire, set up as a herbal practitioner. Despite continued persecution from official doctors, his practice survived and his ideas were imported into Britain in the nineteenth century and became the forerunners of today's medical herbalism in this country. This is the reason that our present-day medical herbalists use many North American, rather than solely native British, plants.

In-fighting between the exponents of botanical medicine, as well as bitter rivalry with the orthodox medical profession, continued well into the nineteenth century and culminated in the Medical Reform Bill of 1852, which attempted to outlaw the practice of herbal medicine. Such was the popular outcry against this act that it was defeated and herbalism struggled on. Its survival was aided by the shortage of imported drugs during the First World War and in 1927 the Society of Herbalists (now called the Herb Society) was formed.

There followed decades of wrangling between the herbalists and Parliament, but from these fraught years there eventually emerged the modern British Herbal Medicine Association, which provided far more rigorous, scientific training. Today the National Institute of Medical Herbalists provides a thorough grounding for its students in many medical disciplines and produces the official *British Herbal Pharmacopoeia*, which ensures the high quality of its practice.

In Britain today, there are three strands to medical practice: official medicine, using mostly modern drugs that are no longer derived from plants; official herbalism, which uses some of our native plants and many others as well; and folk medicine, now largely vestigial, and existing largely in forgotten books and in the minds of relatively few, elderly country people. In this book, I have focused on some individual plants that are native to Britain and tried to show how they have been used in these three separate traditions.

Folk medicine has come in for a lot of scorn and has often been grossly misrepresented. To redress the balance, I have attempted to show that at least some of the valuable medicines currently in use owe their discoveries to folk medicine. So-called 'alternative medicine' in Britain today is a real hotchpotch of sense and nonsense drawn from many continents and cultures. Such remedies can be worthless or even harmful if taken out of context. The preferred term of 'complementary medicine' implies that the best from all the different branches of healing may be brought together, but we need first to disentangle some of the threads in order to evaluate the individual remedies.

Obviously modern medicine is here to stay, but it is increasingly clear that we have not yet learned all that we can and should about the potential of our own common-or-garden plants. It is said that the inventor of Velcro was inspired by burdock's hooked bracts, which stick to anything and anyone they come into contact with – we need to look at our other native plants with as fresh an eye. The untapped natural treasures of the plants of the rainforests now form a familiar story, but here on our very doorstep are humble native plants that are as yet unstudied and unappreciated.

Some of these will almost certainly prove valuable in the future. Even a plant as common as the dock has yet to be thoroughly investigated scientifically. Yet I know from personal experience how valuable a dock leaf can be in binding a bleeding cut. Likewise a plantain leaf quickly rubbed on a horse-fly bite can prevent the swelling and irritation completely. Tansy juice rubbed on the skin deters midges. A fresh leaf of peppermint chewed for indigestion is as effective as any bought remedy and chewing one single fresh leaf of yarrow reduces the severity of a heavy period. These are small examples drawn from my own experience; there are countless others.

COLLECTING FOLK REMEDIES

Folk medicine is primarily an oral tradition, so how can we find out about it? Some historical records are to be found in manuscripts and printed books, in the herbals and floras, in poetry and literature. In addition to these sources, the living memories of those who have used such remedies in their childhood form a gold-mine of information. The last generation of country people who have actual experience of using the remedies is now very elderly and, in many cases, their knowledge has not been written down nor has it been passed on to a younger generation. The reasons for this are various. It is very striking that many elderly country people disclaim all knowledge of 'herbal remedies' but, if asked what their grandmothers did for them when they were ill, will often tell of plant remedies that they regarded just as part of ordinary life – things that 'everybody knew'. Alas, this is no longer common knowledge and it is of urgent importance that the remaining body of knowledge of folk medicine is not lost.

In my own studies, I have spoken and written to many individuals in my quest for information. Actually finding people who have such knowledge is in itself a challenge. Articles in local newspapers and local radio programmes have been very helpful. But most useful of all has been the proverbial 'leaning on gates' approach, simply striking up a conversation with someone who has lived in the country all his or her life. Time and again, I have been told, 'You should have spoken to old Mrs X/Mr Y. She/he knew all about the plants and what the old folk used them for. But she/he died last year.'

When I have been lucky enough to meet someone who possesses a fund of knowledge, the next challenge has been to record the information. Best practice in oral history is to record interviews. In reality, this is often not easy to achieve. Fired with enthusiasm by a seminar in oral history, I set out one day to 'interview' an old man who had worked all his life with shire horses. I approached and knocked on the door, tape-recorder in hand, but couldn't make myself heard above the noise of barking. Eventually the door opened, just a crack. When I went in, the dog continued to bark, there was a clock with a very loud tick and the man whom I had come to see had a dreadful-sounding cough. I shamefacedly hid the tape-recorder, sat down and listened.

THE FUTURE OF PLANT REMEDIES

What I have found in my own small studies has imbued in me a sense of urgency: this part of our heritage is on the brink of extinction. Together with other, like-minded people, many of them botanists and herbalists, I belong to a group called Ethnomedica, which has come into being in order to record plant remedies used within living memory. Readers are very welcome to contribute memories of any plant remedies that they have used to Ethnomedica's growing database (www.rbgkew.org.uk/ethnomedica), based at the Royal Botanic Gardens, Kew. This mass of information should become an invaluable tool for future research.

It is, at last, becoming recognized that man's usage of plants may be viewed as a long-standing clinical trial; remedies that have stood the test of time are likely to be worth further investigation. One might argue that such remembered remedies are more likely to be effective than the copied, re-copied and garbled versions of early medical practice that have survived in the literature.

One remedy, described to me by a Norfolk lady who has since died, has been the subject of pharmacological studies at Kew and its mode of action is now beginning to be understood. The next challenge is to gather sufficient clinical evidence of its efficacy to persuade the medical profession to adopt it. For this to happen we need a whole new mind-set.

We need to rid ourselves of the idea that a single 'active ingredient' must be the holy grail of plant medicine, since it is now becoming increasingly clear that the vastly complex chemistry of a plant means that an extract of the whole plant acts very differently on the human body from any single ingredient taken from the plant. As we learn more about plant chemistry, we are also beginning better to appreciate that the distinction between food and medicine is a largely artificial one. Every week the press has stories that concern the health-giving properties of some of our ordinary fruits, seeds and vegetables. We need to combine our knowledge of modern technology and science with the simpler attitude of our forbears, who knew by trial and error which plants were good for them.

In the pages that follow, I have chosen to include all kinds of facts about the 185 plants described and not to limit myself to their purely medicinal uses. In this I am in good company. Turn to the sixteenth- and seventeenth-century herbalists such as Gerard and Pechey and you will find evocative descriptions alongside information about the plants' other uses. Modern science has added an extra dimension: the historical uses and mythology of a plant can now often be explained in the light of recent discoveries. For instance, hawthorn flowers have long been regarded as having a deathlike smell and thus as extremely unlucky indoors – analysis has shown that they contain trimethylamine, one of the first products of putrefaction.

I have tried to describe the qualities of some of my favourite native plants, but there is so much more to be said about all of them that this can serve only as the briefest of introductions. I hope that it will whet the reader's appetite to find out more. My entries are full of quotations from other people's work and recorded knowledge, from poets and botanists to farriers and farmers. The best way I can thank all these people is to share their insights with you.

Farewell, deare flowers, sweetly your time ye spent,
Fit, while ye liv'd, for smell or ornament,
                    And after death for cures.

George Herbert, *Life* (1633)

Acknowledgements

I would like to extend my heartfelt thanks to the numerous people who have contributed to this book. Jennifer Westwood first suggested the idea and was instrumental in introducing me to Penguin. Over the years, she and other members of the Folklore Society have been immensely supportive and encouraging. The individuals who have shared their knowledge with me also over many years are too numerous to name here; I thank them all. The staff at Penguin have been unfailingly kind and helpful. Georgina Laycock has nurtured the project and I am very grateful for her unwavering support and enthusiasm. The editorial staff have done their utmost to ensure accuracy in the text; any faults remaining must be mine.

Finally, I would like to thank Roy Vickery for allowing me to use the bistort recipe, Grace Corne for the quotation from *Flora, Facts and Fables*, and Dr David Allen for allowing me to refer repeatedly to the book that we wrote together.

The author and editor have made every effort to contact all copyright holders but are, of course, delighted to receive any emendations.

Hatfield's Herbal

Agrimony
(*Agrimonia eupatoria*)

Agrimony was once a common sight in our pastures and verges but, like many of our wild flowers, its numbers have dwindled with increasing urbanization, pollution and use of pesticides. When stumbled upon, what a striking plant it is. It has pinnate leaves resembling those of MEADOWSWEET, except that agrimony leaves are more slender. In early midsummer, it produces a single, slender spire of bright yellow flowers; in honour of this, one of its descriptive country names is 'church steeple'.

The flowers are succeeded by small, bristly fruit of very characteristic shapes, like little spinning tops in motion. The bristles readily stick to animal fur and people's clothes, thus earning the plant another name, 'sweethearts'. The herb has aromatic qualities too: the smell of the flowers has been likened to that of apricots, and the leaves are lightly fragrant when crushed. The plant used to be hung indoors, in bunches, as an air-freshener.

In the past, the plant was regarded as powerfully magical. Its older country names include 'fairy's wand'. In the Scottish island of Arran in 1716, a Ferquhar Ferguson was tried for witchcraft and admitted using agrimony to cure people who were 'elf-shot', that is to say, suffering from an unexplained illness. Perhaps there is no connection but agrimony was also believed to promote sleep, a tradition that persisted until the sixteenth century.

> If it be leyd under mann's heed,
> He shal sleepyn as he were deed;
> He shal never drede ne wakyn
> Till fro under his heed it be takyn.

Old English medical manuscript

Agrimony has been used to cure a multitude of ills. In Saxon times, the plant was recommended as a good treatment for wounds and sore eyes. The Greeks also believed in its usefulness to the eyes, and thought that it made them bright and shining. The plant was originally named *argemone* by the Greeks. In Chaucer's time, *egrimoyne* was used as a wound-healer. Official medicine recommended it especially for jaundice and for kidney trouble. Gerard describes agrimony in 1597 as 'good for them that have naughtie livers' and Salmon too, in 1693, promotes the herb as a liver-strengthener, but also as a wound-healer and as good for coughs. In addition, the juice 'is diuretick, and causes one to piss clear'. A recipe in an eighteenth-century, East Anglian kitchen book suggested using dried agrimony 'as much as will lye upon a shilling' to help those that cannot hold their water, and recommended it steeped in ale to treat rickets in children.

Kemsey in 1838 recommends the plant for cleansing the liver and other vital parts and also reveals that: 'the green herb (or a less quantity of the dry) well beaten, and boiled with an equal quantity of hog's lard, is good for old sores, cancers and inveterate ulcers, and draws forth thorny splinters of wood, or any such things, from the flesh, if outwardly applied.' In this, he is repeating Culpeper's information from two centuries earlier.

Medical herbalism also used agrimony. A twentieth-century anonymous pamphlet from Yorkshire recommends for despondency equal parts of agrimony and rosemary made into tea. Present-day medical herbalists use the plant as a digestive and a wound-healer, as well as a diuretic for cystitis and incontinence.

What about those who had access neither to official medicine nor herbalism, the 'folk' of folk medicine? They used agrimony too, but we have few written records of their uses, a pattern that applies to nearly all the plants in this book. We do know that it was formerly used in folk medicine to treat burns and wounds, diabetes, dropsy, kidney and liver complaints, as well as rheumatic complaints; agrimony ointment was used to treat ulcers and wounds in horses and cattle. In the form of a 'tea' it was still a popular tonic in the mid-twentieth century, given to keep the complexion clear and the eyes bright, according to Mary Thorne Quelch in 1946.

It was once a principal ingredient in home-brewed whisky, and wine is still made from it today. Its Somerset name of 'tea-plant' suggests that it may have been drunk in that county as a tea substitute, as it still is today in France.

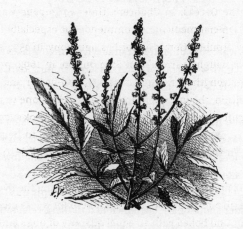

Alder

(*Alnus glutinosa*)

The alder grows where few other trees can survive, fringing lakes and streams, and can flourish both in and out of water. Its large, shining, dark green leaves and its surprisingly delicate, cone-like fruit make it a very ornamental tree. In Derbyshire, the decorative qualities of the fruit (known there as 'black knobs') have been put to good use in traditional well-dressing ceremonies. Well-dressing was once a widespread activity in the days when people relied absolutely on a local source of water, of which the constant flow could never be taken for granted. In gratitude, once a year, wells would be decorated with flowers, or floral tableaux would be created, and it seems most apt that the water-loving alder should have been included in these celebrations.

It is its timber, however, that has made the alder so invaluable in Britain as a source of fuel, building material and fencing. Because it is impervious to moisture, the wood is slow to rot, which makes it particularly suitable for immersion in water. Alder has been used for shoring up riverbanks, especially in the Norfolk Broads, and the famous, Scottish Iron-Age loch houses – crannogs – were built of alder wood. Venice was practically built on alder. The wood underpins, for example, the famous Rialto Bridge over the Grand Canal. In more recent times, alder was used to make the clogs worn by the mill-workers of the industrial North. It is still used today, in Scotland, in the manufacturing of garden furniture.

Some superstitions surround the alder tree: in Scottish folklore, the alder, or 'aller tree', was regarded as sacred and a sanctuary for lovers and outlaws. In Ireland, in particular, cutting the tree is regarded as unlucky. This superstition sprang from the fact that the wood when first cut is white but changes to a startlingly bright reddish-orange that is suggestive of blood. And so the tree cannot be cut because it 'bleeds'.

In folk medicine, alder leaves have served as a comforting dressing on minor burns and been placed in shoes to avoid soreness on long walks. A decoction of the twigs was used to treat gout and, in Scotland, alder was used as a gargle and a treatment for green wounds and ulcers. An early nineteenth-century horseman had this recipe for 'Stoping the Wind':

> A Quart of Milk, 2 handfuls of the inside bark of Alder and cut it fine – pint of honey. Boil the bark in the milk and put the Honey in after it Boiles give him no water after it.

In official medicine, alder was used to treat a variety of complaints. Culpeper in 1653 recommends alder for burns and inflammation but finds an additional use – the leaves attract fleas so may be scattered on the floor and then swept away, together with the offending creatures. A hundred years later, alder was still being used in the war against fleas. Sir John Cullum made a note in his own copy of his *Flora Anglica* (1762) that carrying alder wood protected the bearer against them. Later in the century we learn that alder leaves were rubbed on horses to repel flies.

John Pechey in 1694 vividly describes the leaves as 'indented, green, shining, and clammy' and 'being put into Travellers Shooes, they ease Pain, and remove Weariness'. Parson Woodforde, in his diary entry for 7 March 1767, records how: 'I have taken for these last three mornings one hour before breakfast the second Rind of Alder stick steeped in Water and I do really think that I have found great benefit from it half a Pint each morning; it must be near the colour of Claret Wine. N.B. Very good to take every Spring and Fall.'

In modern medical herbalism, the commonest use for alder is as a gargle and mouthwash.

Other uses for alder have varied – as a source of charcoal for gunpowder, for example. The bark, twigs, catkins, wood chippings and leaves have all yielded dyes of various colours, including green, brown, pink and black. Both bark and leaves have been used to tan leather and the bark was an essential ingredient in the preserving of nets and cordage. In Hereford the alder is called 'aul' and there exists a useful proverb for the county's fishermen:

> When the bud of the aul is as big as the trout's eye,
> Then that fish is in season in the river Wye.

quoted Britten and Holland, *A Dictionary of English Plant Names* (1886)

Alexanders
(*Smyrnium olusatrum*)

Since the introduction of Celery into the garden, the Alexanders is almost forgotten ... It is a warm comfortable plant to a cold weak stomach.

Charles Bryant, *Flora Dietetica* (1783)

This is a Mediterranean plant, now naturalized throughout the British Isles. Its bright green, celery-like leaves and umbels of greenish-yellow flowers have a pungent smell that is reminiscent of myrrh. It is especially common around the coast and on the sites of ancient monasteries, where it was grown specifically for the monks' dinner table.

Alexanders was a potherb, that is, it was used in cooking as seasoning or eaten as a vegetable; one of its alternative names is 'black potherb'. This name originates from the fact that the seeds when ripe are black, ridged and have a sharply spicy smell. The young shoots, before flowering, were steamed and eaten like spinach, but were sometimes earthed up in the same way as celery and blanched. Parkinson in 1629 described other culinary uses: 'The tops of the rootes, with the lower part of the stalkes of Alisanders, are used in Lent especially, and Spring of the yeare, to make broth, which although it be a little bitter, yet it is both wholesome, and pleasing to a great many, by reason of the aromaticall or spicie taste, warming and comforting the stomack, and helping it digest the many waterish and flegmaticke meates [which] are in those times much eaten. The rootes also either rawe or boyled are often eaten with oyle and vinegar.'

In folk medicine, alexanders was valued as an aid to health generally, particularly by sailors, and Quelch in *Herbs for Daily Use* (1941) reported that: 'stories were told of crews being allowed to go ashore at Anglesea that they might gather and cook the herb'. In Dorset, the plant was known as 'helrut', thought to be a corruption of 'health-root'. Alexanders was used in the Isle of Man to treat toothache in humans and mouth sores in cattle. In the Hebrides in the eighteenth century, Martin recorded that a broth made from lovage and alexanders was 'found by experience to be good against Consumptions'.

In official medicine, Culpeper in 1653 recommended alexanders for warming a cold stomach, to 'move women's courses, to expel the afterbirth, to break wind, to provoke urine, and help the stranguary [painful urination]'. Pechey in 1694 advocated it for strengthening the stomach and cleansing the blood. Moncrief in his eighteenth-century *Poor Man's Physician* recommends the seed of *Smyrnium* for febrile convulsions; others found them to be a carminative (remedy for flatulence) and a stimulant. During that period, in Covent Garden Market the plant was called 'Horse-Parsley' and the root was sold for boiling in water as a cure for the gravel (small urinary stones).

By the mid-nineteenth century, the plant had fallen from use and subsequent herbalists have paid it little attention. Today's medical herbalists do not use the plant. Now it grows in unharvested abundance along field edges and beside ruins, its presence a dim reminder of the sites of earlier monastic kitchen gardens.

Ash

(*Fraxinus excelsior*)

An even-leaved ash,
And a four-leaved clover,
You'll see your true love
'Fore the day is over.

quoted James Mason, 'The Folk-lore of British Plants',
Dublin University Magazine (1873), vol. 82

The ash tree has been held sacred in many cultures including our own. In Norse mythology, the first man was said to have been carved from ash wood. The ash is still regarded as a source of divine food and strength. In Scotland, it was traditional for the midwife to give ash sap as its first food to a newborn baby to ensure that the child would be protected from witchcraft and have a long and healthy life. The sap was obtained by placing one end of an ash twig in the fire; the sap that bubbled out of the other end was collected on a spoon. This method of collecting the sap, in use since Saxon times, was still current in parts of Britain as recently as the mid-twentieth century. The technique was identical; the use that was made of the sap however was rather different – it was dripped into the ear to treat earache.

> 'My grandfather ... would gather a bundle of green ash saplings, about half a metre in length, one end of which he would place in the fire. From the other end he would collect the liquid which fell drop by drop into a container. He would then pour the liquid into a bottle with a dropper to use when necessary, having placed the bottle in a warm place before use.'

Mrs M. B—, Lancashire (2002)

Native Americans use an identical remedy for earache, although they use a different species of ash.

Superstition in abundance surrounds this tree. The ash leaf was used in love divination, in a very specific way. Usually the compound ash leaf has a terminal leaflet; if it lacks this, then it is an even leaf; a girl carrying one was likely to meet her true love, as the Devonian rhyme (see top of this entry) implies. In the same county, ash seeds were said to have aphrodisiac properties. They are still today occasionally pickled or added to a salad.

The entire tree was once believed to have curative powers. At one time, many people believed that shrews could cause lameness or paralysis in humans and animals by scampering over their bodies. In a bizarre cure for lameness, a hole was bored in an ash tree and a live shrew imprisoned in it. The shrew soon died, and the tree was then called a 'shrew-ash' and deemed to have the power to cure lameness in cattle and humans as well as other ailments such as 'bewitchment' and whooping cough. The touch of its leaves was sufficient to achieve a cure. A famous shrew-ash stood until 1987 in Richmond Park. The first director of the Natural History Museum, Sir Richard Owen (1804–1892), lived nearby and observed many children being brought to the shrew-ash to be cured.

In a cure for childhood hernia, a split was made in an ash sapling and the afflicted child passed through the hole. The tree was then bound up and, as it healed, so would the child. Such trees must be cared for thereafter and it was an offence to cut them down; it was felt that if the tree died, bad fortune or even death would come to the patient.

The ash tree was also invoked in the cure of warts. The wart was crossed with a pin, and the pin then pushed into the ash tree, with a request to the tree to take the wart away. This is an example of transference of an illness, a phenomenon particularly associated with wart treatments; the ELDER was used similarly. In unpublished notes from the 1920s, held in the Norfolk Records Office, it states:

If a person has warts, a friend of his should stick into a green ash tree as many pins as there are warts. This should be done secretly. As the pins rust away so the warts will disappear.

At least since the time of Pliny the Elder (AD 23–79), it has been suggested that snakes will not come near an ash tree and would rather pass through fire than through its branches. Consequently, one stroke with an ash stick was believed to bring death to an adder, and ash sap was regarded as a cure for snakebite. In a more practical mode, ash leaves could be boiled and the resulting liquid given to an animal or human that had been bitten; the boiled leaves were then placed on the bite.

Other uses of ash in folk medicine were many and varied. In Ireland, ringworm was treated with the smoke of burning ash twigs and rheumatism treated with ash leaves. The bark was used in burn treatments and, in Wiltshire, a rural remedy to stop a nosebleed involved dipping an ash stick into the blood. In Norfolk in the early twentieth century, it was said that 'An ivy leaf grown on an Ash tree is a certain cure for a corn.' The buds have been used as a slimming aid.

In official medicine, Culpeper suggests in 1653 that ash leaves, not the buds, are a slimming aid. Pechey in 1694 repeats this use. He claims that 'the Juice of three or four Leaves taken every Morning, makes those lean that are fat.' A seventeenth-century receit from Midlothian for gravel (small urinary stones) recommends taking the inner bark of the ash, dried and powdered, in wine. Burnt ash bark was also recommended for scabby heads and, in the eighteenth century, the ashes of green ash were recommended for jaundice.

For a weak child, ash is the cure – an early eighteenth-century manuscript gives a recipe for a health-restoring drink. The constituents are AGRIMONY, hart's-tongue fern (*Asplenium scolopendrium*), DANDELION and the 'rind' (bark) of green ash, all dried in the sun and then soaked in small beer. There seems to be no end to the tree's uses and yet by 1838, when Kemsey's *The British Herbal* was published, it receives no mention and nowadays the tree is seldom used by medical herbalists in this country.

Ash has, however, always been prized for its strong timber. Its botanical name, *Fraxinus*, is thought to be derived from the Greek *phrasso* meaning 'to fence', alluding to its usefulness in that role. But even practical uses of the tree are shot through with superstition – the handle of a witch's broom was said to be made of ash, conferring upon the wood a dark reputation. More benevolently, shepherds' crooks used to be made of ash, a wood which it was said could never hurt sheep. A wagon with an ash axle could, it was believed, go faster than any other. Ash branches were burned around Christmas time as a protection, to keep the occupants of the house safe for the following year – a custom observed in Derbyshire, Devon and Somerset. But only green ash burns well; when dried, it does not make good firewood.

Burn ash-wood green
'Tis a fire for a queen;
Burn ash wood sear,
'Twill make a man swear.

James Orchard Halliwell, *Popular Rhymes and Nursery Tales* (1849)

In a more romantic era than ours the ash was revered for its beauty as well as for its usefulness. Hamerton writing in 1885 has this to say about the tree:

The ash is one of the most graceful trees we have, especially when ornamented by her 'keys' in the early months of the year. The toughness and strength of her wood, and its extraordinary weight, are not at all suggested by the elegant outward appearance of the tree, as the same qualities are by the stout and rugged character of the oak. The ash resembles some deceptive feminine organisations that attract admiration for beauty, whilst nobody suspects the toughness and resisting power with which the graceful being is armed against the difficulties of existence. The foliage of the ash is light and pretty in small quantities, and masses handsomely when there is an abundance of it.

Philip Gilbert Hamerton, *Landscape* (1885)

Betony

(*Betonica officinalis*)

For wo[u]ndys in ye hed
Betonye and verveyn per[r]-to you take
With swinys grees a plaster you make
And bynde to ye wounde faste
And it shall be hol in haste

Old English medical manuscript

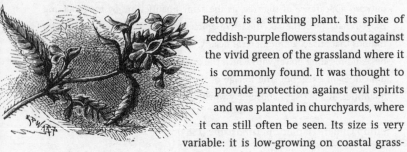

Betony is a striking plant. Its spike of reddish-purple flowers stands out against the vivid green of the grassland where it is commonly found. It was thought to provide protection against evil spirits and was planted in churchyards, where it can still often be seen. Its size is very variable: it is low-growing on coastal grassland but, in lusher conditions, it will grow much taller. The basal leaves have long stalks and characteristic, lobed leaves that are oval in shape. Betony is a cousin to WOUNDWORT.

It has been suggested that the name of betony comes from the Celtic 'ben' (head) and 'ton' (good). Since betony is comparatively rare in the highlands of Scotland, this has led to the suggestion that it may have been cultivated there especially for medicinal use.

Betony was a great heal-all, effective in a variety of ills. In the eighteenth century, a wound ointment was prepared from betony, ST JOHN'S WORT and GOLDENROD. Betony was used in Sussex to heal burns as well as wounds. An infusion of betony has also been drunk as a tonic and, within living memory, to treat a headache. The leaves may be made into a green 'tea', and were once a common constituent of herbal tobaccos and snuff – the latter was used to relieve headaches or simply taken for pleasure.

Betony was still planted in many a cottage garden in England in the early twentieth century, to be used for 'rheumatism and all aches and pains'; an Essex man recalls that, 'In the 1920s, I used to gather betony for my grand-father who used to boil it and drink the water. I think this was for his kidneys or urine.'

In official medicine, Culpeper, quoting Emperor Augustus' physician Musa from the first century AD, also recommends betony in 1653 for headaches, as well as for many other complaints, including colds, coughs, epilepsy, fevers, indigestion, labour pains and wounds. 'It is a very precious herb, that is certain,' he adds.

Gerard quotes in 1597 a proverb, 'Sell your coat and buy betony', to sum up his feelings for the plant. A hundred years later, Pechey states that it is good 'for the Gout, Head-ach, and Diseases of the Nerves' and, intriguingly, Johnson in 1862 states that in the past it was used to drive away 'devils and despair'. But by then betony had fallen largely from favour.

Today's medical herbalists continue the centuries-old tradition of using betony to treat headaches, as well as 'frayed nerves', indigestion and nose-bleeds. Perhaps our modern frayed nerves are the same devils and despair of our forbears.

Bilberry
(*Vaccinium myrtillus*)

Bilberry grows in beautiful and romantic places, as a very low shrub on moorland and mountains throughout the north and west of Britain. Its small, neat, bright green leaves hide the tiny, blush-pink bells of its flowers. The dark purple fruit ripen in late summer, and have been a valuable source of food in upland areas where it was difficult to grow crops. Also called 'blueberries' and 'blaeberries', they were, and still are, gathered in season. In Victorian times, the Board School in one Dartmoor village would close for a week every bilberry season so that the children could harvest the berries. In the early twentieth century, the bilberry became a commercially important crop on Exmoor. In Ireland, the rural poor would gather them to sell in Dublin's markets and streets. The Gaelic name for bilberry is *fraghan*, meaning 'growing among the heather'.

Bilberries were used in cooking in a variety of ways: to flavour bread, as an ingredient of pies and puddings and as a constituent of 'moorland tea', a mixture of bilberry leaves, heather tops and other herbs. According to one nineteenth-century writer, bilberry-leaf tea, if made properly, was indistinguishable from ordinary tea. Lightfoot in 1777 recorded that in the Scottish Highlands bilberry jelly was mixed with whisky for a treat. A delicious country wine can be made from bilberries and the blossoms of bell heather.

In folk medicine, bilberry has been used especially to treat kidney stones. A fourteenth-century cattle drover in one of the glens of Scotland was known to use it as a cure for kidney stones. In Ireland, too, bilberry was a treatment for kidney complaints, as well as jaundice and measles. Colds, diarrhoea and sore throats as well as rheumatism have all been treated using bilberries and, in the early twentieth century in the Scottish Highlands, a bilberry infusion was taken to soothe pain. In Cornwall, those afflicted with blocked sinuses were given an inhalant made from the stems, leaves and roots of bilberry together with cowberry (*Vaccinium vitis-idaea*) and BOG MYRTLE.

In official medicine, the illnesses treated with bilberry were different from those in folk medicine. Culpeper recommended it in 1653 for diarrhoea, spitting of blood and excessive menstruation. Pechey in 1694 also favoured bilberries for treating diarrhoea and, in addition, 'bloody flux' and vomiting. Sir John Hill in *c.*1820 tells us that syrup of bilberries 'taken for a week before the time' is good for moderating heavy periods.

Present-day medical herbalists in this country use the dried berries of bilberry to treat diarrhoea, especially in children. They also recommend an infusion of the berries as a mouthwash, and a preparation of the leaves for treating urinary tract infections.

During the Second World War, it is rumoured that British pilots noticed that eating bilberry jam seemed to improve their night vision, but there is little actual documented evidence. Research into the possible value of bilberry in various eye conditions is ongoing, but results so far are contradictory. However, bilberry has been shown to contain provitamin A, which is known to be good for vision.

Birch
(*Betula* species)

I dreamed a dreary dream last nicht;
God kee us a' frae sorrow!
I dreamed I pu'd the birk sae green
Wi' my true love on Yarrow.

I redde your dream, my sister dear,
I'll tell you a' your sorrow;
You pu'd the birk wi' your true love;
He's killed, – he's killed on Yarrow.

Scottish ballad

The birch is native throughout Britain, forming open woodland on light soil. It is sometimes called the 'lady of the forest' and is one of our most graceful trees. Yet traditionally, in Somerset for example, the birch is regarded as evil; it is from this tree that witches cut their brooms, and the birch is often associated with death, as in the ballad quoted above. Yet, conversely, birch has protective powers and has been used to decorate houses, churches and streets, especially at Rogationtide, an ancient country festival held to bless fields and crops. In Hereford, a maypole was made each May Day from a decorated birch sapling and it was placed against the byres to protect the animals over the coming year.

In folk medicine, birch was valued for its laxative properties. Tapped from the tree in spring, the sap was made into birch wine, a celebrated country drink still made in rural areas, even commercially. The Gunton Household Book (compiled in the seventeenth and eighteenth centuries) gives a recipe for birch wine, which is described as 'A good drink made of ye birch tree by boreing a hole and put in a quill in March and tye a bottle under it.' The recipe includes honey, cloves and lemon peel. We are told that 'this wine Exquisitely made is soe strong yt the Comon Sort of Stone bottles canot contein ye spirits, so subtile they are and valuable and yet its very gentle and harmless in operation within ye body, and exceedingly sharpens ye apetite being drunk before meales, its most Powerfull opener doeing wonders for Cure of the Ptisick.'

In subsequent centuries, birch wine was considered a tonic and especially good for the kidneys and bladder. It was also found to be useful for rheumatism and in the Scottish Highlands a birch-leaf tea was said to ease rheumaticky pains. Birch bark had its uses too, and in Ireland was recommended for a number of ailments including eczema.

In official medicine, Pechey prescribed birch sap for kidney and bladder complaints, as well as jaundice and skin blemishes in 1694. *Delightes for Ladies* (1609) by Sir Hugh Platt has this recommendation for improving the complexion:

To take away spots and freckles from the face and hands.

The sap that issueth out of a birch tree in great abundance, being opened in March or April with a receiver of glass set under the boring thereof to catch the same, doth perform the same most excellently and maketh the skin very clear. This sap will dissolve pearls, a secret not known to many.

Today, medical herbalists in this country also use birch for treating skin conditions, but it is the bark and leaves that are used and not the sap. They do, however, use birch sap as a mild diuretic.

The practical uses found for birch timber have been many and varied. The toughness and flexibility of the branches made it ideal for building, and the frames of Scottish shielings (temporary huts on high grazing and pastures) were constructed from birch. In parts of Scotland, the birch was one of the few local trees and was used for practically everything. Many household items were made of birch, including the shuttles used in weaving in the Scottish Highlands. The finer twigs were used to make ropes. Lightfoot in 1777 mentions that birch ropes were used to tie down thatches in the Scottish Highlands. Brooms, hurdles, baskets and cask-hoops were all made from birch, and the bark could be used in tanning leather or as writing paper, or could be rolled into the shape of candles and burned. Pechey describes this particular use:

Fishermen in Northumberland fish a-nights by the Light of this Bark: they put
it into a cleft Stick, which serves for a Candle-stick, and so they see how to use
their Three-teeth'd Spear for killing fish.

Of course, infamously, the 'birch' was once much used for punishment,
being the implement of choice for hundreds of years. Gerard tells us in 1597
that 'in times past the magistrats rods were made thereof; and in our time
also Schoolmasters and Parents do terrifie their children with rods made of
Birch.' But there were other ways of looking at it. Coles in *Adam in Eden*
(1657) relates that the birch 'hath an admirable influence upon [children] to
quiet them when they are out of order, and therefore some call it
makepeace'.

Bird's-foot Trefoil
(*Lotus corniculatus*)

Thy dainty petals, tipp'd with red,
By sunbeams of the springtime fed,
Are quick in yellow beauty spread –
Lotus Corniculatus!

James Rigg, *To the Bird's-Foot Trefoil* (1897)

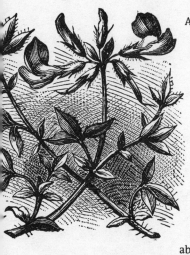

Abundant on grassland, heaths and dunes, this member of the pea family bears bright yellow flowers tipped with crimson that are borne in an inflorescence shaped rather like a miniature bunch of bananas. The dried seedpods resemble the clawed feet of a bird. It is the unusual flowers and fruit that have given rise to a great variety of country names – about seventy in total – such as 'egg and bacon', 'fingers and thumbs,' and 'lambtoe'. This plant's distinctive appearance means that it is readily recognizable and we can be reasonably sure of its identity in historical records. The converse applies to many of its near cousins, the vetches, which tend to be lumped together.

In folk medicine, an infusion of bird's-foot trefoil was made in the Outer Hebrides as an eyewash. The plant was used to staunch bleeding from wounds in Somerset and was still being used to treat cuts on horses' legs in the 1960s.

In Culpeper's time, official medicine utilized the plant externally to treat wounds and internally as a wound drink and to help expel gravel and stone (urinary stones). A century later, Salmon in 1693 describes similar properties for the 'codded trefoil', and adds that the juice is good for eye complaints.

The plant seems to have fallen from favour in official medicine and modern medical herbalists do not use it. Instead, it has continued to fascinate the imagination and attract even more local names. It was recorded at the end of the nineteenth century that children in the south of Ireland called the plant 'no blame' and they competed with each other to gather pieces of the plant, which at school would make them immune to punishment.

Bistort
(*Persicaria bistorta*)

3 good handfuls of Easter ledges

3 good handfuls of nettles

1 good handful of cabbage or broccoli or dandelion leaves with a few raspberry, blackcurrant and/or gooseberry leaves

1 onion

1 large cup of barley – previously soaked overnight in water

Salt and pepper, or sometimes parsley

Method: Wash greens, and chop with onion. Put in a muslin bag and boil for one and a half hours. Empty bag into a bowl and beat in three eggs, bacon dripping and about two ounces of butter. Reheat in oven.

Cumbria (1985), collected by Roy Vickery

This member of the dock family is named from its strangely shaped, spirally contorted root: *bistorta* means 'twice twisted'. It grows in grassland throughout Britain, but is commonest in the northwest of England, and it is here that the plant has been used for centuries to make Easter puddings. In Cumbria, the plant is called 'Easter ledges'; in Yorkshire, it is known as 'passion dock'. The pudding recipes are varied, but all use the shoots of bistort with a selection of other ingredients including nettles, onions, oatmeal and dandelions. This tradition is still continued, and the puddings are regarded as a good tonic for the blood.

The plant is eaten in other ways and at other times, as a salad or cooked like spinach, apparently tasting best if soaked in water overnight before cooking. According to Johnson in 1862, steeping the root in water and then roasting it makes for a very nutritious vegetable.

The *Grete Herball* of 1526 describes the plant as an aid to conception. It is possible that this, rather than nutrition alone, was the origin of the north of England's Easter puddings, Easter being a celebration of, among other things, the continuity of life. Culpeper in 1653 confirms this use of the plant and adds many more; he recommends it for 'any fluxes in the body', for treating wounds, toothache and for killing worms in children. Pechey in 1694 prescribes similar uses, and mentions its ability to prevent miscarriage. By the nineteenth century, bistort is described by Kemsey in 1838 as 'rather binding. It is given in fluxes, also in intermitting fevers. A strong tea of it is used for spongy gums and foul ulcers', but by this date its association with fertility has completely disappeared.

In folk medicine, bistort was used for headaches, urinary problems, worms and toothache and in Norfolk the juice was rubbed on horses' gums to prevent tooth decay.

Present-day medical herbalists use the plant for externally treating mouth ulcers, sore gums, burns and slight wounds, vaginal discharge and piles. Bistort is taken internally for peptic ulcers and ulcerative colitis, dysentery and irritable bowel syndrome. Bistort is described by a leading medical herbalist in this country as one of the most astringent of all medicinal herbs, a property which makes it useful in contracting tissues and in staunching blood. And bistort puddings are highly recommended!

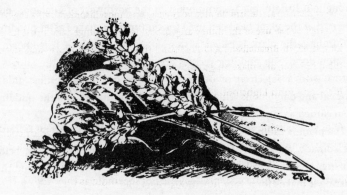

Bitter Vetch
(*Lathyrus linifolius*)

This vetch has pretty, purple, pea-like flowers that fade to blue as they age. The stems are winged and the leaves, unlike those of many of its cousins, do not end in a tendril. The plant has tuberous rhizomes that are edible.

Bitter vetch occurs throughout much of Britain, but it is in the Scottish Highlands that the plant has been most exploited. There it was known as *cairmeille*. The tuberous roots were eaten raw to dispel hunger, or roasted and ground and used as a bread substitute. They have a sweetish taste like liquorice. At the end of the seventeenth century on the Isle of Mull, people chewed the raw roots after drinking whisky, both to sweeten their breath and to prevent themselves from becoming drunk. There were other uses too:

> The highlanders . . . affirm them to be good against most disorders of the thorax and that by the use of them they are enabled to repel hunger and thirst for a long time. In Breadalbane and Ross-shire they sometimes bruise and steep them in water, and make an agreeable fermented liquor with them.

Reverend John Lightfoot, *Flora Scotica* (1777)

Official medicine seems to have largely ignored this plant but Gerard in 1597 was aware of its food value: 'The Nuts of this Pease being boiled and eaten, are hardlier digested than be either Turneps or Parsneps, yet they do nourish no lesse than Parsneps: they are not so windie as they, they do more slowly passe thorowe the belly by reason of their binding qualitie, and being eaten rawe, they yet be harder of digestion, and do hardlier and slowlier descend.' 'Bitter vetch' is described by Pechey in 1694 as useful for expelling kidney stones – this may or may not be the same plant.

Herbalism too seems to have found little use for bitter vetch. However, its nutritive value has been appreciated until much more recent times. Writing in the 1920s, the Reverend Angus MacFarlane records this chewing gum substitute: 'For chewing purpose I consider them superior to and far less deleterious than the common chewing gum. The taste lingers in the mouth for long after the last shred is chewed.' Undoubtedly another benefit would be that it is much easier to clean off city pavements!

Black Bryony
(*Tamus communis*)

The black bryony is called in Wales 'Serpent's Meat' ... an idea is there prevalent that those reptiles are always lurking near the spot where the plant grows.

W. A. Bromfield, *Flora Vectensis* (1856)

This is a twining plant with shiny, heart-shaped leaves and tiny, green, six-lobed flowers borne on very short stalks. It has a fleshy, black rhizome and bright red berries, both of which have featured in folk medicine. The rhizome was found to ease rheumatic complaints and the berries were used to treat chilblains. In the nineteenth century on the Isle of Wight, chilblains were treated with bryony berries only after they had been soaked in gin.

Black bryony's efficacy in clearing skin discoloration has been much feted. In France, this ability to remove bruising has been acknowledged in its name, *herbe aux femmes battues*, or 'the plant for battered wives'. A similar appreciation is recorded in an old English country name for the plant – black-eye root.

Botanically, this plant is unrelated to its namesake WHITE BRYONY but, like white bryony, it is a climber and, similarly, male and female flowers are borne on separate plants. So it is not surprising that some of its uses have overlapped with those of white bryony and therefore several records are undoubtedly confused as to which plant is meant. Salmon in 1693 tells us that bryony is of two kinds: white and black 'of which the White kind ... is the best'. Culpeper in 1653 also lumps the two together.

To add to the confusion, white bryony roots and black bryony tubers have both been used as counterfeit mandrake (see WHITE BRYONY). In Lincolnshire, black bryony was actually called mandrake although that name strictly applies to the Mediterranean plant *Mandragora officinarum*, whose tuberous root was prized in medicine as a painkiller and an anaesthetic. The resemblance of the root to the body of a man led to the legend that the plant shrieked when it was torn from the ground, so that dogs were used to dig them up. Real mandrake was valuable and so difficult to grow in Britain that a thriving trade developed in the making of counterfeit mandrake roots, usually from bryony. By association, many of the dark and dangerous powers of the 'true' mandrake were also attributed to bryony, and doubtless its connection with snakes, the embodiment of the sinister, arose in this way.

The whole plant does need to be treated with caution – in particular the shining red berries, which are toxic. In Devon, it is called 'adder's poison', but this name is probably derived from the Old English *attor*, meaning poison – a name giving a double warning.

Despite the nervousness surrounding this plant, Bryant in 1783 states that 'its young shoots are frequently boiled and eaten in the spring, the same as those of Hops, and are by many much esteemed.' Apparently the tuber is also safe to eat once boiled, but perhaps it would not be sensible to champion its revival as a vegetable.

Blackthorn
(*Prunus spinosa*)

At the end of October go gather up sloes,
Have thou in readiness plenty of those,
And keep them in bedstraw or still on the bough
To stay both the flux of thyself and thy cow.

G. Clarke Nuttall, *Wild Flowers As They Grow* (c.1920), vol. IV, p. 8

The snowy-white flowers of the blackthorn against its striking, black, leafless stems provide a lovely, early-springtime sight, inspiring one of its names, 'the lady of pearls'. It blooms so early in the year that generations of countryfolk have always called a spell of cold weather at the end of early spring 'the winter of the blackthorn'. Traditionally the blackthorn in full bloom was an indication that the time was right to sow barley.

As an ancient plant, blackthorn has magical associations. There is a proverb in Scotland 'better the blackthorn than the devil' and, in the same country, there is a tradition that the blackthorn sprang from the blood of slain Norse invaders. As with many white-flowered plants, there is an old superstition against bringing it into the house when it is in flower: to do so can bring about misfortune or even death. Yet on the other hand, blackthorn has been seen as protective against the forces of darkness. In nineteenth-century Hereford, a blackthorn branch would be cut before daybreak when the wheat crop was just showing, and part of it ceremonially burned in the field to prevent mildew and smut from developing on the crop. The remainder of the branch was then hung in a barn. In Sandwich, Kent, for the past seven centuries a blackthorn 'wand' has been part of the civic ceremonial surrounding the appointment of a new mayor.

The small rounded fruits, the sloes, have a characteristic blue bloom on them. A heavy crop was believed to forecast a harsh winter; 'many sloans, many groans' was a Devonshire saying. Sloes, slaes, or sloans, as they are sometimes called, are very bitter and must be left until late autumn to be reasonably palatable; badgers, birds and foxes will all eat them late in the season, helping to disperse the seeds. Robert Bloomfield (1766–1823) in 'The Farmer's Boy' describes roasting sloes over a bonfire and the Victorian writer Anne Pratt recalls that in her childhood, in the early nineteenth century, she and others used to collect sloes and bury them in a bottle until winter 'when it forms a very pleasant preserve'. The combination of sloes and alcohol is centuries old, as testified by this seventeenth-century recipe:

> Take very ripe sloes with their stalks, and put thereto two parts of honey and one part of wine, and let them seethe so long until the wine be thoroughly sodden away; afterwards lay the sloes in a pot with the stalks on high, and pour the same honey upon it and cover with a trencher, and lay some heavy thing on them to the end that they may be covered with the liquor, and set them in a cellar.

Sloes are still used to flavour liqueurs and to make sloe gin, and can even be added to ice-cream. The vibrant colour of the juice is impressive, and it is no surprise that a dye was once obtained from it, and was used as a marking ink for linen.

Perhaps it is their acidity that first gave rise to the idea of using sloes to burn off warts: a sloe is rubbed on the wart and then tossed over the shoulder. Another method is to rub the warts with a black snail and then impale the poor creature on a thorn; as the snail perishes, so the wart will wither. Other ailments have been treated with blackthorn, especially diarrhoea – in folk medicine this particular use was widespread in Britain until relatively recent times. It was still current in twentieth-century Ireland, where the thorns were boiled to provide a remedy for people as well as animals. In the Scottish Highlands, the blackthorn blossoms were used as a laxative, an apparent paradox that will probably be resolved only when the plant is more thoroughly investigated.

In official medicine, Gerard in 1597 recommended the juice of sloes to 'stop the belly, the laske and the bloody flixe, the inordinate course of womens termes, and all other issues of blood in man or woman'. Early herbalists used the plant to treat diarrhoea and excessive menstruation, but it does not figure in present-day official herbalism in Britain.

Blackthorn wood is tough and strong and has been used to make walking sticks and the famous Irish shillelaghs (cudgels). Some thorns can be so hard and sharp that they can puncture a car tyre, so it is no surprise that they were once used to make the teeth of rakes. Blackthorn continues to be planted, as it has been for centuries, to form traditional farm hedges, and hopefully this wonderful harbinger of spring will grace the countryside for generations to come.

Bluebell
(*Hyacinthoides non-scripta*)

A bluebell wood in spring is one of the great delights of the British countryside and has been the inspiration for numerous poems and paintings. Since the twentieth century, as more and more woodland disappeared, the English bluebell has come under threat. It thrives on just the right amount of shade; too little and it dies out because of competition with other plants, too much and it begins to suffer. Most new woodland plantings of the last fifty years or so have been of coniferous forest and its dense shade is highly unsuitable for bluebells, which thrive only at the very edge. Hopefully, now that more mixed woodland is being planted, the sight of a bluebell wood will become more common once again. There are still many bluebell strongholds: Norsey Wood in Essex is said to have the highest concentration of bluebells anywhere in the world, and in some places, notably the Isle of Man, there are large tracts of bluebells that mark the sites of former woodland.

Apart from its sheer beauty, the bluebell has served man in a number of ways. Its bulbs and leaf bases are full of a white slime that was used as glue, for example in bookbinding, and as a source of laundry starch. This latter use was still current, at least in Norfolk, in the early years of the twentieth century. Gerard in 1597 says 'The roote is Bulbus, ful of a slimy glewish juice, which will serve to set feathers upon arrows in steed of glew, or to paste books with: whereof is made the best starche, next unto that of wake robin rootes.'

In folklore the bluebell had some unexpected associations. In some parts of Scotland, it was considered unlucky to pick bluebells, which were called 'the aul' man's bell' and in Devon likewise it was thought to be unlucky to bring bluebells into the house, especially if the owners kept poultry (see also DAFFODIL, PRIMROSE).

The bluebell seems to have been little used in folk or official medicine, although in Inverness-shire a plaster was made from the roots to aid wound-healing, while in Ireland the plant has been used to treat whitlows and throat ailments.

Insects, however, especially bees, find the bluebell invaluable. Bees will often 'cheat' on the flower by biting through the base of the bell, rather than entering by the front door and pollinating as they go (see also COMFREY). They are attracted by its scent, described by Parkinson in 1629 as 'sweetish, but heady'. Bees will doubtless find themselves disappointed by the Spanish bluebell (*Hyacinthoides hispanica*), which is currently hybridizing with our native species and producing plants that do not smell as sweet. Being more vigorous than our English bluebell, this hybrid could endanger our native bluebell.

Bog Myrtle
(*Myrica gale*)

The aromatic smell of bog myrtle is strongly evocative of the wide and wet open spaces of the north and west of Britain. It was once also common in the old East Anglian fens before they were drained.

This small shrub with upright, red, catkin-like spikes borne in the spring is the only British representative of the fragrant family (*Myricaceae*) to which it belongs. Its association with wet and boggy areas is surely no coincidence. The Scottish midge, abundant in such habitats, finds bog myrtle to be its worst enemy, and the plant's insect-repelling properties are legendary. Bunches of it were hung in houses and used as a strewing herb to keep insects at bay, and it was laid between layers of linen for the same reason.

Recently, a repellent based on the plant was developed under the name 'Myrica', and although it is not yet commercially viable, the research continues. Studies are also under way on the Isle of Skye into developing bog myrtle as a 'green' way of controlling such pests as aphids, fungi and house mites.

Magical powers were once ascribed to bog myrtle. In the Scottish Highlands, it was said to keep away mischievous fairies. There is a story of a young child in Moray in the nineteenth century who was failing to thrive. A local wise woman put this down to her being 'overlooked' (bewitched) by a wandering beggar-woman to whom the child's mother had refused money. The child was passed through a burning hoop, then put to bed with a sprig of bog myrtle hung over the bed and left to recover for a month. By this time the child had 'already very visibly improved in health and temper'. In a similar story, a sprig of bog myrtle hung over the bed for a month was said to have helped restore an eighteen-year-old who had had the 'evil eye' cast upon her.

Bog myrtle has not been widely used in folk medicine although children were sometimes given an infusion of the leaves to rid them of worms, and an inhalation could be prepared to clear blocked sinuses (no doubt its aromatic smell came into play here). In Ireland, bog myrtle was prescribed for measles, sore throats and kidney troubles and, on the Scottish island of Barra, it was a traditional remedy for ulcers. Interestingly, we now know that the plant contains substances that can kill fungi and some bacteria.

The plant has largely been neglected by official medicine and is little used by modern medical herbalists in this country.

Bog myrtle had numerous practical uses. The waxy scum skimmed off from the boiled flowering spikes was used to make candles in the Scottish Highlands, and no doubt a similar practice existed in Somerset, where the plant is known as 'candleberries'. The leaves have been used to improve the foaming of beer and, recently at the West Highland Brewery, a new version of heather ale has been developed from an old Gaelic recipe. This new brew is made from heather and bog myrtle leaves, and is marketed under the name of *Fraoch*.

It looks likely that there may be a commercial future for bog myrtle in Scotland. It is already harvested on a large scale for the florist industry, and studies are under way to see whether it can become a sustainable crop for this and for its essential oils.

Bogbean
(*Menyanthes trifoliata*)

Like silvered candelabra round the lake,
Thy fairy lights illume the rushy mead;
While cherub larks above thee music wake,
And, flushed, Aurora to the Day doth Speed!

James Rigg, *To the Bog-bean* (1897)

Just as its name suggests, this plant grows in boggy regions throughout Britain where its beautiful, star-shaped flowers with delicately fringed petals grace many a shallow pond and fen. In 1838 Kemsey rightly claimed that 'this is one of the most beautiful of our indigenous plants', and Gerard described the flowers very poetically in 1597, as 'of a white colour, dasht over slightly with a wash of light carnation'. Bogbean's flowering period is said to last a month; its botanical name of *Menyanthes* derives from the Greek *men*, meaning 'month', and *anthos*, or 'flower'. It is the only widespread member of its family, Menyanthaceae, to grow in Britain.

Wherever bogbean has grown, both its rhizomes and shoots have been widely used in folk medicine. In official medicine, its reputation was nationwide.

In folk medicine, bogbean was prescribed for numerous ailments. An infusion was recommended as a treatment for dropsy, scurvy, stone and gravel (urinary stones), as well as a tonic. A spring tonic was made in the Glencoe region, within living memory, by simmering bogbean in a stone jar; alternatively, 'the stems were boiled for two hours, pulped, left to cool, the liquid strained and bottled for winter. A teaspoon three times a day for a persistent cough was most effective.' The Irish too knew of its value as a pick-me-up: they pulled the 'bogbine' in the springtime and boiled the roots with treacle and sulphur to make their own tonic; this concoction was still made in the late twentieth century.

In Scotland, where bogbean is commonly found, it was widely used.

Tuberculosis, heart and skin disorders, constipation and headache were treated, and arthritic conditions were eased. An extract of bogbean was found to be useful for arthritis in Wales and Ireland too. In Shetland, where the plant's name means 'yellow sickness', it was used to treat jaundice. Wounds and sores were treated with its leaves and, as with many other plants, the rougher lower side of a leaf was used to 'draw', the smooth upper surface of the leaf to heal.

In the herbals, the name often given for bogbean is 'marsh trefoil'. Under this name, Pechey recommended it in 1694 for scurvy and pains in the limbs. Dr Sutherland grew bogbean in his eighteenth-century Edinburgh physic garden, but along with a number of other herbs he also collected it from the wild in an area known as the Guills of Scalpa. In Kemsey's *The British Herbal* (1838), bogbean was still being advocated to treat rheumatism and gravel as well as 'intermittent fevers, and breakings out of the skin'. Present-day medical herbalists have continued to prescribe the plant for rheumatoid arthritis and digestive problems.

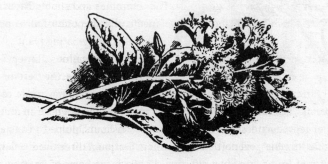

Bramble or Blackberry
(*Rubus fruticosus*)

The flora of the year is past–
Adown the lanes I ramble,
The faded leaves are falling fast,
Yet jetty hangs the Bramble.

Its blossoms still are silken white,
And black, and red, and green,
Its berries dangle with delight–
Fit jewels for a queen.

James Rigg, *The Bramble in October* (1897)

This is such a familiar hedgerow plant in Britain that it needs no introduction. It is commonly found in town and country and is generally ignored and scorned until its fruit comes into season. The bramble's very ubiquitousness means that we often fail to notice that it is a fascinating plant.

Its five-petalled flowers are beautiful and, like the rest of the plant, extremely variable in size, colour and detail. The bramble is one of our few native plants that have an unusual form of reproduction, known as apomixis, which enables it to constantly reshuffle its genes, even without cross-fertilization. This has led to a huge diversity of forms, each one differing slightly in appearance, fruiting time and flavour of berry.

The bramble's powers of entanglement are impressive. Its strong, backward-pointing thorns on long trailing stems enable the plant to scramble through vegetation, and make it extraordinarily difficult to detach from other plants (or clothes). 'As cross as a bramble' is a proverb in Scotland, while in parts of England thorny bramble stems are called 'lawyers' because 'when once they get a holt an ye, ye doänt easy get shut of 'em'. Bramble was deliberately planted as hedging in the past. An Elizabethan writer, Thomas Tusser, advises:

To plot not full
Ad Bramble and Hull
For set no bar
Whilst month hath an R.

This indicates that the plant will successfully root throughout the year except in the months May through to August.

Sometimes the bramble's long shoots bend over and root at the tip, forming a natural arch. This arch has been used in folk practice as the basis of ceremonies for treating hernias, boils and rheumatism. The sufferer is passed through the arch, symbolizing a new beginning. Such 'passing-through' ceremonies were also performed with split ASH trees.

There are many down-to-earth folk uses for the plant. The fruits were recommended for treating sore throats and frozen blackberries can still be very helpful in soothing an irritating night-time cough; both the cold and the fruit contribute to the cure. In Scotland, asthma and bronchitis were treated with bramble root. For diarrhoea, the young, juicy growing tips were stripped of their spines and chewed. The leaves were also chewed to alleviate toothache and used as plasters to remove thorns. In addition, they were used for burns and scalds, spots, boils and shingles.

Official medicine recommended the leaves too, but for treating fluxes, for example diarrhoea. Gerard in 1597 adds another use: 'The leaves of the Bramble boyled in water, with honey, alum and a little white wine added thereto, makes a most excellent lotion or washing water, and the same decoction fastneth teeth.' Other treatments included the roots for kidney stones and the berries for sore mouths and vomiting. Modern medical herbalists use the plant for treating sore mouths and throats.

Almost everyone has been blackberry picking, and it is a tradition that goes back many generations. There are numerous local names for black-berries; the names recorded in Lanarkshire alone include 'blackbides', 'blackbutters', 'bumblekites' and 'scaldberries'. In the West Country where 'mooching' means 'playing truant', blackberries are called 'moochers'; in blackberry season many a country child has been late for school – if they've turned up at all. There is a widespread belief that blackberries should not be eaten after a certain date, because then the devil spits on them; the actual date given varies from place to place. Presumably this idea arose from the fact that late-season blackberries have little flavour.

Blackberries picked at the right time are delicious and are used to make jams, jellies and pies. They also make a delicious country wine. Salmon in 1693 gives it an honourable mention: 'A Wine made of the fermented juice ... is of a deep Red ... and is as pleasant as *Canary*.' In the springtime, wine can also be made from young bramble buds. It comes as no surprise to learn that numerous dyes can be obtained from the juice, ranging through pink and purple to red and orange.

Practical uses of the plant included, in Scotland, using the wood to make pipes for smoking and making traditional skeps for beekeeping from rushes and bramble stems. In Devon, an ingenious idea was to use a bramble shoot like a fishing rod to unearth young rabbits from their burrows.

Brooklime
(*Veronica beccabunga*)

To cure the Scurvy ...

Take of the juice of Brooklime, Water-cresses and Scurvy-grass, each half a Pint; of the Juice of Oranges, four Ounces; fine Sugar, two Pounds; make a Syrup over a gentle Fire: Take one Spoonful in your Beer every time you drink.

John Pechey, *The Compleat Herbal of Physical Plants* (1694)

The piercingly blue, tiny flowers of this succulent cousin of SPEEDWELL adorn the edges of many of our ponds and streams. The 'lime' in its name is thought to be derived from the Anglo-Saxon word for the mud in which it grows. The plant has been eaten as a wholesome, although not pleasant-tasting, vegetable. Its specific name, *beccabunga*, means 'pungent'.

In official medicine, the plant has served one major purpose: the prevention and treatment of scurvy.

In country medicine, brooklime has been used in a variety of ways: for treating coughs and colds, as a diuretic, a tonic and for the treatment of burns and wounds, as well as for scurvy. 'Country-people cure Wounds with Brook-lime, mix'd with a little Salt and a Spider's Web, and applied to the Wound, wrapped about with a double Cloth.'

The plant has been used to treat animals too. Parkinson in 1640 writes: 'Farryers do much use it about their horses to take away swellings, to heal the scab, and otherlike diseases in them.'

In the eighteenth century, a famous 'doctress' from County Cork, Elizabeth Pearson, made her fortune with the prescription of this plant for treating glandular tuberculosis, known then as scrofula. Elizabeth Pearson was the daughter of an English farmer in County Cork and well connected through marriage to the son of Archdeacon Pearson of York. She was known as 'The Big Mrs Pearson' and her great-great-great grandson describes her as 'broad of bosom, masterful in the extreme, and very self-willed'. It was her father-in-law who first aroused her interest in herbal matters, and she learned much from a gypsy whom she befriended. Soon she was brewing up the potion for which she became famous. This was apparently prepared behind locked doors in a stillroom.

With her new-found wealth, she began taking her family to London for the 'season' every year, and later bought a house in Park Lane. She evidently took fright there and, in 1815, petitioned parliament to recognize her cure officially, lest she be tried as a witch. Here is the recipe, preserved by her family, of 'Pearson's Celebrated Cure for Scrofula':

> Take two large handfuls of Brooklime, cutting off the roots. Pound it as fine as you can, pour it into an old iron saucepan, with a pint of grounds of beer, a piece of salt butter, the size of a walnut, and as much rust of iron as would cover a penny. Let all boil, till the leaves sink to the bottom, then thicken with bran, or oatmeal, until it is quite the right consistency for a poultice.
>
> The poultice to be applied night and morning, first washing the sore with warm soap and water.

By the nineteenth century, official practitioners were still using the plant as an antiscorbutic. Kemsey in 1838 suggests that it can be eaten like watercress to prevent scurvy. Although it is still mentioned in the twentieth century as a diuretic and blood purifier, it has now largely fallen from use since scrofula and scurvy have long been consigned to the history books, and today's medical herbalists do not often employ it.

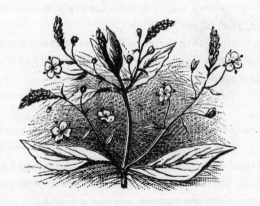

Broom
(*Cytisus scoparius*)

Then out it speaks an auld witch wife,
Sat in the bower aboon:
'O ye shall gang to Broomfield Hills,
Ye shall not stay at hame.
'But when ye gang to Broomfield Hills,
Walk nine times round and round;
Down below a bonny burn bank,
Ye'll find your love sleeping sound.
'Ye'll pu the bloom frae off the broom,
Strew't at his head and feet,
And aye the thicker that ye do strew,
The sounder he will sleep.

Peter Buchan, *Ancient Ballads of the North of Scotland* (1828)

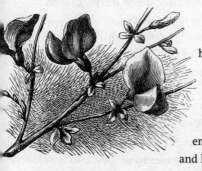

Broom has a narcotic property, claimed to have been noticed originally by shepherds observing its effects on their grazing sheep; first they became intoxicated, then extremely sleepy. It was this effect that was utilized in the ballad quoted above; the sprigs of broom ensured that the knight would stay asleep, and his lady would win her wager.

Famously, the broom is the badge of the Plantagenets, who took their name from the mediaeval Latin name of the plant, *Planta genista*. The plant has further royal connections: Henry VIII was said to drink the distilled water of broom flowers after over-indulging. Gerard noted in 1597: 'That woorthie Prince of famous memorie Henrie the eight King of England, was woont to drinke the distilled water of Broome flowers against surfets, and diseases thereof arising.' Broom buds were served as a delicacy at the coronation of James VI of Scotland.

Everything about the broom plant is evocative. In summer, its straggling, wind-bent branches are transformed into a mass of fragrant, bright yellow blossoms. Then come the silky, grey-green seed pods, which dry out slowly until they are black; finally the pods explode on dry days with an audible pop, expelling the small, black, pea-like seeds quite a distance from the mother plant, which is once again left to sit out the winter in its evergreen livery. The plant's tough wiry stems gave the plant its common name: the original household broom was a simple affair, just a cluster of broom stems.

The plant's natural habitat is windswept heathland with acid soil, and it is especially common in the north of England and in Scotland. It is from these areas that most of the lore surrounding the plant has grown up.

When the bloom flowered profusely, it was considered a good omen. But to sweep the house with a branch of flowering broom could spell disaster: 'If you sweep the house with blossomed broom in May, you are sure to sweep the head of the house away.' In parts of northern Scotland, it was traditional for the bride-to-be on the eve of her wedding to keep a broom staff in the house as a symbol of future fertility.

Every part of the broom plant has been used in the service of man. Its branches have been used as thatch and to make baskets; its wood has been made into beautiful veneer; its fibre was exploited in cloth and paper; its leaves and flowers provided green and yellow dyes; its flower buds were used as a delicacy as well as an appetizer; its roots went to make rope. In Ireland, broom was used as a fumigant, in much the same way that JUNIPER was used elsewhere.

The commonest use for broom in folk medicine was in the treatment of dropsy, but it has also been used for jaundice and rheumatism. A lovely Cornish remedy for rheumatism, recorded by Freethy in 1985, is to sprinkle broom flowers in the bath.

In official medicine, broom was used to treat dropsy, gravel and stone (both urinary stones), and liver complaints. In addition, according to Salmon in 1693, 'the flowers or buds pickled, being gathered in April before they are blown, they are pickled with Vinegar and Salt, like Capers for Sawce, and called German Capers; they are a good Stomacick'.

Herbalists continued to use broom for dropsy and liver troubles throughout the nineteenth and early twentieth centuries, but in modern-day herbalism the plant is treated with caution. In addition to being a powerful diuretic (that is, it increases the flow of urine), it is known to slow and regulate the heart rate, and so should be used only under professional supervision.

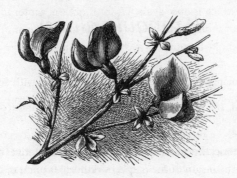

Buckthorn
(*Rhamnus cathartica*)
Alder Buckthorn
(*Frangula alnus*)

A medicine more fit for clownes, then for civill people.

John Gerard, *The Herball or Generall Historie of Plantes* (1597)

Our two native buckthorns are the only British representatives of their family, Rhamnaceae. The origin of the name 'buckthorn' is unclear, but, according to Watts, may be a translation of the mediaeval Latin *cervi spina*, meaning 'stag's thorn'. In fact only one, *Rhamnus cathartica*, also known as the purging buckthorn, has thorns.

They are attractive shrubs, with smooth, slightly shining leaves, that are toothed in the case of the buckthorn and entire in outline on the alder buckthorn. The larvae of the yellow brimstone butterfly feed almost exclusively on alder buckthorn leaves. The flowers of both buckthorns are small and inconspicuous and greenish-white in colour; in the case of the purging buckthorn, the male and female flowers are usually borne on separate plants. The berries ripen to a deep black colour, and are an important source of winter food for birds.

Medicinally, buckthorns have been highly valued for one reason – they are extremely effective in clearing the bowels. As its specific name implies, *Rhamnus cathartica* is a violent purge, the more efficient of the two, and can also cause vomiting. Authors of early herbals urged great caution; Dodoens in his *Herball* describes the berries of buckthorn as 'not meet to be ministered but to lustie people of the country, which doe sett more store on their monie than on their lives'. Salmon in 1693 says that buckthorns 'are one of the best of strong Purgers'. He recommends gathering the ripe berries in early or mid-autumn. Both the black berries and the bark were used as purgers in official medicine as recently as the late nineteenth century. Whether or not they featured in folk medicine too is unclear, but if so it is probable that the milder alder buckthorn was the one administered. Even this is still a fierce purge and can be dangerous if the fresh plant is used. It is safest to dry the bark for at least a year before use.

Confusingly, the early herbalists sometimes refer to alder buckthorn as 'black alder' and Gerard recorded it under this name as growing in various localities including Hampstead Heath. Sir John Hill in 1820 states: 'In Yorkshire they bruise the bark with vinegar, and use it outwardly for the itch, which it cures very safely.' Today's medical herbalists continue with the traditional use of buckthorn as a treatment for chronic constipation, but prescribe only the alder buckthorn.

Buckthorn berries are not always to be regarded with caution. Here is what Pechey says about them in 1694:

> The Berry of this Shrub yields three sorts of Colours. Those that are gather'd in Harvest-time, and dried, and powder'd, and infus'd with Water and Allum, make a yellow or rather a Saffron-colour; and [it] is now in use for painting of Playing-Cards and leather. Those that are gather'd in the Autumn, when they are ripe and black, being pounded, and kept in a Glass-Vessel, afford a delicate Green, which is called Sap-Green, and is much used by Painters. Those that remain on the Trees till the Feast of St Martin make a red Colour.

Sap-green was in use in Gerard's lifetime and was still being used in the nineteenth century by many watercolour artists.

Buckthorn wood, especially that of alder buckthorn, makes extremely good, fast-burning charcoal. Its suitability for small-arms powder was pre-eminent, and in the nineteenth century the tree was grown for this purpose in Sussex and Kent. Over the years, the wood was made into walking sticks and umbrella handles and fashioned into skewers, and for this reason alder buckthorn was often known quite succinctly as 'butcher's prickwood'.

Bugle
(*Ajuga reptans*)

It is put in drinkes for woundes, and that is the cause why some doe commonly say, that he that hath bugle and sanicle, will scarce vouchsafe the chirurgion a bugle.

R. Surflet's *Countrie Farm* (1600)

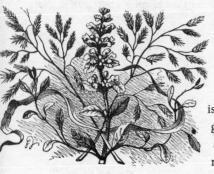

With shining, bronzed leaves and spikes of flowers 'of a Sky and change-able colour, and of a sweetish Taste', as Pechey described it in 1694, bugle thrives in shady places on light soil. It is a wild flower that is often grown in gardens for its beauty and for its value as ground cover. Among its country names are 'middle consound', a name derived from the Latin *consolida*, implying its ability to unite broken and wounded tissue and, especially in Ireland, 'wood betony'.

In medicine, bugle's prime use has been as a wound-healer. Folk medicine throughout Britain and Ireland championed bugle for this and for healing bruises and infected fingers.

In official medicine, Gerard in 1597 recommends it for treating wounds and ulcers. Culpeper valued it so highly that he advises in 1653 to 'keep a syrup of it to take inwardly and an ointment of it to use outwardly always by you'. Pechey knew of its value as a wound-healer too, but also prescribed it for jaundice and for relief of the suppression of urine. He records that it is one of the ingredients of a wound drink listed in the London Dispensatory under the name 'The Traumatick Decoction'. Bugle was still in use in the nineteenth century, and Kemsey in 1838 describes an ointment made from the leaves and flowers that 'is good for all sorts of sores and old ulcers. A decoction, with honey and alum, cures foul sores in the mouth and gums'. Thereafter bugle fell into disuse in official herbalism, but modern medical herbalists still occasionally use it in the way it is known best, as a wound-healer.

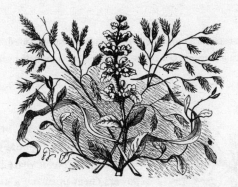

Bugloss
(*Anchusa arvensis*)

The flowers are of great use in melancholy … A person was cured of the Falling-Sickness by the Constant Use of the Flowers in Wine for half a year.

John Pechey, *The Compleat Herbal of Physical Plants* (1694)

Bugloss is native to Britain and is commonly found, especially on cultivated and waste ground where its bright blue flowers cheer up many a dreary site. The name bugloss is derived from the Greek for 'ox tongue', which its rough, bristly leaves were thought to resemble. It has proved a useful plant to humans in a number of ways; we have eaten it, worn it and used it to lighten our mood when we are feeling low.

Culpeper in 1653 recommends bugloss 'to comfort the heart and spirits', as does Pechey. Culpeper also suggests that nursing mothers take the seeds and leaves to increase their milk. He recommends the leaves to help mend wounds and broken bones, and the root to be made into a 'licking electuary' for a cough. Gerard in 1597 tells us that the root boiled with wine and butter is good for healing injuries, and the leaves can be eaten in salads. In official medicine in England, wild bugloss and the cultivated borage (*Borago officinalis*), a close relative, seem to have been used interchangeably, but it is the borage leaf that has the more refreshing taste and is the more likely to be used in the kitchen. Both Culpeper and Gerard maintain however that the 'vertues' of bugloss and borage are the same.

It was reported by Gerard that the gentlewomen of France painted their faces with the juice of bugloss roots. It seems a strange practice to indulge in but, to confound the sceptic, it is worth noting that in some areas of Britain the closely related alkanet (*Anchusa officinalis*) is called 'painting root'; this suggests that the plant may also have been used for similar cosmetic purposes, or even in the painting of pictures. Further confirmation comes from the generic name *Anchusa*, which is derived from the Greek word *anchousa*, meaning 'a cosmetic paint'.

Yet another unusual use for bugloss is recounted in an eleventh-century narrative poem composed by a monk in southern Germany that tells the tale of a knight errant, Ruodlieb, exiled from his own land. He accompanies the king on a fishing trip and scatters bugloss seed on the water. The fish float up to the surface, and the king is so impressed with his hunting skills that he takes Ruodlieb into his service.

It is worth mentioning the closely related viper's bugloss (*Echium vulgare*), illustrated on the previous page; it is a relatively scarce plant which grows on heathland, particularly in East Anglia. Its reddish-purple flowers are borne in a tight, snake-like coil that may have given the plant its name. In folk medicine an infusion of the leaves has been used to treat headaches. In official medicine it was used in the same ways as bugloss, but in addition was given as a treatment for snakebite.

In recent times, the use of both bugloss and viper's bugloss in medical herbalism has largely lapsed, due to the presence of toxic alkaloids in the plants. Today, medical herbalists still sometimes recommend using these plants externally as a poultice for treating boils and some other skin conditions.

Burdock
(*Arctium lappa*)

... they are burs, I can tell you;
they'll stick where they are thrown.

Shakespeare, *Troilus and Cressida*, III, ii, 108–109

It is said that the inventor of Velcro was inspired by what is perhaps the burdock plant's most memorable feature – the hooked bracts surrounding the flowerhead which stick to anything and anyone they come into contact with. Any dog owner will be familiar with this superb dispersal method. Children love the game of throwing the burrs at each other, now and even in Culpeper's day. Such games have inspired the strange annual ritual of the 'Burry Man' which takes place every August at South Queensferry near Edinburgh. The Burry Man's costume is covered in a layer of burrs, and he goes from house to house collecting money and gifts. At the end of the day, he is released from his costume, which is then burnt. The origin of this tradition is not known, but it seems to be of relatively recent origin; there are no records of it before the nineteenth century.

Medicinally, the burdock has been of great importance and has a reputation for being a superb cleanser and purifier. The root was – and still is – the most valuable part. Both folk and official medicine have used a decoction of the root as a cleansing tonic, reputed to be good for the liver and for rheumatic conditions and renowned especially for treating skin conditions, including acne. In official medicine, the seeds were used for treating kidney stones. This seventeenth-century recipe was recommended for both gout and kidney stones:

Take burdock Leaves gather' in June and wn ye sun is hot and ye are very dry, and still yem in a Cold Still and drink a quarter of a pint of ye water every morning fastin, and fast an hower after it, and for yer breakfast, take a burdock root and wash it clean and wipe it dry and eate it wth some bread and butter as you doe a raddish ys is very good for pains in ye back or reains doe yt till you are well, and after some time drinke ye water and be sure always keep some by you to drink, if you find it return.

In folk medicine, burdock leaves, which are among the largest of any of our native British plants, have been used to wrap around wounds and bruises, like dock leaves. Burns too were soothed using the biggest and softest of the leaves. Skin complaints (especially boils), rheumatism and urinary complaints were also treated in folk medicine using burdock.

Present-day medical herbalists still use the plant, often in combination with others, for treating skin conditions, arthritis and infections such as mumps and measles. Studies have recently shown burdock to have antibiotic, antifungal and antibacterial properties. There is clearly still a great deal to learn about this plant.

In the spring before the plant flowers, the stems of burdock may be peeled, chopped and boiled and eaten as a vegetable. They have an asparagus-like flavour. The stems may also be eaten raw in salads or pickled in vinegar as an accompaniment to meat. In earlier times, the stems were candied just as angelica (*Angelica archangelica*) is today.

A mixture of dandelion and burdock is still commercially available, especially in the north of England. It is not drunk just for its taste. Burdock is regarded as a tonic to the kidneys and dandelion as a liver tonic, so a combination of the two plants provides a healthy, as well as pleasant, drink. Some proprietary versions of 'dandelion and burdock' contain no trace of either plant, but the natural version can still be obtained in at least one teetotaller's 'pub' – the last of the so-called temperance bars founded in the 1830s – in Rawtenstall, Lancashire.

This versatile plant has been used in yet another way too. Salmon in 1693 states that a cataplasm of the plant will make the hair yellow.

Butcher's Broom
(*Ruscus aculeatus*)

> Now it is used by few unless it be Butchers who make cleane their stalls, and
> defend their meat from the flyes therewith.
>
> William Coles, *Adam in Eden* (1657)

Butcher's broom is a tough and spiny shrub, native throughout Britain on
heaths and the edges of woodland. It is a strikingly unusual evergreen, and
what appear to be its leathery green leaves are in fact flattened stems,
called cladodes, on which minute flowering shoots are borne. The male
and female flowers are separate, with the female producing bright red
berries in the autumn. It is hard to believe that it is a member of the lily
family.

The plant's tough and prickly characteristics make it ideal, when dry, for
sweeping away flies and for brushing down butcher's blocks, hence its
common name of butcher's broom. The butcher also made further use of
the plant by decorating his meat with it. Strangely enough, crowned heads
were decorated with it too: the 'laurel' wreath worn by Caesar was made
from a related species.

In Devon, the plant is called 'knee-holly' and it was used there to thrash
chilblains to speed up their healing, in just the way that HOLLY is used elsewhere in the country. Also in folk medicine, the plant was chopped and dried
and an infusion made from it to treat gravel (small urinary stones) and
jaundice.

In official medicine, the rhizome of the plant was recommended for
treating dropsy and kidney complaints. Culpeper in 1653 confirms these uses
and others, including provoking menstruation, soothing a headache and
clearing the chest. In addition, he suggests that a decoction of the root drunk
and a poultice of the shoots applied will help mend broken bones and dislo-
cations. Pechey in 1694 recommends butcher's broom for other ailments:
'Obstructions of the Liver, the Urine, and the Courses'. Salmon's *English*

Physician says of the powder of the root that 'strewed into Wounds, it cleanses them, and prevents a Gangreen'.

Despite its great usefulness in the past, butcher's broom is not often prescribed today by modern herbalists. However, recent chemical analysis has shown the presence of some interesting and potentially useful compounds called glycosides. Some of these cause the contraction of blood vessels, which could explain the observed beneficial effect of the plant on varicose veins and haemorrhoids, so the plant may yet come back into use and resume its former importance.

Until then, it would seem that the plant is still appreciated only in Devon. There the young edible shoots are sometimes eaten, in the same way as asparagus shoots – a practice that also existed in Classical times.

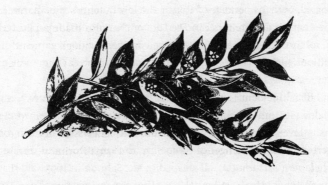

Butterbur
(*Petasites hybridus*)

Butterbur once had a particular reputation as a plague remedy. Lyte in 1578 described it as 'a soveraigne medicine against the plague' and Gerard endorsed this opinion in 1597, adding that it works by causing sweating. In one Cornish village, it still grows on the graves of plague victims and it is said that nothing else will grow there.

Butterbur is unusual in many ways. The male and female plants are not only separate but different in appearance and in distribution, the male being larger-leaved and more vigorous. As with the COLTSFOOT, the flowers, which look like large, pink cones, appear in spring before the leaves. Butterbur's botanical name derives from *petasos*, the Greek word for a wide floppy hat worn by shepherds and refers, as do its English names of 'flapperdock' and 'umbrella leaves', to its unusually large leaves. These were once used to wrap butter, keeping it moist, as the name suggests. It is a rather magical-looking plant and, perhaps because of this or the lovely sound of its name, J. R. R. Tolkien named an innkeeper in *The Lord of the Rings* Barliman Butterbur.

In folk medicine, the plant was used mainly for the treatment of skin conditions such as shingles, sores and spots, but also for rheumatism and scurvy.

In official medicine, in addition to its value as a plague cure, Gerard in 1597 also recommended it for less worrying ailments such as worms and ulcers. A seventeenth-century recipe from Norfolk consists of fresh roots of butterbur, roots of angelica (*Angelica archangelica*) and masterwort (*Peucedanum ostruthium*), all steeped in ale. Salmon in 1693 said that this was used not only for 'pestilential fevers' but also for 'swoonings' and 'vapors'. Nineteenth-century physicians used a decoction of the root in wine for 'short wind and wheezing' and an ointment prepared from the root to treat sores, according to Kemsey in 1838. Nowadays butterbur is not taken internally because of its toxicity but medical herbalists still recommend it in an external application for skin complaints.

Butterbur seeds were once used in love divination. In one method, the instructions were very precise. They had to be sowed in a lonely place half an hour before sunrise on a Friday morning, and the maiden sowing them meanwhile had to say:

I sow, I sow!
Then, my own dear,
Come here, come here,
And mow and mow!

She would then have an apparition of her future husband. In the late nineteenth century in Scotland, a charm was still in use for ensuring a husband's faithfulness. It was difficult to prepare and tricky to apply, and consisted of sprinkling on the man's chest a mixture prepared from butterbur, FOXGLOVE, ROYAL FERN (see FERNS) and an old man's bones.

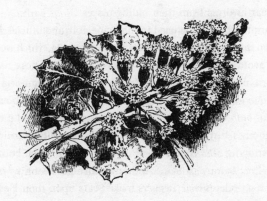

Buttercup
(*Ranunculus* species)

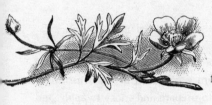

For many people, the buttercup is a sweet reminder of childhood. Everyone knows the game where a buttercup flower is held under the chin; if a golden reflection shows on the skin, then that person is said to like butter. On Midsummer's Eve, dairymen used to garland their cows with buttercups, to bless the milk, and yet cows usually avoid the plant when grazing unless they are very hungry. Swathes of meadow buttercup (*Ranunculus acris*) growing in lush grassland are surely one of our loveliest sights, but one that is becoming increasingly scarce.

The name buttercup is a relatively recent one, uncommon in print before the eighteenth century. Gerard in 1597 does refer to 'butterflower' but the plant was then more often known as 'crowfoot' or 'gollan'. Thornton tells us in 1810 that a strong infusion of meadow buttercup poured onto the ground will force earthworms from their hiding-places.

The plant has been little used in medicine, folk and official, for the very good reason that its sap is caustic and causes blistering, which would explain why cows avoid them so assiduously. Its main use therefore has been as a counter-irritant to relieve the pain of gout and rheumatism, and as a caustic application to warts. The species most used for this is the bulbous buttercup (*Ranunculus bulbosus*), whose swollen leaf bases have earned it the name of 'Saint Anthony's turnips'. This saint is associated with burning, and the intensely stinging skin condition of erysipelas used to be known as Saint Anthony's fire. 'Beware of Saint Anthony's turnips' warns an old proverb. Pechey in 1694 relates that 'Beggars make Soars upon their Flesh with this Plant, to move Compassion.'

In folk medicine, in the Scottish Highlands, the water buttercup (*Ranunculus flammula*) was crushed, placed in a limpet shell and clapped to the face to treat toothache, blistering the face in the process. However, not all uses of the plant had to be this painful. A twentieth-century recipe from Northumberland suggests simmering buttercup flowers and vaseline together for three-quarters of an hour to make an ointment for all skin troubles. In Ireland, buttercup and garlic were combined and rubbed on the skin to keep midges away, and the plant was also recommended there to treat heartburn, mumps and tuberculosis, as well as black leg and red water fever in animals.

Medical herbalists in the recent past have used this plant to treat shingles; in modern-day herbalism, it is little used.

The creeping buttercup (*Ranunculus repens*) is the least caustic species, and has in some parts of the country been used to remove the marks in eyes formerly known as 'kennings'. It is more widely known as a troublesome weed of gardens and allotments, and has the apt name in Cumbria of 'Meg-many-feet', in reference to the readily rooting stems. Unusually, its flowers are rain-pollinated: perhaps one reason why it does so well in a typical British summer. Water collects at the base of the shiny petals and is drawn by capillarity up to the stigmas; the flower is, quite literally, a cup.

Perhaps as a cautionary tale, it was said that to smell a buttercup could cause madness, and one of the plant's country names is 'crazy'; yet it was held to cure madness, too. According to the Latin Herbarium of Apuleius Platonicus (*c*.AD 600), if the plant were hung around the neck when the moon was on the wane, a person would be restored to their right mind.

Butterwort
(*Pinguicula vulgaris*)

> A magic hoop was made of milkwort, butterwort, dandelion and marigold. It
> was from three to four inches in diameter, and it was bound by a triple cord
> of lint – for lint also had magical properties – in the name of the Father, the
> Son and the Spirit, and placed under the milk-vessel, to prevent the substance
> of the milk from being spirited away.
>
> Alexander Carmichael, *Carmina Gadelica* (1900–1971)

Butterwort grows in shallow streams and on the edges of bogs throughout
Britain; an alternative country name for it is 'bog violet'. Its characteristic
star-shaped rosette of yellow-green leaves produces a single flowering stem
with a blue-purple flower of great beauty. The leaves are sensitive to touch
and roll up lengthways, trapping small insects inside. It is one of our two
native insectivorous plants, the other being SUNDEW. It has been suggested
that it is the greasy feel of the leaves that has earned the plant the name of
butterwort. Similarly, the botanical name comes from *pinguis*, meaning 'fat'
or 'greasy'.

In common with sundew, butterwort was thought to have certain magical
powers. Carrying it protected the wearer from witches; cows fed on it were
immune to 'elf-arrows'. In the Inner Hebrides, it was believed that if a mother
partook of butter made using butterwort, her children would be safe from
the fairies. Furthermore, wearing it made one secure 'from all despite; from
the sorrow of love ungiven; from a foeman's stroke; from the gnaw of hunger;
or from drowning, the doom of the sea'. Magical indeed.

In some areas, it was said to have additional powers and was called
'Valentine's-flower' because 'If you put one under your pillow and think of
someone you would like to see, you will be pretty likely to dream of him.'

Butterwort has a long association with the dairy, more specifically with
butter-making, and this could provide another explanation for its common
name. It was used to curdle milk and help in butter-making, and in

Lanarkshire was known as 'earning grass', 'earning' being a North-Country word for rennet.

The plant did have some medicinal uses. In folk medicine, it was used in Wales to treat the liver and as a purge. Elsewhere, it was made into an ointment to treat chapped skin and bruises. Within living memory, an infusion of butterwort was used in Cornwall to make the skin smooth. Pechey in 1694 refers to these uses in folk practice and adds that the leaves, beaten before being applied, are good for pain, and to treat ruptures in children.

Thereafter the plant seems to have fallen out of favour and was seldom mentioned by later herbalists. It is little used in modern medical herbalism in this country.

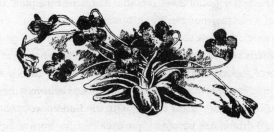

Centaury
(*Centaurium* species)

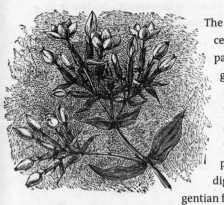

The pretty pink, star-like flowers of centaury are a fairly common sight, particularly near the sea and on dry grassland. The flowers open only on sunny days. The plant has a very bitter taste and is rarely eaten by grazing animals. It may have been this observation that first led humans to use this plant as a 'bitter' – a stimulant to the digestive juices. It is a member of the gentian family, several of which are famous for this property, and in parts of Scotland it is actually called 'gentian'.

In folk medicine, centaury has been used not only as a tonic and a digestive but also as a wound-healer. Official medicine too used the plant in this way: it is named after the Greek centaur Chiron, who was said to have cured himself of a mortal wound using this plant.

There were other folk uses for centaury. An infusion was considered good to remove freckles, and to destroy body lice; in Uist 'a tonic was made from a tincture of pink centaury in whisky and pronounced "excellent".' The tradition continues: a twentieth-century book of homemade wines includes a recipe for centaury wine and adds that 'in the Hartlepools, centaury is just scalded and drunk. It is known as "pink tea".'

Sir John Hill in 1820 stated that 'country people cure agues with it' and Quelch in 1941 records a gypsy's description of centaury as 'one o' they blessings as God put on the earth to make us well ... 'Tis powerful good for consumption and poor blood.'

In official medicine, centaury was used to treat snakebites and fever as far back as Saxon times. An early-seventeenth-century manuscript found in Suffolk includes a recipe for using 'Senteway' for 'pain in the loins, breast and heart'. By the mid-seventeenth century, Culpeper was continuing these recommendations, as well as prescribing it for treating wounds, gout and jaundice and for improving the complexion. He alludes to its bitterness, saying that the plant is 'very wholesome, but not very toothsome'. Salmon in 1693 states that 'the whole Plant, is a great Vulnerary', meaning it is a wound-healer.

By the nineteenth century, Kemsey was still recommending centaury as a 'stomachic' and for dropsy, gout and jaundice. Today's medical herbalists use the plant as an aid to digestion.

Chamomile
(*Chamaemelum nobile*)

Chamomile is native to the whole of Britain but is much more commonly found in the south, where it favours short grassland on sandy soil. When crushed, its fragrant foliage smells slightly of apples; in Spain, it is known as *manzanilla*, meaning 'little apple', and both its botanical and common name are derived from the Greek *khamaemelon*, meaning 'earth apple'. Over the centuries, chamomile has been much in demand for use in both folk and official medicine, and so popular was its domestic use that it could be found in abundance in many a cottage garden. It featured in Beatrix Potter's *The Tale of Peter Rabbit*, when Peter Rabbit ate far too many lettuces and had a stomach-ache. His mother made him chamomile tea which settled his digestion and he was able to get off to sleep.

With the current, renewed interest in herbal medicine and aromatherapy, the plant is being cultivated as a crop in parts of East Anglia. One lady who worked in the chamomile fields noticed how much her psoriasis improved after handling the flowers. The factory owner gave her the sludge left from the oil-extraction process and she used it to keep her psoriasis at bay. This twentieth-century cure is just one in a long line of successes for chamomile.

Medicinally, the plant has been valued at least since the time of the ancient Egyptians. The Anglo-Saxons called it *maythen*, and in pre-Christian times it was known to them as one of their nine sacred herbs, celebrated in the Lay of the Nine Healing Herbs:

Remember, maythen, what you made known

What you ordained at Alorford:

That no one's life be given up to infection

After anyone has prepared him maythen as food.

Chamomile has been widely used in folk medicine. Apart from its value for upset stomachs, it has been used to treat coughs and colds, earache, neuralgia, period pain and toothache. Mrs L. P— of Suffolk relates that it was also used for treating gallstones, in an infusion of the flowers that was drunk cold morning and evening. To treat asthma, the fumes from a hot infusion could be inhaled, or the plant smoked. In Wales so great was the faith in the plant that the dew shaken from its flowers was said to cure tuberculosis.

Practitioners of folk medicine used the native species of the plant, but the related German chamomile (*Matricaria recutita*) was often used in official medicine, and many records do not distinguish between the two. In Culpeper's words, 'Camomile takes away weariness, eases pains, to what part of the body soever they be applied', confirming the plant's reputation as a great 'soother' of many ills. But clearly there were more specific uses.

Pechey in 1694 tells the story of a man who cured himself of the stone using a strong decoction of chamomile flowers: 'By the use of this simple Medicine (God be prais'd) the dreadful symptoms were mitigated, and the Ureters relaxed; so that some Stones came away with the Urine, without any great Pain.' The man went on to treat several other sufferers successfully in the same way. Salmon in 1693 lists similar properties, adding that it 'provokes Urine and the Terms, facilitates the Birth, and brings away the dead Child and After-birth'. The seventeenth- and eighteenth-century kitchen book from Suffolk, the Gunton Household Book, gives the following unusual instructions:

To Stay a Cough or Rhume

Take brown Paper and Cut it like a Cap yn quilt wooll within it and take Camomile flowers beaten to Powder and strow it thick upon ye wooll soe let ye child wear it till ye Paper wears out then renew it.

Modern-day herbalists recommend chamomile for headaches, indigestion and skin irritations. Chamomile also still has ordinary domestic uses. Bunches of the plant keep insects away (it was once used as a strewing herb in the Middle Ages), and an infusion of chamomile makes a good rinse for blonde hair. Its ability to withstand trampling has also led to its being planted in gardens as an ornamental chamomile lawn; as the saying goes: 'The chamomile bed; the more it is trodden, the more it will spread.'

Finally, this wonderful herb has been called the plant's physician, as Frances A. Bardswell relates in her book, *The Herb Garden*: 'Nothing is thought to keep a garden so healthy as plenty of Chamomile about; it will even revive drooping and sickly plants if placed near.'

Chickweed
(*Stellaria media*)

Everyone knows this plant as a weed of cultivated land. It grows and flowers all through the year (even in winter), wherever the soil is rich enough to support it. Chickweed makes an excellent addition, with its gentle lettuce-like flavour, to a salad and is also good in sandwiches or steamed like spinach as a vegetable. Cage birds, as well as poultry, feast on it, and this of course is where the plant gets its common name. It has also been called, more poetically, 'starwort', which is a very apt description of the tiny white flowers; the generic name *Stellaria* means much the same.

Chickweed is also a weather forecaster. When its flowers and leaves open fully, good weather can be expected: 'If it should shut up, the traveller is to put on his greatcoat.' Even the seed capsules close up tightly in wet weather. Withering, famed for his work on the FOXGLOVE, noted the tastiness of chickweed as a vegetable in *A Botanical Arrangement of the Vegetables naturally growing in Great Britain* (1776). He went on to say:

> This species is a notable instance of what is called the Sleep of Plants; for every night the leaves approach in pairs, so as to include within their upper surfaces, the tender rudiments of the new shoots; and the uppermost pair but one at the end of the stalk, are furnished with longer leaf-stalks than the others, so that they can close upon the terminating pair and protect the end of the branch.

A number of our native plants exhibit movements of their leaves at night or under adverse weather conditions. WOOD SORREL is one obvious example, where the leaflets fold in such a way as to minimize exposure to cold or heat. Periodic movements of leaves had been noted by natural historians, from Pliny the Elder (AD 23–79) onwards, but it was not until the eighteenth century that their study provided the first evidence for the existence of 'biological clocks'.

Chickweed's medicinal uses have been many and varied but it enjoys a reputation, as does chamomile, for its 'soothing' qualities. Its juicy leaves and mat-like growth make it an ideal plant to use as an old-fashioned poultice. In folk medicine, it has been used to ease the pain of burns, chilblains, leg ulcers, rashes and other skin irritations, including eczema. As a poultice, it had the ability to bring boils to a head and to soothe the swellings of mumps. Martin after his travels in Scotland reported in the early eighteenth century a cure from the Isle of Skye. A person who had suffered from fever was washed with warm water in which chickweed had been soaked, and was then put to bed with warm parcels of the herb between the shoulder blades and on the neck.

Chickweed juice has been used to ease insect stings, and an ointment prepared by boiling it in lard was used as a general healer and for the treatment of rheumatism. In the Highlands, it was used to treat insomnia, and an infusion of it was used for slimming. Ireland had numerous uses for it, including the treatment of burns, colic, coughs and sore throats, and jaundice.

In official medicine, the weed was used as a cooling application for inflammation; Pechey in 1694 recommended it for sufferers from consumption. Echoing Gerard from the previous century, Pechey also tells us, 'Birds that are kept in cages are much refreshed by this Herb, when they loath their meat.' Salmon recommends in 1693 the distilled water of chickweed for soothing sore eyes, a treatment confirmed in the seventeenth- and eighteenth-century Gunton Household Book, where there is a recipe for treating wounded eyes with 'starwort' that has been rotted: 'If this medicine be a year old its never the worse.'

Kemsey writing in 1838 is full of praise for chickweed: 'The juice is good for pains in the ears; and the bruised herb for heat, inflammation, and swellings, in any part of the body, also for piles, ulcers, and sores.'

In present-day medical herbalism, chickweed is used mainly to soothe skin irritations including rashes and eczema; when added to the bath, it can help to ease rheumatic pain.

Chicory
(*Cichorium intybus*)

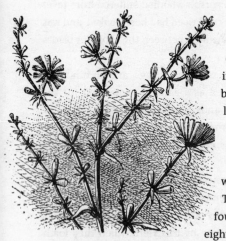

The unforgettable sky blue of chicory flowers in late summer is a sight more common in continental Europe than in this country but, nevertheless, it can be spotted, scattered on chalky grassland throughout Britain. Pechey in 1694 noticed this fascinating feature: 'The Flowers of this Plant open and shut at Sun-rising and Sun-setting, whether the Heavens are clear or cloudy.' The plant is also known as 'succory': the founder of the Linnean Society in the eighteenth century, Sir James Smith, recalls in his childhood 'tugging ineffectually with all my infant strength at the tough stalks of the wild Succory, on the chalky hills about Norwich'.

In folk medicine, the plant has been used in the treatment of rheumatism. A market gardener in Norfolk in the early decades of the twentieth century was renowned for his treatment of this disease, and the plant he used most was chicory. He prided himself on the fact that many patients who came crawling to see him the first time, returned later on their bicycles. A very different use altogether was adopted by the gypsies who used the root of chicory to treat jaundice.

Official medicine regards the plant as tonic, laxative and diuretic. It is described by Parkinson in 1640 as 'a fine cleansing, jovial plant'. Pechey fifty years later tells us that 'the Water distill'd from the blue Flowers is an excellent Remedy for Inflammations and Dimness of the Eyes'. However, a manuscript of notes taken down by an eighteenth-century Peebles-shire woman recommended a very different use altogether. Cosmetic surgeons, take note.

For a Woman that hath great breasts.

Oftentimes anoint her Paps with the juice of Succory, it will make them round and hard: If they be hanging or bagging, it will draw them together, whereby they shall seem like the Paps of a Maid.

Chicory was also recommended to ease childbirth by John Moncrief in *The Poor Man's Physician* (1731):

Take a little castile Sope, temper it in the Hand until it be soft, then make it into little Pills, whereof the Party may swallow down five, being a little rolled in Sugar; then let there be in readiness a good Draught of Posset-drink, wherein some Succory hath been boiled. Let the Patient drink it as hot as she can suffer it, and it will work the Effect.

In modern medical herbalism, chicory is used as a mild digestive tonic, much like DANDELION, recommended for liver and kidney complaints and for rheumatism.

Most of us are familiar with chicory as an ingredient in salads, and it is often cultivated on allotments for this purpose; the leaves are nicest if blanched to remove some of their bitterness. The root itself can be boiled and eaten, and for many years now the seeds have been used as a coffee substitute, or as an additive to coffee to make it go further. Country folk have often made country wine from chicory, using both flowers and leaves.

Clubmosses
(*Lycopodiaceae*)

The club-moss is on my person,
No harm or mishap can me befall;
No sprite shall slay me, no arrow shall wound me,
No fay nor dun water-nymph shall tear me

Alexander Carmichael, *Carmina Gadelica* (1900–1971)

Clubmosses are such strikingly different-looking plants that they simply cannot be mistaken for anything else. They grow mainly in uplands and mountains, and their low-growing branches resemble miniature trees. They are related to the FERNS and, like them, produce spores rather than seeds. It is these spores that have attracted human interest for hundreds of years.

Pliny the Elder (AD 23–79) named clubmoss as one of the herbs important to the Druids, who believed that it should be carried as an amulet against accidents. The 'smoke' of its extremely fine spores was believed to be a good treatment for eye diseases. The unwettable or water-repellant quality of the yellow spores has earned the plant the name of 'vegetable sulphur'. The spores have been used as face powder in Scotland and they were still in use in the twentieth century as a dusting powder and in the manufacture of pills to prevent them from sticking together. They are still used today in the coating of condoms. Because the spores ignite explosively, they have also been used in the production of fireworks and stage lighting.

Clubmosses had a very important country use in the Scottish Highlands, as mordants for dyeing, before the use of alum was widespread. (A mordant was a substance that had the ability to 'fix' the colour of the dye.) This was an ancient practice that extended back at least to the twelfth century.

Other parts of the plant have been found to be useful medicinally. Dyer in 1889 tells us that clubmoss was considered in Cornwall to be good for diseases of the eye. There were very specific instructions for gathering the herb; this was to be done kneeling down, at sundown, on the third day of the moon. An incantation accompanied the cutting of the herb:

> As Christ healed the issue of blood,
>
> Do thou cut what thou cuttest for good.

The cut herb was gathered in a white cloth and boiled in water from the nearest spring. It was then used as a fomentation or made into an ointment with butter.

Clubmoss was used in other ways too in folk medicine. An infusion was used as recently as the early twentieth century in Sutherland as a lotion for soothing and softening skin. There the plant was known, in Gaelic, by a name translated as 'little rough one of the moors'. In the Scottish Highlands, an infusion was also taken internally as an emetic and emmenagogue (menstrual stimulant), but the dose had to be regulated, otherwise its action was found to be too drastic. James Robertson after his tour of the West Highlands in 1768 found clubmoss in use for suppression of the menses. He states: '*Lycopodium selago* is said to be such a strong purge that it will bring on an abortion.' In recent years, one of the plant's alkaloids, lycopodine, has been demonstrated to produce uterine contractions in rodents, giving a possible scientific explanation for its use in this way.

Official medicine seemed largely to ignore clubmoss. Gerard grouped it with the true mosses and described them as all having the same properties. Salmon describes 'earth Moss' as being used to 'break the stone and expel it . . . it also fastenes loose teeth and draws up Ulcers and Wounds being laid on'. The name 'wolf's-foot' is a direct translation of the current generic name *Lycopodium*.

In the nineteenth century, clubmoss was still used by herbalists to treat urinary disorders, and this use has continued to the present day.

Coltsfoot
(*Tussilago farfara*)

It grows in pleasant moist places and near Rivers which make a Noise.

William Salmon, *The Compleat English Physician* (1693)

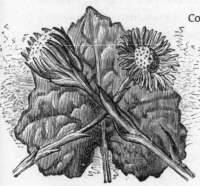

Coltsfoot is usually said to get its name from the shape of its leaves, but an alternative explanation is to be found in the shape of the flower bud. Pick a stem and turn it upside-down – the likeness to a foal's slender leg and hoof is quite striking.

The flowering stems appear before the leaves and each produces a single golden blossom as rich in colour as the yolk of a free-range hen egg. The large basal leaves do not appear until late in the spring when the flowers are over. It grows often on clay banks and brightens up many patches of waste ground. Traditionally, it is said that where coltsfoot grows in profusion there will be coal underground.

Since the time of Pliny the Elder (AD 23–79), and probably earlier than that too, the plant has been used medicinally to treat bronchitis and coughs, including tubercular coughs. In the sixteenth century, a Scottish archbishop who suffered greatly from asthma was restored to better health with coltsfoot soup. Far from appreciating the skill of his Italian healer, the archbishop ascribed the effects to witchcraft. As well as its main role as a remedy for coughs and asthma, other folk applications of coltsfoot have included treating sprains and swellings (with an ointment prepared from the root) as well as, in Ireland, earache and neuralgia.

Several accounts testify to the supreme power of coltsfoot in curing respiratory ailments. John Clerk of Penecuik in Midlothian, Scotland, in the eighteenth century, kept a detailed diary of his own health. After suffering for months with a cough, he decided to try coltsfoot because it was said to be effective in the works of Pliny. Evidently he couldn't bring himself to give up smoking tobacco, but he mixed it with dried coltsfoot, half and half 'as near as I can guess by little heaps', and he soon found the benefit from it.

In Scotland in the 1980s, I came across a gardener in Lanarkshire who regularly treated his coughs with what he called 'dishyluggs', a name that puzzled me until I recognized it as a corruption of the botanical name, *Tussilago*, itself derived from the Latin *tussis*, meaning 'cough'.

During the Second World War, coltsfoot was used as a substitute for tobacco – not for medicinal reasons but because it was free and readily available, at least in rural areas. In general, it has been a regular constituent of British herbal tobaccos. 'Old Bill's cough cure' from the north of England is made from coltsfoot flowers, barley, sugar and water, and flavoured with the old-fashioned mint sweets known as 'black bullets'. Another combination of confectionery and medicine was coltsfoot rock, a popular treatment for sore throats and coughs that was still being made in England in the 1970s. Here is a recipe taken from a nineteenth-century 'Consult Me', owned and annotated by a Norfolk woman:

Coltsfoot Lozenges

To 1 pint of water add one handful of coltsfoot leaves. Boil down to 1 gill [a quarter pint], strain, add ½ lb sugar. Boil to a syrup. Strain. Add as much common liquorice as will give it consistency. Then form into any shape you please.

Official medicine, like folk medicine, used coltsfoot mainly for respiratory conditions. An infusion was also recommended by Gerard in 1597 for erysipelas, a painful skin condition; in early-twentieth-century Yorkshire, coltsfoot was still used in a poultice as a folk remedy for this affliction.

Today's medical herbalists are still prescribing coltsfoot for chest conditions, taken as an infusion of the leaves.

The fine down which covers the plant has been found to have many practical uses. The down easily rubs off, and in the past it was collected onto cloths and used, with the addition of a quantity of saltpetre, as tinder for starting a fire. Goldfinches choose to line their nests with coltsfoot 'down' and, in the Scottish Highlands, people sometimes used it in lieu of feathers for stuffing pillows and mattresses – a laborious process, one would imagine.

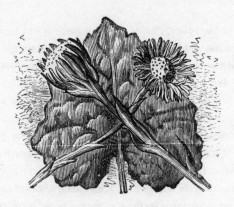

Comfrey
(*Symphytum officinale*)

The water of the Greater Comferies druncke helpeth such as are bursten, and that have broken the bone of the legge ...

George Baker, *Jewell of Health* (1576)

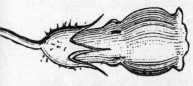 Comfrey is easily recognized when it is in flower. The whole plant is rough and hairy, and the bell-like, red-purple flowers are borne in characteristic crosier-like spikes. Sometimes the flowers are cream-coloured. The flower has a long corolla tube and some insects have learnt to bypass this; look at a number of flowers and you are likely to find some with small holes bitten in the bases of the tubes, where a nectar-thief has been (see BLUEBELL). It is one of relatively few native plants that have been cultivated in gardens for medicinal use.

Its generic name *Symphytum* means 'to make whole', or 'heal' and refers to the quality that has made the plant so medicinally valuable in the past. The name comfrey is thought to derive from the Latin *con firma*, meaning 'making [bones] firm'. The plant has a long taproot, which when scraped yields a white liquid described by some as nature's putty. This has a remarkable effect on fractures when applied as a poultice, easing the pain and promoting healing. Culpeper in 1653 goes so far as to claim that if the roots 'be boiled with disseevered pieces of flesh in a pot, it will join them together again'. In this, he was repeating an assertion of Pliny the Elder (AD 23–79). Salmon in 1693 is more cautious: 'In Shops is Used ... A Cataplasm thereof which outwardly staunches Blood in Wounds and heals them, heals Broken bones and Cures the Gout being applied, so as it never returns any more to that part.'

Early herbalists also recommended comfrey for respiratory complaints. 'The roots are glutinous and mucilaginous and have been used for coughs', says Withering in 1841. As the nineteenth century progressed, the medicinal use of comfrey declined and by 1862 it was not much used, but was good as fodder. Comfrey has been widely exploited in folk medicine too:

'My husband has reminded me that when he was a Casualty Officer in the Royal Hospital, Sheffield in the 1950s, it was not uncommon for patients suffering from suspected breakages and sprains to arrive at hospital with the affected bones swathed in comfrey leaves, held in place by bandages.'

Mrs M. T—, Staffordshire (2002)

Folk medicine has also used the plant for treating sprains, for healing wounds and ulcers, for the pain of arthritis, and to treat boils:

Comfrey and its uses

'Obtain the 7lb toffee jar and pack the leaves as tight as you can in it. Then forget them for at least six months. The leaves will have become a ball of "goo" and I add, stink to high heaven. Pour the liquid into a much smaller jar for immediate use as a cure for sprains and the like. Leave the old stuff in the old jar and top up with new leaves the following year . . . Next on the agenda is the certain cure for the "Boil". Dig down to the root and cut the end off one, it is similar to the end of the Parsnip. Wash it, then with a knife scrape the root and place the creamy texture on to a piece of lint. Apply to the boil and believe me the soreness has gone in a matter of minutes, and the boil in a day.

'Number 3. Boil the leaves along with an amount of "chickweed" and drink as a medicine. This remedy not only acts as a tonic, but is purported to have been the chief remedy to curing Sugar diabetes.'

H. G—, Manchester (1985)

Among other compounds, the plant contains allantoin (remarkably, this is also found in human foetal membranes, which have themselves been used in healing). Allantoin has been shown to stimulate the growth of epithelial cells and promote healing. However the plant also contains so-called pyrrolizidine alkaloids which are toxic to the liver.

If applied externally, preparations of wild comfrey root were probably harmless as well as healing; nevertheless, use of the plant is now restricted by law as a result of scares over liver toxicity. This is a prime example of a traditional remedy which, if applied correctly and with the necessary knowledge, can be very helpful. But drinking large quantities of comfrey-leaf tea is certainly not to be recommended, nor is internal use of the root. It is for this reason that past applications of comfrey in treating pulmonary complaints have now largely been discontinued: modern medical herbalists still use the root and shoots externally for treating fractures, minor wounds and sprains.

Comfrey has been and continues to be utilized as food and medicine for animals too. One Norfolk lady keeps cats, chickens, geese and ponies. When any of them are out of sorts, she feeds them comfrey, which she grows in her garden in large quantities. Apart from its use as a tonic, the plant was also given to animals for sprains, fractures, sores and swellings as well as coughs and digestive problems.

Comfrey makes an excellent manure for the garden; its deep roots access minerals from layers of the soil that are untapped by many other plants. It begins to be clear why some people say, 'no one knows the value of comfrey ... it is so great!'

Corn Marigold
(*Chrysanthemum segetum*)

My fancy never groweth old
To meet thee 'mong the ripening corn,
Arrayed in thy gay garb of gold
Where Plenty fills her Autumn horn:

And when the sickle steals thy crown,
And all the barns are big with grain,
Among the tubered fields so brown
Thy beauty hails me once again:

James Rigg, *To the Corn Marigold* (1897)

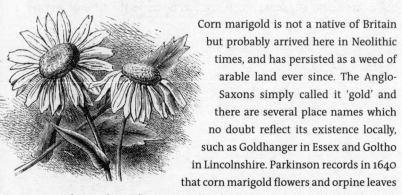

Corn marigold is not a native of Britain but probably arrived here in Neolithic times, and has persisted as a weed of arable land ever since. The Anglo-Saxons simply called it 'gold' and there are several place names which no doubt reflect its existence locally, such as Goldhanger in Essex and Goltho in Lincolnshire. Parkinson records in 1640 that corn marigold flowers and orpine leaves were used to make midsummer garlands.

Grigson notes that there are records of orders in the fourteenth-century court roll that call upon tenants to uproot 'the plant called Gold'. However, the plant persisted, to annoy future generations of farmers including one Irish farmer who apparently could grow nothing else on his land. In the eighteenth century in Scotland, heavy fines were extracted from tenant farmers who had corn marigolds on their land. To the non-farmer, the flowers are a beautiful sight in midsummer – a rich golden colour among the corn and poppies – although in most parts of Britain it is now a relatively rare sight.

The plant's role in folk medicine seems to have been minor, but in the Hebrides it was used to treat 'throbbing pains'. Official medicine, it seems, ignored it altogether and it is not utilized by modern medical herbalists.

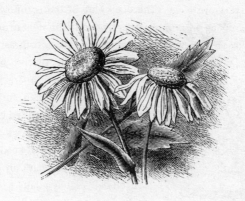

Cornflower
(*Centaurea cyanus*)

The deep blue of the cornflower was until recently a common sight in our cornfields, providing a striking contrast to the blood-red poppies: its specific name *cyanus* means 'dark blue' in Greek. It is often called 'bluebottle'. In some areas, its tough stems have earned it the name of 'hurt sickle'. Like the CORN MARIGOLD, it has been a victim of pesticide use and now it is to be seen only where it has been deliberately planted.

In East Anglia, the flower was, quite literally, a sight for sore eyes. Mixed with chamomile flowers, it was used within living memory as a compress for tired eyes. In the seventeenth century, a preparation called 'break spectacles water' was used, and in the seventeenth- and eighteenth-century Gunton Household Book, we read:

> Take blew bottle that Grow in ye Corn gathered with their Cups and bruise as many as you please, steep them in a good quantity of snow water for 24 hours then distill them in an ordinary still very moderately and keep ye water. This is most wonderfully efectuall . . . to Clear ye Sight and Strengthen it and preserve it especially of old women for that reason it's called break spectacles water for they that use it need no spectacles, some few drops into ye eye morning and evening.

Gerard in 1597 refers sceptically to this use, but is enthusiastic about its quality as a wound herb. Culpeper does, however, endorse its use in 1653 as a soother of inflamed eyes, but also claims that the 'Blue-bottle' is good for bruises, bleeding and pestilential fevers. Pechey in 1694 likewise recommends it for inflamed and 'bleared' eyes, as well as for putrid ulcers.

Nearly 150 years later, Sir John Hill's herbal dismisses the infusion of the flowers but endorses the use of the freshly gathered leaves, which when bruised 'will stop the bleeding of a fresh wound, even if a large vessel be cut', and he goes on to remark that the plant 'may save a life where a surgeon is not to be had in time'. Despite such enthusiasm, the cornflower seems to have been largely ignored in medicine from then on. In present-day herbalism, it is little used in this country, although an eye lotion prepared from it is still used in France.

In addition to their use as colourful ingredients of potpourri, the blue cornflower petals readily produce blue ink or a vividly coloured dye. In a late eighteenth-century manuscript, there is a recipe for producing such a dye. The juice of the petals 'will yield an excellent colour that by the experience of 2 or 3 years has not been found to fade. From a sufficient quantity ... press the juice: add a little alum, which will give a lasting transparent blue scarcely inferior in brightness to ultramarine.'

Couch Grass
(*Elytrigia repens*)

Silvius says, that Sheep and Oxen that are troubled with the Stone in the Winter-time are freed from it in the Spring by eating Grass.

John Pechey, *The Compleat Herbal of Physical Plants* (1694)

Every gardener in the land has at one time cursed this plant. It spreads throughout vegetable and flower gardens by means of an efficient system of fast-growing rhizomes, and it is hard to eradicate, because it can regenerate from the smallest piece of rhizome. It thrives in open areas of soil, but in pastures is soon defeated by other species.

The names 'couch' and 'quickgrass' are derived from the Old English *cwice*, meaning 'alive'; these names doubtless refer to its vigorous and almost unstoppable growth. Other country names include 'twitch' and 'speargrass'. Many of its vernacular names, such as 'dog grass' and 'foul grass', are far from complimentary. But this plant's properties are not all negative. The same rhizomes that are so tiresome to the gardener have for centuries been the source of a valuable remedy for urinary infections which is still used today. This remedy is from 1990:

'For cystitis: take a good handful of speargrass roots (speargrass is the wild kind which grows in most people's gardens). Boil the handful in two and a half pints of water, drink a cupful straightaway, then another cupful after one hour, another three hours later, and a wine-glassful about four times a day, for four to five days.'

L. W—, Norwich (1990)

Within living memory in Suffolk, an infusion of couch grass has also been used to treat rheumatism and bee stings.

In official medicine, following Classical tradition, Gerard recommended couch grass in 1597 'for it openeth the stoppings of the liver and the reins [kidneys]', and Salmon a hundred years later gives additional uses for the grass: killing worms in children, as a headache remedy, and in the treatment of diarrhoea.

Dogs seek out the grass when they are ill, and chew it to make themselves sick; hence the name 'dog grass'. Culpeper was aware of this and in 1653 wrote 'watch the dogs when they are sick and they will quickly lead you to it ... and although a gardener be of another opinion, yet a physician holds half an acre of them to be worth five acres of carrots twice told over.'

By 1838, Kemsey also appreciates its worth and describes couch grass as 'deobstruent; it eases pain and inflammation. The seed powerfully expels urine. The roots, bruised and applied, consolidate wounds.'

The plant is used mainly for treating urinary infections and kidney stones in modern herbalism in this country.

The practical uses for couch grass are numerous and give us further reason to revise our opinion of this plant. The roots have a sweet taste and were once dried and ground as a flour substitute, and the boiled stems were often fed to pigs for extra nutrition. In Ireland in the early twentieth century, the grass was collected by people of the poorer districts and used as fodder for the donkeys in the winter.

And if the gardener needs convincing yet further, the plant is known to be a rich source of minerals and makes a good liquid fertilizer, which seems to have the surprising effect of deterring growth of the weed. Couch grass is also a good consolidator of unstable ground. Where it grows along the coast its rhizomes help bind the sand and soil, in much the same way as marram grass (*Ammophila arenaria*), thus helping to prevent coastal erosion.

Cow Parsley
(*Anthriscus sylvestris*)

Without this common wayside plant we would have no white lanes of summer. Road after road is edged with it and it plays an important role in the British landscape. The name of cow parsley hardly does justice to its loveliness – although cows, along with pigs, sheep and rabbits do like eating it. Pechey wrote in 1694: 'In the Spring, when the Leaves are tender, Cows eat them greedily; wherefore our Country-People call it Cow-weed.' In Sussex, it is 'rabbit meat'. 'Queen Anne's lace' is a more evocative name, suggestive of the froth of white surf along the edge of a country road.

In some areas there was a ban on picking cow parsley; bad luck, misfortune or even death could follow and among its country names is 'mother die'. Other local names such as the Yorkshire 'devil's meat' also suggest negative associations. Could this have been a prohibition put in place to guard against the picking of some of its poisonous relatives such as hemlock? Certainly, hemlock shares many of cow parsley's country names.

The plant has been little used in folk medicine; those records that do exist are uncertain since many plants in the umbellifer family (Apiaceae) share the same country names. It may be the plant used in Gloucestershire for treating kidney trouble and in the Outer Hebrides as a sedative. It is definitely the plant used within living memory, as a strong infusion, for treating laminitis in horses. Official medicine has largely ignored the plant, and it does not feature in modern herbalism.

Cow parsley does have several practical uses however. In the Scottish Highlands, bobbins were sometimes made from cow parsley stalks. Children have fun making whistles out of the dried stalks, which are known in many areas as 'kecks'. Again, in Scotland, the flowering tips were the source of a yellow-green dye used in making the famous Harris tweed. Believe it or not, a range of colours may be produced from cow parsley – yellow, green, orange and bronze.

Cowslip
(*Primula veris*)

I play'd with you 'mid cowslips blowing,
When I was six and you were four;
When garlands weaving, flower-balls throwing,
Were pleasures soon to please no more.

Thomas Love Peacock (1785–1866), *Love and Age*

These beautiful flowers have suffered greatly from the changes in agricultural practice and increased use of pesticides. Once a common sight, they are now making a come-back on some unsprayed motorway verges and as a result of deliberate planting schemes.

It is hard now to imagine a time when cowslips were so common that cowslip wine was a regular farmhouse brew and a popular children's game was to make 'totsies', balls of cowslip flowers, as mentioned in the poem above. A girl could use a cowslip flower-ball to determine her future husband, by tossing the ball into the air and singing, 'Tisty, tosty, tell me true, who shall I be married to?' She then would list all the possible candidates, and the ball would fall to the ground when the correct person was mentioned.

There were numerous country uses for cowslips: the leaves and flowers were eaten in salads and a tea was made from the blossoms, as Margaret Plues recalls in *Rambles in Search of Wild Flowers*:

There were some fields near Hewick, in the Ripon neighbourhood, which afforded a plentiful harvest of these flowers ... we used to make Cowslip tea of the petals, adding sugar and lemon-juice.

Wine made from the flowers also was particularly valued in folk medicine
– as a gentle treatment for insomnia and a soothing drink during childhood
fevers. Here is a recipe for a delicious, lemony cowslip wine from 1842:

> Take twelve pounds of sugar, the juice of six lemons, the whites of four eggs
> well beaten, and six gallons of water. Put all together in a kettle and let it boil
> half an hour, taking care to skim it well. Take a peck of cowslips, and put them
> into a tub, with the thin peeling of six lemons. Then pour on the boiling liquor,
> and stir them about, and when it is almost cold, put in a thin toast, baked hard,
> and rubbed with yest [sic]. Let it stand two or three days to work. If you put in,
> before you turn it, six ounces of syrup of citron or lemon with a quart of
> Rhenish wine, it will be a great addition. The third day strain it off, and squeeze
> the cowslips through a coarse cloth. Then strain it through a flannel bag, and
> tun it up [put it in barrels]. Leave the bung loose for two or three days till you
> be sure it has done working, and then bung it down tight, let it stand three
> months, and then bottle it.

Other country uses included a cowslip cosmetic, particularly recommended to give bloom to the complexion of those unfortunate girls who
live in town; jaundice, too, was treated with an infusion of cowslip flowers.
Oscar Wilde's mother in 1898 described an Irish remedy for deafness which
used the juice of the cowslip flowers, leaves and roots with honey added;
the mixture was placed in the nostrils while the patient was lying down.

In official medicine, the cowslip was valued as a treatment for insomnia,
headache and joint pains as well as paralysis (hence another common name,
'palsywort'). Infusions prepared from the cowslip, Pechey tells us in 1694,
'are very proper Medicines for weakly People'.

The plant has continued to be used by herbalists as a mild sedative and
in present-day medical herbalism the root in particular is recommended for
insomnia and for relieving coughs.

The cowslip has a whole host of vernacular names: 'cowflops', 'golden
drops', 'freckled face', to name but a few – and such a quantity hints at the
flower's ubiquitousness in the past. The plant's single flower stalk, bearing
a head of drooping golden bells, was thought to resemble a bunch of keys
and gave rise to the name of 'key flower'.

The flowers themselves are small and very beautiful, and each one is
enclosed in a papery calyx, which later expands to cover and protect the

seeds. It is worth examining one closely to see the unexpected cluster of tiny red spots within:

In their gold coats spots you see;
Those be rubies, fairy favours,
In those freckles lie their savours:

Shakespeare, *A Midsummer Night's Dream*, II, i, 11–13

It is also worth becoming acquainted with the delicate scent of the cowslip. One writer, Roy Genders, has compared it to that of a baby's breath. There is a strange tradition that nightingales sing only where cowslips grow abundantly. How this (untrue) idea originated is not clear, and is a puzzle to this day.

Crab Apple
(*Malus sylvestris*)

The crab of the wood is sauce very good for the crab of the sea,
But the wood of the crab is sauce for a drab that will not her husband obey.

T. F. Thiselton Dyer, *The Folk-lore of Plants* (1889)

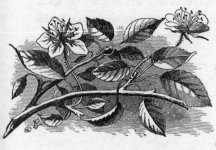

The crab apple is native in ancient woods throughout lowland Britain. It is a parent of the domesticated apple, but unlike our cultivated apples its branches bear thorns.

There are a number of disparaging sayings and strange practices in connection with crab apples, since they are considered smaller, sharper and inferior to cultivated ones. A woman who chooses an inferior husband is said to have gone through the orchard and selected the crab. On the other hand, in the nineteenth century in the west of England, crab apples were used to divine which of several possible suitors was the most eligible. In Scotland a girl could put a crab apple under her pillow on St Andrew's Eve; on the following Sunday she had to take it with her to church, and the first man she saw standing in the porch would be her husband. Britten and Holland report that in the nineteenth century the inhabitants of Mobberley in Cheshire were called 'Mobberley Crabs' and it was the custom there, on the Sunday after St Luke's feast day, to pelt the parson with crab apples.

In folk medicine, crab apples had numerous uses. The juice, known as 'verjuice', was widely used in the eighteenth century for treating sprains and was also prescribed as a laxative. It was realized very early on that apples are extremely easily digested, and good for the bowels. Hence the saying:

'To eat an apple going to bed
Will make the doctor beg his bread.'

In Ireland, crab apples mixed with buttermilk were used to treat hoarseness. In the Scottish Highlands, crab apples were crushed to treat sprains and cramps. Rotten apples were applied as a poultice to sore eyes, a remedy still in use in Lincolnshire in the nineteenth century. Boils and earache were also treated with rotten apples. Apples, of any kind, were rubbed on warts and then buried, in the hope that they would take the warts with them. It was believed that other diseases too could be transferred to an apple. In Norfolk, there was a belief that an apple placed in the bedroom of a sufferer from smallpox would itself become spotty and then the patient would recover.

On the whole, crab apples were ignored in official medicine, and the innumerable varieties of cultivated apples were probably the ones generally used. However, Salmon in 1693 has this to say about 'Crabs or Wildings'.

> They are cold and astringent, but boyled or scalded, and eaten with Butter and Sugar, they strengthen the Stomach, quench thirst, and cool the heat of Fevers.

John Pechey in 1694 recommends apples for melancholy as well as fevers; the variety he favours is 'fragrant pippins'. In Parkinson's day, a pomatum was prepared from apple pulp and used as an astringent cosmetic and for treating chapped skin; again, this would almost certainly have been prepared from cultivated rather than wild crab apples. Sir John Hill in his early-nineteenth-century herbal recommends verjuice for sore throats but, in accord with the general feeling, crab apples were largely ignored in official medicine. Later herbalists used them rarely.

As a foodstuff, crab apples were invaluable and there is no shortage of recipes, for wine for example or for an excellent jelly to accompany meat or to eat as a jam. In the past, where grain was scarce, crab-apple pulp was dried and mixed with flour for breadmaking. The crab-apple fruit had another use, too; drawing a knife through one repeatedly etches the edge and sharpens it, hence the name 'Grindstone Apple'.

Here is where the crab apple beats the ordinary apple hands down – it is claimed that crab-apple wood is superior to all other sorts of apple wood for cabinet-making.

Cuckoo Pint
(*Arum maculatum*)

They have eaten so much of wake-robin
That they cannot sleep for love.

John Lyly, *Love's Metamorphosis* (1601)

This plant is unmistakable in leaf, and surprising in flower. A long, pointed, green spathe, or modified bract, surrounds the flower spike, and opens to reveal the long, cylindrical spadix that bears numerous tiny flowers. These emit a foul smell, which is attractive to the tiny midges that pollinate them.

The plant's phallic appearance has given rise to a large number of bawdy country names, some more obvious than others. Any names with cuckoo in them tend to have amorous associations, and the 'pint' comes from 'pintle', the old word for penis. Another name, 'wake Robin', has been explained as meaning 'alive' or 'erect penis' (from an old French word, *robinet*). In Dorset, it was said that a girl could get pregnant simply by looking at wild arum. Not surprisingly, cuckoo pint was considered to have aphrodisiac properties and Turner called the plant 'rampe', meaning 'wanton'. Wild arum is a more decorous name for the plant, suggesting the lovely white lilies so often used to decorate churches.

The folklore and country tales connected to this plant are many and varied. Its bright, shiny red berries are poisonous, and there was a legend that the adder got its poison by eating cuckoo pint. In the fens around Ely in Cambridgeshire, there was a story that St Withburgha's body was stolen from East Dereham by the monks of Ely. On its passage down the Little Ouse river, the arum flowers with which the body was covered fell off and floated to land, where they carpeted the river bank with blossoms which glowed at night. Cuckoo-pint pollen does glow faintly at night, a fact which led Irish incomers to Cambridgeshire to name the flowers 'fairy lamps'.

In folk medicine, the cuckoo pint was occasionally used. A poultice of it was used on swellings; the juice was used to burn off warts; the dried powder of the root was used to treat rheumatism; and in Ireland, a small quantity of the powdered root was placed under the tongue for palsy.

In official medicine, arum juice was considered to be useful against the plague. Culpeper in 1653 mentions its use for treating plague sores and other skin conditions but had little to say about taking it internally. 'I know of no great good they do inwardly taken, unless to play the rogue withal, or make sport: outwardly applied they take off scurf, morphew, or freckles from the face, clear the skin, and ease the pains of gout.' Pechey in 1694 tells us that 'the Country-People around Maidstone, in Kent, use the Herb and Roots, instead of Soap.'

In the eighteenth century, the distilled water of cuckoo-pint juice was said to be good for wrinkles in the face, and the juice of the root was recommended for treating asthma, ruptures, scurvy and wind. By the mid-nineteenth century, its uses had changed to those of stimulant and diuretic until its usefulness finally died out in the twentieth century. Today's medical herbalists find no use for this plant.

One surprising use of cuckoo pint is as a source of starch for laundry. Lawn was introduced as a fabric in the sixteenth century and, being fine and limp, it needed a strong starch to make it into satisfactory ruffs for Elizabethan aristocrats. Gerard commented in 1597 that this was 'most hurt-full to the hands of the laundresse that hath the handling of it'. Presumably because of its corrosive nature its use was discontinued, but its fortunes revived at the end of the eighteenth century when a Dorset woman won a prize for her rediscovery of the starch, known as arrowroot. This purified starch does not contain the volatile acrid compounds that were present in the whole corm, and the arrowroot was valued as food for invalids as well. The arrowroot that we use today in cooking comes from quite a different plant, the South American *Maranta*.

Cudweed

(*Filago* species, *Gnaphalium* species)

This is a white, woolly, low-growing member of the daisy family, formerly common in cultivated land and coastal areas. Although it is small, it stands out by reason of its all-over 'wool', which gives the whole plant a white appearance. The generic name *Gnaphalium* comes from *gnaphalon* meaning 'soft down'. According to Mascal in 1662, the plant was bruised with fat and given to cattle that had lost their cud or quid; hence it became known as cudweed.

There are various types of cudweed, some of which are native to Britain and others that have been brought to this country and have naturalized. The commonest is *Filago vulgaris*. In the sixteenth century, it was noted that the people in the West of England used the plant, gently crushed in oil, for treating spots, cuts and bruises. Pechey in 1694 confirms that the West-country people 'use the Herb infus'd in Oyl, to take off Black and Blue Bruises and Stripes'. Its soft leaves were sometimes used to prevent chapped or chafed legs in horseriders. More recently in the Scottish Highlands, the plant was used to treat sciatica.

In official medicine, there is more than the usual confusion over which type of cudweed is referred to in the herbals. Gerard in 1597 describes cudweed or 'cottonweede' which 'boiled in strong lee, clenseth the hair from nits and lice: also the herbs being laid in wardrobes and presses, keepeth apparel from mothes'. He also suggests *Gnaphalium* to treat coughs, insect bites and worms. Culpeper in 1653 reported the use of cudweed for stopping the bleeding of 'immoderate courses' as well as wounds, and Pechey recommended the distilled water of cudweed for the treatment of cancers, especially breast cancer.

Nineteenth-century medical herbalists valued cudweed for treating sore throats and for stopping bleeding but at the present time the plant is little used by medical herbalists in Britain, although related North American and European species are still in favour.

Daffodil
(*Narcissus pseudonarcissus*)

Daff-a-down-dill
Has now come to town
In a yellow petticoat
And a green gown.

Country rhyme, quoted T. F. Thiselton Dyer,
The Folk-Lore of Plants (1889)

Our native wild daffodil grows in England and Wales, and although not a common plant is often very abundant where it does occur. Daffodils growing in profusion are thought to indicate the site of an old monastery. Such a strikingly beautiful flower has attracted attention from poets and gardeners alike and, when it was more widespread, it excited enormous interest generally. People would travel great distances to see a display of the wild daffodil in its natural setting. Our innumerable garden daffodils are descended from this native species and from various other European species.

The plant has attracted its share of folklore. In the south and west of England, it is sometimes considered unlucky to bring the flowers into the house of anyone who keeps poultry, because it would prevent the eggs from hatching. This idea has earned the plant the name of 'gooseflop'. On the other hand, sometimes it is believed to be acceptable to bring a large number of flowers indoors, as their number will then equal the number of eggs in a successful hatch.

The daffodil is one of the national emblems of Wales, said to flower for the first time on St David's Day. In Elizabethan times, it was called the Lent lily and, at that time of the year, the Cheapside marketwomen would carry baskets of daffodils on their heads for sale. Daffodils were called 'Leny cocks' in Somerset and used instead of 'cock shies' (targets for throwing games). A more dignified use comes from the Isles of Scilly where the Prince of Wales is paid one daffodil annually as rent for the untenanted parts of these islands.

Surprisingly, it seems that daffodils have been little used in folk medicine in Britain. In official medicine, the picture is confused. Parkinson in 1629 describes a very large number of garden daffodils, as well as the native one. He states that he does not know of anyone who uses the daffodil as 'a remedy for any griefe, whatsoever Gerrard or others have written'. Gerard himself was only quoting the famous Greek physician Galen when he claimed in 1597 that the daffodil is useful in wound treatment and for burns. On the other hand in 1694 Pechey *does* recommend the daffodil and states that 'The Root is Vomitive. The Leaves bruised, are proper in an Erisipelas.'

Was the daffodil used or not? It is known that the bulbs are poisonous and can cause paralysis and even death, and maybe it is this very risky aspect that discouraged use. Perhaps the daffodil was more written about than actually used in medicine. Recently the substance galanthamine has been isolated from daffodil bulbs as well as other interesting and hitherto unknown compounds. Galanthamine is now produced synthetically and is showing promise in treatment of Alzheimer's disease, so the full story of the daffodil still remains to be told.

Daisy
(*Bellis perennis*)

> Of all the flowers in the meadow I most love those white and red flowers which men in our town call day's-eyes. For them I have such affection, as I have said, that when May is come, no day dawns upon me in my bed, but I am up and walking in the mead to see these flowers opening to the sun when it rises, in the bright morn, and through the long day thus I walk in the green.

Geoffrey Chaucer, *The Legend of Good Women* (1385–86)

The daisy is the 'day's eye', 'opening to the sun when it rises', as Chaucer wrote in his lovely little homage to one of our most common and abundant flowers. With their characteristic, spatula-shaped leaves flattened against the grass, they shade out and so prevent the growth of other, competing plants, which is doubtless one reason for their successful colonization of our lawns. Grazing animals tend to avoid them, presumably on account of the bitter taste of their leaves, and so they survive too in our pastures. Endless generations of children have made daisy chains; so much so that in Scotland the plant is called 'bairnwort'. In Devon, there is a belief that wearing a daisy chain protects against being kidnapped by fairies.

Our common daisy is not used in medical herbalism today, but in the past it was known as 'brusewort' and was used in official medicine not only for treating bruises but also to help heal wounds. Gerard in 1597 records the strange belief that puppies fed on an infusion of daisy flowers in milk will remain small.

In folk medicine the daisy was used in different ways. A daisy ointment was used to treat burns and, in Wiltshire, an infusion of the flowers was recommended for coughs and colds. In Dorset, a touch of magic enters into their use: for treating boils, one should eat either seven or nine daisy blossoms, growing close enough together to be covered by one foot. These are not as difficult to collect as it sounds: daisies do not have the wind-dispersed seeds (parachutes) of many of their family, and the seeds (and eventually, new plants) therefore tend to remain a short distance from the parent. As the old saying goes, when you can place a foot on seven daisy plants, you know that summer has come.

If the sight of a daisy-strewn meadow gladdens the heart in spring and summer, whisky prepared from daisies can serve the same purpose in the winter:

1 gallon of [daisy] flowers	1 gallon of boiling water
1 lb wheat	1 lb large raisins
2 lemons	2 oranges
3 lb best white sugar	1 oz yeast

Pour boiling water onto daisies and allow to stand for twenty-four hours, then squeeze out the flowers. Add the sugar to the liquid, and chopped raisins, the wheat and the thin yellow rind (no pith) and juice (no pips) of the fruits. Stir until the sugar is dissolved, then warm to lukewarm a little of the liquid and sprinkle in the yeast. When it froths, add it to the wine and leave the vessel covered with clean cotton cloth, for twenty-one days, stirring daily.

After this, strain twice and pour into fermentation jar; store in a warm place for two weeks and then in a cooler one for another two weeks or until bubbles cease to rise. Siphon off, clear and bottle.

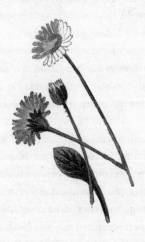

Dandelion
(*Taraxacum officinale*)

Her treading would not bend a blade of grass
Or shake the downy blow-ball from his stalk ...

Ben Jonson, *The Sad Shepherd*, I, i

If this, one of our best-known wild flowers, were not so common, we would probably compete to have it in our gardens. In Gerard's words, the flower turns into a 'round downy blowbal that is carried away with the wind'. In Somerset, the name of 'fluffy puffy' is given to the plant. The name 'dandelion' has never been satisfactorily explained, but it has been suggested that the toothed leaves (the *dent-du-lion*, or lion's tooth) have been the inspiration behind it.

Nowadays, the dandelion is regarded as a nuisance, to be dug up and eradicated from gardens nationwide, yet this was not always the case. It was respected as a powerful medicine used by many, and effective in easing a number of ailments from kidney complaints to jaundice.

It is hard now to imagine the time, not so long ago, when it was possible to make a living digging up roots of medicinal plants in the wild, yet as comparatively recently as the 1930s, teams of root-diggers in East Anglia did just that. Dandelion roots were one of the main herbs collected and this benefited both the farmers and the collectors. So common was this practice that a special 'green-herb' rate was charged for transporting them by train to London. Nowadays, the dandelion root used by herbalists is mostly imported.

In folk medicine, dandelion roots were dug up, dried and infused as a tonic and for treating kidney complaints and rheumatism. The dandelion was often recommended for kidney ailments. It is in fact a powerful diuretic; eating it or drinking an infusion increases the flow of urine. This led to several superstitions against picking the plant. Perhaps because the juice from the plant stains hands and clothes brown, children were sometimes prohibited from picking it by being warned that they would wet the bed. A Norfolk remedy from the early twentieth century for treating dropsy calls for 'dandelion wine from the flowers, made with cold spring water and no yeast. Teetotallers consider wine made with cold water and no yeast is not an intoxicant and drink it.'

The dandelion's other principal use was in removing warts: the juice from any part of the plant is rubbed on the wart and allowed to dry; this is repeated until the wart shrivels and disappears. Innumerable other ailments, ranging from heart conditions (in Ireland) to jaundice and indigestion, were treated using dandelions. In Ireland, it was regarded as a plant that was good for all ills; to be effective as a tonic, the leaves with white veins had to be used by a man, those with red veins by a woman.

In official medicine, the plant was used mainly as a tonic, a digestive and for treating kidney and liver complaints. Culpeper in 1653 adds to this list: 'It helps to procure rest and sleep to bodies distempered by the heat of ague fits.' By the nineteenth century, the dandelion was still being recommended for 'jaundice, dropsy and diseases of the liver and lungs' and was still included, as a tonic and a digestive, in the British Pharmaceutical Codex of 1914. Modern medical herbalists use the plant as a purifying tonic to treat arthritis, constipation, gall-bladder problems and skin conditions.

In the kitchen, the dandelion may one day come back into fashion and be appreciated once more. The leaves, blanched, may be added to salads. They can also be steamed and eaten like spinach. The root, roasted and ground, serves as a coffee substitute but, unlike coffee, it has a sedative effect and may be used to promote sleep.

The flowers make a delicious country wine – if the flower bracts are meticulously removed from the blossoms. Dandelion beer can be made from the whole plant, if it is gathered before it flowers, and should be ready to drink in a week. It is reassuring to know that the traditional drink of dandelion and burdock is still produced commercially in the north of England.

Deadly Nightshade
(*Atropa belladonna*)

Robed in her Autumn dress of brown and sere,
The dark-eyed Belladonna glanced at me
With her wild wondrous eyes so clear:
And, charm'd, I thought can aught more glorious be?

James Rigg, *Atropa belladonna No. 2* (1897)

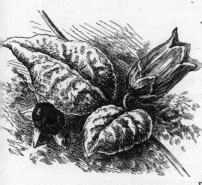

This is a highly poisonous member of the family Solanaceae, which also includes familiar edible plants such as the potato, tomato and sweet pepper. Deadly nightshade is native in Britain and occurs especially on chalky soils, although it is not commonly found. The bell-shaped flowers are brownish-purple, and open in early summer. Its petals wither and fall as soon as the flower is pollinated. The flowers open at slightly different times, so that at any one moment there may be berries, buds and flowers on one plant. The berries are large, very shiny and black.

Most of its country names, including of course deadly nightshade, relate to its poisonous nature. Such a toxic plant not surprisingly was associated with witches, and was claimed to be one of the plants that made them avoid detection. It has been called 'banewort', 'devil's berry' and 'mad berry'. In Chaucer's time, it was called *dwale*, a Middle English word meaning 'dulling' or 'stupefying'; our word 'dull' is the same. Its generic name *Atropa* derives from Atropos, one of the Three Fates in Greek mythology who cut the thread of life.

Throughout the centuries, there have been tales of tragic deaths from this plant. When King Duncan I ruled Scotland, it was said that an entire army of Danish invaders was poisoned using the berries of this plant in wine, offered to them during a truce. Here is a first-hand account of the effects of the plant from William Salmon, who survived to tell the tale and became a well-known seventeenth-century physician:

> The berries being eaten, bring present death in an hour or two at most; I speak by sad experience, for my part when very young, with some other Children, going into a Garden where this plant grew with ripe black berries, we all gathered them, and eat them. I eat but 3 or 4 as I remember, being too luscious for me, and so escaped, but not without vehement Vomiting, sickness at Heart, and loss of my Hair, Nailes, and Skin; the other Children who eat more of them, all died in an hour or two raving Mad, and extreamly swell'd, as if they would burst, &c. But enough of this unpleasant and sad Subject, these lines being only written to give others warning.

No wonder that the plant was not used in folk medicine. Country people would have been well aware of its poisonous nature and would have steadfastly avoided it. It was used in official medicine however, externally, to relieve pain. Gerard's advice in 1597 though was uncompromising: 'But if you will follow my counsel deal not with the same in any case, and banish it from your gardens and the use of it also, being a plant so furious and deadly.'

The ladies of ancient Rome are said to have used its juice as a cosmetic: when dropped into the eyes it causes the pupil to dilate; hence the Latin specific name of *belladonna*. Even rubbing the eye after handling the plant can produce this effect. The drug atropine, derived originally from this plant, is still used by eye surgeons.

Approached carefully, deadly nightshade has had other medicinal uses. In the nineteenth century, it was prescribed as a remedy for whooping cough, and was cultivated for medicinal use in Hertfordshire and Suffolk in the 1940s. Belladonna plasters were bandages that were impregnated with belladonna and used to relieve rheumatic pain; they were still available commercially in this country until the 1950s. Deadly nightshade and compounds derived from it are used in modern medical herbalism as well as in orthodox medicine. The plant contains chemicals that relax the involuntary muscles, making it useful in treating intestinal and renal colic. It may be prescribed only by a qualified practitioner because of its highly poisonous nature.

Devil's Bit
(*Succisa pratensis*)

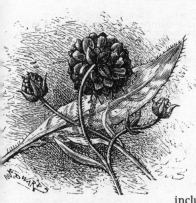

This pretty, little early-summer flower of heathland has a strange, thick root that ends abruptly and is supposed, according to legend, to have been bitten off by the devil, who was angry because the plant had such medicinal value for mankind.

Certainly, in official medicine, the list of ailments treated with devil's bit, or devil's bit scabious, is a long one, and includes wounds and skin conditions. Culpeper in 1653 writes: 'The herb or the root (all that the devil hath left of it) being boiled in wine and drank is very powerful against the plague … poisons also, and the bitings of venomous beasts.' In 1838 Kemsey recommends devil's bit for inward bruises, sores and ulcers as well as for treating worms and provoking menstruation. The root was still being recommended for 'pestilential fevers'.

In folk medicine, the plant has been used to treat dog bites: the wound was bathed in water in which the plant had been steeped, then devil's bit leaves were placed on the wound to complete the healing. Other wounds were treated in this way too. In the Scottish Highlands, it was used to treat scabies; in Scotland generally, to treat toothache and boiled in wine for the plague; in the Isle of Man, it was applied to scurvy sores.

Devil's bit continued to be used by medical herbalists well into the twentieth century, for coughs and fevers and as a wash for skin conditions. Recently, at least in Britain, it has been little used.

Whether its place in local folklore will endure remains to be seen. Its association with the devil produced many a superstition. The root has been used on the island of Colonsay in a children's game. If it is twisted at the point of constriction, it can appear to move on its own when released, indicating magical power on the part of the person holding the root. In Fife in Scotland, the plant was called 'curl-doddy' and children would chant this rhyme:

> 'Curl-doddy, do my biddin
> Soap my house and hool my midden.'

It seems that the chant could enable them to summon a brownie-like being who would do their household chores for them. At the other end of Britain, though, in Cornwall, if a child picked devil's bit, the devil would come to their bedside.

Dock

(*Rumex crispus, Rumex obtusifolius* and other species)

Nettle out, dock in –
Dock remove the nettle-sting.

Traditional

Dock is a rough, tough plant of waysides and cultivated land, unprepossessing and overlooked. Yet its uses have been manifold and it is the subject of what is probably the country's most widely remembered plant remedy.

It has proved to be of service to mankind in a number of ways. Its edible leaves were cooked as a vegetable in times of hardship. It was used especially in Scotland in this way, added to a stew to give much-needed vitamins: indeed, it was regarded in some areas as a specific treatment for scurvy. Also in Scotland, where the dock was more usually called 'docken', the leaves were fed to cows to keep them still when they were milked.

In the Shetlands, baskets were made of docken stems, which were softened by immersion in seawater and interwoven with marram grass; in Orkney, the stems were sometimes woven into 'doors' for poorer dwellings. Butter for the market would be wrapped in the large cooling leaves of docks (*Rumex obtusifolius* in particular) and, with a similar aim in mind, the leaves were often tucked into tobacco pouches to keep the tobacco moist. Water-dock root was used to clean teeth in the Scottish Highlands.

As any gardener knows, docks have long and very tough taproots and these were greatly prized in folk medicine. Liver problems, cancerous sores and heart trouble were all treated with dock root, and in the Scottish Highlands the root was made into a healing ointment by combining it with beeswax and fresh, homemade butter.

Dock roots were often boiled and the liquid drunk to 'purify the blood' and, more specifically, to cure boils, as this twentieth-century remedy testifies:

'This is a cure for boils, which has been proved in my own family. Dig up five dock roots, wash them so that they are very clean, put two cupfuls of clean water in a saucepan, also the five dock roots, and let them boil for thirty minutes. Strain with a fine muslin, and put into a bottle. Drink one teaspoonful night and morning.'

F. H—, Bedfordshire (1985)

This same liquid could also be used to treat dermatitis, and, specifically, the rashes produced by childhood vaccinations.

'My grandmother ... used to gather the roots of marsh docks – why marsh docks I don't know, but the garden ones wouldn't do. She washed them and boiled them up and the liquid was bottled and rubbed on anything from gnat bites to measles rashes. It was very soothing and we were never without a bottle in the house.'

Mrs G. R. F—, Norfolk (1989)

The use of dock leaves to relieve the itch of nettle stings is familiar to all, but it represents only a vestige of much wider use in the past. Sometimes the leaf was simply rubbed on the sting; sometimes it was recommended to spit on the leaf first. Interestingly, this small piece of folklore has been shown to be very valid: the enzymes in saliva actually release some of the anti-inflammatory properties of the leaf. Dock leaves were also wrapped around minor wounds; they effectively stop the bleeding. As a readily available remedy throughout the year, they were used in Norfolk to wrap around chapped legs in winter, and on aching heads in summer. Dock's soothing and cooling properties gave relief to insect bites and stings, minor burns, scalds and blisters too. They were also found to be useful for sprains: 'First aid for a strained ankle – wrap in dock leaves tightly' (Mrs D. M. P—, Sussex, 1996). Even dock seeds have their uses: boiled, they will, like linseed, 'draw' a wound or sore and, on Tiree, an infusion of dock seeds with barley sugar was used to treat coughs. The white, slimy base of a young unfurling leaf was used to treat ringworm, stings and sores.

In official medicine, the preferred type of dock was the non-native variety, monk's rhubarb (*Rumex alpinus*); the name reveals its use – the roots were an effective purge. The native dock was sometimes used as well: Pechey in 1694 recommends it for treating scurvy and jaundice.

In modern herbalism, dock, especially yellow dock (*Rumex crispus*), is used to treat constipation, sluggish digestion, arthritic conditions and a wide variety of skin conditions.

There were all kinds of other uses for dock. Water-dock root was used to clean teeth in the Scottish Highlands. A yellow dye was obtained from the shoots, and a black from the roots. Dock leaves were used to enhance colours during dyeing. They could be wrapped around the paste of dye-stuff.

In Orkney, it was on docken stems that the 'trows' (trolls) were said to ride.

Dog Rose
(*Rosa canina*)

The dog rose, sometimes also called the 'wild rose' or 'briar', is one of our longest-living plants; a bush growing in Hildesheim in Germany was said to have been planted there in AD 850 by Emperor Charlemagne's son. Viewed from a distance, a flowering English rosebush looks as though a flock of pink butterflies has perched on it. The delicacy of the flowers makes a startling contrast to the harsh, thorned stems. Look into the heart of any wild rose and you see a jewel-like beauty, with a golden crown of stamens protected by delicate petals that fade from pink at the edges to the merest blush near the centre. No wonder this flower has inspired our poets.

Rosehips are one of the best sources of vitamin C, a fact exploited during the Second World War when they were collected up and down the country and turned into rosehip syrup. The collection was organized at county level by schools, voluntary groups and branches of the Women's Institute. By the end of the war, 2,000 tons of rosehips had been collected for syrup manufacture! Mary Thorne Quelch in 1945 described use of rosehips as 'a patriotic duty' and supplied the following recipe:

Wash four pounds of ripe hips in lukewarm water and put into an enamel pan. Cover well with water and bring to the boil. Simmer till tender and mash with a wooden spoon. Put into a flannel jelly-bag and squeeze out the juice. Return the pulp to the pan and add the same quantity of water as you did at first. Bring to the boil and simmer for from five to ten minutes. Put into the jelly bag again and squeeze. Empty the jelly-bag and wash it thoroughly. Mix the two lots of juice and pour into the clean bag. This time do not squeeze but hang up over a basin and leave to drip all night. By this method perfectly clear juice is obtained, free from all harmful seeds and hairs. It is very important the juice should be thus carefully strained. Return the juice to the saucepan and boil till it is reduced to three pints. Add two and a quarter pounds of sugar, sir till dissolved, then boil for five minutes. Bottle while hot and seal down immediately. Store in a dark cupboard. Fifteen drops divided into two portions is the daily dose for a baby. Older children should take a teaspoonful at least twice daily.

This delicious drink is laborious to make because all the fine, irritant hairs surrounding the central seed must be excluded, but the resulting syrup is wonderful and has been used to treat coughs and colds as well as being given to children during the winter months as a preventative tonic. The hips themselves may be nibbled carefully – eating just the outer layer – and along with other edible berries were probably an important source of vitamin C in the winters of the past.

Other uses of the hips have included being turned into wine, carried in the pocket as a safeguard against piles and in Dundee, where the hips are called 'itchy-coos', children love the mischief they can get up to with their very effective, rosehip itching powder.

Other parts of the rose have proved useful in folk medicine. The shoots have been fed to goats to treat indigestion; the leaves were used in first-aid in the country to treat cuts; in Ireland, the juice of the plant was said to relieve coughs. CHICKWEED and rose leaves boiled together have been used as a lotion for eye troubles, and even the spherical, red, mossy gall, known as robin's pincushion, that grows on the wild rose stems has had its uses. An infusion of the gall was used as a treatment for whooping cough and, in Yorkshire, schoolboys carried rose galls as a charm against flogging, thus earning the plant the vivid name of 'save-whallop'.

In official medicine, the garden rose has been favoured over the wild variety, red roses in particular being seen as medicinal. Pechey in 1694 wrote that the 'red rose is astringent and bitter: It comforts the Heart and strengthens the Stomach'. Among its uses, he lists headache, fluxes and coughs. A mid-eighteenth-century physician's notebook recommends conserve of red roses 'to prevent abortion and comfort the foetus'. This conserve was also recommended for rheumatism. A century later in 1838, Kemsey states that 'the infusion of red roses is astringent, cooling, and drying, either used as a gargle for a sore mouth, or taken inwardly with compositions, all serving to sundry uses.' In the *British Pharmacopoeia* for 1914, red rose petals are listed as medicinal; they are to be gathered specifically from *Rosa gallica*.

A remedy collected by the Women's Institute in the 1920s uses syrup made from red rose petals for coughs and spitting of blood, while an ointment for chilblains involved seven different kinds of roses, together with rosemary (*Rosmarinus officinalis*) and southernwood (*Artemisia abrotanum*). Red roses steeped in vinegar provided a rub for a headache.

Medical herbalists in this country recommend the dog rose as an excellent source of vitamin C and also as a gentle remedy for diarrhoea, while *Rosa gallica* is prescribed as an infusion for sore eyes. Both the essential oil and the petals of *R. gallica* have a cholesterol-reducing action; a leading medical herbalist considers that 'it is probably time for a re-evaluation of its medicinal benefits'.

In the domestic household, rose petals have been invaluable. They have been made into wine and rosewater, used to flavour and perfume butter, and coated with crystallized sugar to make sweetmeats, as recently as the 1930s. Of course they also form an important constituent of potpourri. Rose petals have often been used as confetti to shower the bridal pathway. And let us hope that all Devonian brides dream of roses – they portend happiness in love.

Early Purple Orchid
(*Orchis mascula*)

No more shall violets linger in the dell
Or purple orchis variegate the plain,
Till spring again shall call forth every bell,
And dress with humid hands her wreath again.

Charlotte Smith, quoted Roy Genders,
The Scented Wild Flowers of Britain (1971)

The early purple orchid was once a common plant of chalky grassland and woodland copses, and its flowering was a welcome sign of spring. A Kentish country name for the plant is 'skeat-legs', derived from the Anglo-Saxon *sceat*, meaning 'sheath' – the stem, or leg, of the plant is indeed partially sheathed by its leaf. Its leaves are splotched with purplish patches that make the plant easily recognizable.

In some areas, it is known as 'Gethsemane', or 'cross-flower', from the legend that the plant grew at the foot of the cross and Christ's blood dripped onto its leaves, giving them their characteristic spots. The flowers have a delicate, vanilla-like scent when they first open, but after they are fertilized this is replaced by a bitter smell. The vanilla we use in the kitchen also comes from an orchid, the tropical vanilla orchid (*Vanilla planifolia*).

From ancient times, the tuberous roots of orchids had a reputation as aphrodisiacs, a belief no doubt originating from the fact that the tubers, of which there are two, look like men's testicles. In Britain, the wild varieties were traditionally used in love charms. The root would be ground into a powder and placed under the pillow to bring on dreams of the person you were going to marry. The two tubers are of different sizes; the smaller was taken to symbolize the woman and the larger the man. To discover whether the outcome of a love affair would be favourable, the orchid roots had to be pulled up before dawn, while facing south. With her lover in mind, the woman would then place the larger tuber in spring water (a man put in the smaller tuber) and if it sank, marriage would be the outcome. In Aberdeenshire, a person could entice another into love by secretly feeding them the powdered root, being careful of course to choose the appropriate tuber. This would apparently make you irresistible.

It is hard now to imagine a time when orchids were so plentiful in the wild that anyone could conceive of starting a business using them. Yet in 1783 that is just what Bryant suggested:

> As most country people are acquainted with these plants, by the name of Cuckoo-flowers, it certainly would be worth their while to employ their children to collect the roots for sale; and though they may not be quite so large as those that come from abroad, yet they may be equally as good, and as they are exceedingly plentiful, enough might annually be gathered for our own consumption, and thus a new article of employment would be added to the poorer sort of people.

There would have been a ready market for such an enterprise, since orchid roots were always in demand as the main ingredient of a popular drink called 'saloop', or 'salop'. This was a celebrated restorative, probably originating in the East, made from the powdered root mixed with honey and spices; it was regarded as such a valuable foodstuff and medicine that it commanded very high prices.

In the eighteenth century, salop cost a shilling an ounce. At one time it was available in London's coffee houses (in Charles Lamb's day there was even a dedicated salop house in Fleet Street), and its use continued right through until the 1950s. Although in official medicine salop was generally imported, in parts of Scotland at least native orchids were harvested to make it. In the Glencoe region, common twayblade (*Listera ovata*) was used to make salop in addition to early purple orchid. As well as providing nourishment, salop was also used as a 'soother of the bowels' and, intriguingly, was said to create a sense of well-being.

Salop came highly recommended by official medicine too. Pechey and Culpeper both prescribed it as a semi-aphrodisiac and an aid to conception, and also for killing worms in children and for treating scrofula. By the end of the eighteenth century, salop was still being promoted for its nutritional qualities and herbalists mentioned it in the 1950s, one book describing it as 'demulcent, highly nutritious. Used similarly to Arrowroot'. After such an illustrious history, it became no longer possible to collect early purple orchids in the wild and herbalists were no longer able to prescribe it, thereby ending a long tradition.

To Prepare the Roots for Salop

Mr. Mault of Rochdale's recipe: Wash the fresh roots in water and separate with a small brush the outer brown skin or dip them into hot water and rub the skin off with a cloth.

Spread the blanched roots on a tin plate and bake them in the oven for from six to ten minutes during which time they will lose their milky whiteness and acquire the transparency of bones. Remove them from the oven and leave them in the air for several days to harden or they can be left to harden for a few hours in the oven. Powder as required.

Salop to Boil

Take a large teaspoonful of the powder and put into a pint of boiling water, keep stirring it till it is like a pure jelly; then put in wine and sugar to your taste, and lemon if it will agree.

Earthnut
(*Conopodium majus*)

Sweet maize I'd give thee
Earthnut, lard and whiting
And the spring tansy I'd give thee
My love, wert thou mine own!

'Croon of the shellfish gathering', recorded Alexander Carmichael, *Carmina Gadelica*, vol. V (1940)

What a surprise it is to dig down and release the fine root of this small umbellifer and, with patience, to be rewarded with an edible nut, about the size of a peanut. Nowadays it is a rare country treat; in the past, it was well-known as a source of free food. In Ireland, the nuts were regarded as the property of the leprechauns and were known as 'fairy potatoes', while in Scotland it was said that eating too many of them caused headlice. When dried and roasted they were made into bread, and when chewed could assuage the feeling of hunger.

Some Victorians disdained the earthnut, or pignut, as food better fitted to pigs than humans, but at least one Victorian, the writer Richard Jefferies, wondered why it had never been cultivated as a vegetable. According to Bryant, writing in the eighteenth century, it will not grow on tilled land. Certainly today it is an indicator of ancient grassland and woodland. Pechey in 1694 tells us:

Our Country-people eat the Root raw; but when it is pill'd, and boyl'd in fresh Broth, with a little Peper, it is pleasant Food, and very nourishing, and stimulates Venery. Being mix'd with Medicines, it helps those that spit Blood, and void a Bloody Urine.

The earthnut has been little used in folk medicine; it was regarded as a blood-cleanser in Ireland, and tea was sometimes prepared from it. In the

Isle of Man, it was employed as a diuretic for horses. Sadly, modern herbalism does not find any role for the plant.

The pollen record shows that this plant was available in prehistoric times as a food for early man. In case any enterprising reader would like to take up Richard Jefferies's challenge and try to grow this plant as a vegetable, here is what Charles Bryant, writing in 1783, had to say:

> The roots, which are of a dirty brown colour, and a little bigger than Hazel-nuts, are as pleasant as a Chestnut . . . the root has a styptic [blood-staunching] quality, and has been deemed serviceable against the laxity of the urinary passages.

Tantalizingly, Margaret Plues, writing in 1892, tells us:

> There was a paper in the *Gardener's Chronicle* some years ago recommending the cultivation of this plant because of the edible properties of the roots.

Another nineteenth-century writer refers to earthnut as 'Caliban's treat and the schoolboy's luxury' [Burgess]:

> I prithee, let me bring thee where crabs grow;
> And with my long nails I will dig thee pignuts,

Shakespeare, *The Tempest*, II, ii, 167–168

All these suggestions: but who will actually grow it?

Elder
(*Sambucus nigra*)

Mistress Jean, she was makin' the elder-flo'er wine:
'And what brings the Laird at sic a like time?'
She put off her apron and on her silk goon,
Her mutch wi' red ribbons, and gaed awa' doon.

Lady Nairne (1755–1845), *The Laird o' Cockpen*

The elder is a tree of contradictions. Its leaves give off an unpleasantly bitter smell, so much so that it is avoided by mammals and insects; its straggling form is neither that of a tree nor a bush; it is often found in graveyards and waste places – yet the drinks and medicines made from its sweet, musky blossoms and purple-black berries have been relied on and highly prized for centuries. This mix of features may explain mankind's ambivalent attitude to the plant. It has been respected, revered and reviled by turns through different cultures and eras, but never ignored. It is said in Leyden that the famous eighteenth-century physician Boerhaave always raised his hat when he passed an elder tree.

Vestiges of these violent reactions remain in British traditions today. Woodsmen regard it as unlucky to cut down elder; if you need to, you should ask the druids first. In parts of East Anglia, within living memory it has similarly been seen as unlucky to burn its green branches: do this and 'you'll die with aching bones'. In Devon, burning elder was also prohibited: to do so was thought to endanger the lives of sheep. All these beliefs seem to have originated in pre-Christian times, but in the Middle Ages its sinister magical reputation was enhanced by the suggestion that Christ's cross had been made from elder wood, or that this was the tree on which Judas hanged himself.

Alongside respect for the elder ran belief in its protective powers. If planted outside cow byres, it protected the livestock inside; near a house, it could protect the occupants from evil. It has even been suggested that an elder tree was safe to shelter under in a storm because it would not be struck by lightning. The very earth from around the tree's roots was thought to have special power in treating toothache, and a spring rising from underneath was believed to cure eye ailments. An amulet composed of nine pieces of elder wood was worn to protect against epilepsy.

Whatever its folkloric reputation, it is no exaggeration to say that in rural Britain the plant has long been regarded as nature's medicine chest, especially good for preventing colds and treating skin conditions. All parts of the elder have featured in folk medicine.

The bark has been used as a painkiller and emetic; the buds as a gentle laxative; in Ireland, the root has been used to treat rheumatism; and even the pith was put to good use in Gloucestershire, to treat ringworm. Coughs and colds, rheumatism, dropsy, toothache, burns and scalds are among the ailments treated with elder.

Elder roots and branches have long featured in wart cures; the wart was frequently 'transferred' by charms and ceremonies to the elder tree. For example, a wart sufferer is advised to take an elder stick and cut into it the same number of notches as there are warts. The twig is then buried, taking the warts with it. In Somerset and elsewhere, the root was rubbed on warts. As many notches as there are warts are then cut in the root, which is buried in the ground. As it rots, the warts should disappear.

The leaves have been used to treat eczema and sores in both man and beast, but have an even greater reputation as an insect repellant. They have been rubbed onto insect bites, and the juice used to repel mosquitoes and flies. Sprays of flowers tied on a horse's bridle have helped keep flies away. The water in which elder leaves have been boiled is still sometimes used as a garden insecticide against mildew and aphids. In nineteenth-century Dumfries-shire, elder branches were laid among gooseberry bushes to keep away the caterpillars that so often devour them.

Elderflowers, despite their sickly-sweet smell, have been highly valued. They were gathered by placing a sheet under the tree and shaking the boughs. The flowers were then made into infusions for fevers, coughs and colds and an elderflower ointment was widely used for skin troubles and cosmetics. Elderflower water was said to be good for removing freckles, as well as sunburn.

From our home-produced lard my mother used to make hand cream. Lard and elderflowers were simmered together and then strained.

Mrs B—, Essex Age Concern essay (1991)

In the Forest of Dean, elderflower wine was regarded as such a good, all-round medicine that it was given for any ailment for a couple of days; if the patient showed no improvement, it was time to call a doctor!

In official medicine, many of these same uses are recorded. Gerard in 1597 recommended elder for dropsy and gout, Culpeper in 1653 suggests in addition the use of the flowers for the complexion and the juice of the leaves for sore eyes and ulcers. Pechey in 1694 tells us: 'My Father makes an Ointment of the Red-Lead-Plaster and Oyl of Elder, which he frequently uses for Burns: and I have found it very successful also in other Inflammations.'

Our modern medical herbalists still find elder to be invaluable and use it in the treatment of allergies, arthritis, colds, coughs and skin infections.

Practical uses for elder have included using the hollowed-out wood to make excellent popguns and whistles, and providing the reeds for Scottish bagpipes. But it is as a source of food and drink that the elder is most celebrated today. Elderflower cordial is a well-known product, even stocked in supermarkets, but there are many other uses. A pickle may be made from the young shoots in late spring, and the buds have been pickled to make imitation capers. The flowers may be dipped in batter and fried as fritters and they impart a delicate taste when added to stewed gooseberries. In the Second World War, elderflowers were packed in barrels with salt, to be used as flavouring. The berries can substitute for blackcurrants in fruit pies and jam, or have been used in Cumbria crushed with honey as a cure for fevers. And a warm glass of elderberry wine at bedtime has long been held to banish colds and influenza.

'When I go out for a walk I look at the elderberries left to rot on the trees. They are really medicine, made into wine – nothing could beat a glass of elderberry wine. The cure for all ills; at least, I think so.'

Mrs E. D—, Taunton, Somerset (1985)

Elder Syrup

Take half a gallon of elderberry juice and put it into a brass pan over a clear but slow fire, adding to it the white of an egg well beaten to a froth. When it begins to boil skim it as long as any froth rises then put to each pint 1lb of cane sugar and boil the whole slowly until it is a perfect syrup which may be known by dropping a particle on your nail and if it congeals it is done enough. Let it stand and when cool put into bottles covered with paper pricked full of holes. It will make elderberry wine in winter and if taken hot is excellent for colds.

From early-twentieth-century notebook owned by S. W—, Norwich

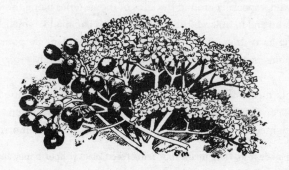

Elecampane
(*Inula helenium*)

Elecampane will the spirits sustain.

Mediaeval saying

This handsome and striking plant, a member of the daisy family, originated in central Asia and probably arrived in Britain with the Romans. In Classical times, it was grown as a root vegetable and was also cultivated in physic and cottage gardens. In the seventeenth century in *The Country House-wifes Garden*, William Lawson wrote, 'Elicapane-Root is long-lasting ... it seeds yearly, you may divide the Root, and Set; the Root taken in Winter is good (being dried, powdered, and drunk) to kill itches.' Elecampane has survived in the wild, especially around the sites of monasteries along the west coast of Scotland and in Ireland. The fresh root has a banana-like smell, becoming aromatic as it dries; it was formerly a component of potpourri. Its old Latin name was *Enula campana*; elecampane is probably a corruption of that.

In folk medicine, it was used mainly for respiratory conditions such as asthma, consumption and whooping cough; but also as a wound herb and, in the eighteenth century, as an interesting remedy for haemorrhoids:

Paste made from Elecampane root, fennel seed, black pepper, honey and sugar. Eat a piece the size of a nutmeg, morning noon and night.

A twentieth-century Suffolk remedy for coughs is 'elicampaign roots dried and grated in a spoonful of sugar'.

In official medicine, the plant's uses were numerous and varied, although it needed to be handled with care because it can cause contact dermatitis. Gerard in 1597 says: 'This Elecampane is marvellous good for many things' and recommends it especially as a counterpoison and for shortness of breath, as well as 'for them that are bursten and troubled with cramps and convulsions'. Culpeper in 1653 gives a long list of its medicinal virtues, covering indigestion, shortness of breath, obstructed menstruation or urination, intestinal worms, loose teeth, sore gums, poor eyesight, spots and sores. The seventeenth- and eighteenth-century Gunton Household Book includes a recipe for a 'fume', which is poured onto a hot brick, to use in times of infection. It includes elecampane roots, angelica roots, herb grace (rue) and JUNIPER berries.

The roots were made into a candy which was sold in London as flat, round cakes. 'A piece was eaten each night and morning for asthmatical complaints, whilst it was customary when travelling by a river, to suck a bit of the root against poisonous exhalations and bad air.'

By the nineteenth century, it was still being recommended for breathlessness and today's medical herbalists continue to recommend it for chest conditions and asthma. It is now known that the plant contains a high proportion of a chemical called inulin, which soothes the bronchial linings. There is also some evidence that the antiseptic terpenes that the plant contains may be active against the tuberculosis bacillus, an interesting discovery which needs further investigation.

Elecampane was well known to be a favourite herb of horsemen, as its alternative name of 'horseheal' suggests, but the usual secrecy surrounding horse remedies means that we do not know precisely how the herb was used. When George Ewart Evans wrote his books about Suffolk villages, he commented on the elecampane, the 'horseman's herb', that still survived in a cottage garden at Helmingham. Such fragmentary records are typical of horsemen's remedies from the past. There was often rivalry among teams, and maintaining the horses' appearance was important to the reputation of each team. This may in part explain the secrecy, but it was probably not the whole story. A postman who died ten years ago recalled that his father, who had been a horseman in Norfolk, made a bonfire of all his notebooks rather than leaving them to his son, who would not be following in his father's footsteps. Undoubtedly much interesting information has been lost in this way.

We do know that elecampane was regarded as a horse tonic in the Isle of Man, and was used to treat lameness in horses in Shropshire. A rare, surviving eighteenth-century horseman's notebook from Norfolk has the following recipe:

For Splent Sparvin or Curb

First apply the Oil Origanum and Haswell Stick then take one handful of
Enulacapany Root chop it fine put it in a Cabage Leaf Roast it in hot Ambers
then Pulverise and apply it to the part warm.

Other domestic uses of this plant have called on its ability to deal with
insect pests. Until the eighteenth century in Britain, the roots were hung in
doorways to trap flies – a use still current in Spain. An insecticide may be
prepared from the dried and powdered plant.

Elm

(*Ulmus* species)

Ellum do grieve
Oak, he do hate,
Willow do walk
If yew travels late.

Somerset rhyme recorded in 1953, Ruth Tongue,
Somerset Folklore (1965)

How different Constable's famous paintings of the Suffolk countryside would have been without the towering elm trees. For our native rooks (for whom the elm was the nesting site of choice) as well as our artists, the death of most of our British elms through Dutch elm disease has brought immense change, and altered the country landscape subtly but profoundly. Though largely unsung, the elm is one of our most magnificent trees, growing to very great heights.

The rhyme quoted above, recorded as recently as 1953, is based on the notion that elm trees grieve for each other; if one of a group is cut down, its neighbours will soon die. Despite its size, elm is particularly subject to wind damage, as another Somerset saying indicates:

'Ellum when cometh a blow
Up with her roots and down do go.'

In the distant past, the elm tree was held sacred, and to pagans and tree worshippers it played a significant role. Also, individual elms became natural landmarks and some of them were locally famous. One tree growing in Somerset is known as the Bleeding Elm. Said to have been planted on the grave of a Saxon warrior bloodily slain, it is claimed that it bleeds when cut with a knife. Anyone foolish enough 'to touch it with anything but iron and steel ... will sooner or later die very bloodily'. Another elm in Bedfordshire was said to have grown from a stake that was thrust through the heart of a murderer. Elm was used as a fever cure until the early nineteenth century. Sufferers nailed hair or nail clippings to the tree, thus transferring the fever from themselves to the tree.

When elm wood was more plentiful, it was used for building the keels of boats and making water pipes because of its ability to withstand wet conditions. It was used also for gunstocks for the military and for fashioning cottage furniture and utensils such as bowls, spoons and stools. In Scotland, the fibrous inner bark has been used to make ropes for tethering livestock.

Surprisingly, the rough, coarse elm leaves and bark have been found to be 'demulcent', that is, soothing to inflammations or irritations. In folk and official medicine, it has been much valued for such properties. Horses will seek out the bark of certain trees, including elm, when they are unwell. In his book *The Pattern under the Plough* (1966), George Ewart Evans quotes a Suffolk horseman:

> I used to watch my horses when they were in the fields. They whoolly liked to eat some trees . . . Some of my horses used to strip the bark off an oak and some would take to the ellum. Chance times I used to give 'em some in their bait. It used to make their coats shine like satin.

Elm was evidently of benefit to animals in other ways too: in Scotland the wych elm was used to assist in expelling the afterbirth of cows.

In our more rural past perhaps we, like animals, were more largely guided by instinct in our choice of remedy. In Wiltshire, people have chewed young sprigs of elm for sore throats and colds or boiled them into a jelly. In Hampshire, they treated eczema with an elm decoction, and in Ireland where the native elm is the wych elm (*Ulmus glabra*), the inner bark was used for a large array of ailments – for burns, inflammation, scalds and swellings. In the Eastern Borders, the elm was known as 'chewbark' because 'the inner bark . . . for a certain pleasant clamminess, is chewed by children'.

In official medicine, Gerard tells us in 1597: 'The leaves of Elme glew and heale up greene wounds, so doth the barke wrapped and swadled about the wound like a band'. Culpeper in 1653 recommends elm leaves and bark for the treatment of burns, ruptures, skin complaints and wounds. The roots when boiled, he says, produce a liquid that is effective as a hair restorer. Pechey in 1694 suggests its use for 'hip gout' [sciatica] as well. By the nineteenth century, Kemsey was still recommending elm for treating hair loss, scurf and leprosy.

In present-day medical herbalism, which for historical reasons uses many non-native species, the elm used is the imported slippery elm (*Ulmus rubra*), a native of North America. Its bark is famous for its soothing and nourishing properties, which are helpful in treating intestinal problems. The Native Americans used this species in much the same way that we once used our own native elm.

Eyebright
(*Euphrasia officinalis*)

This diminutive cousin of the FOXGLOVE is commonly found in short turf on acid soils throughout Britain. Its minute, white flowers with their patterned yellow throats are unmistakable, and as its name suggests, it is famous for one healing property above all others – it soothes sore eyes.

In domestic medicine, the use of eyebright continued right into the twentieth century. The Victorian naturalist Anne Pratt recalls finding bunches of dried eyebright hung up in a small shop in Dover at the very end of the nineteenth century and Doris E. Coates, in her book *Tuppeny Rice and Treacle: Cottage Housekeeping (1900–1920)*, remembers gathering the plant in the wild in the early decades of the twentieth century, for bathing sore eyes. Usually an infusion was used to bathe the eyes, although in Shropshire it was drunk instead.

In Scotland, eyebright was also considered a sedative, and mixed with MEADOWSWEET has been used in the Isle of Lewis within living memory for treating insomnia. The people of Lewis clearly find more alternative uses for eyebright than anywhere else – an infusion has also been used there for treating blocked sinuses.

In official medicine, eyebright was highly recommended both for preserving and restoring the eyesight, even eyesight 'decayed through age'. Culpeper commented in 1653 that it could render spectacle-makers redundant if only it were better used. Pechey stated in 1694 that 'The Oculists in England, and Beyond-Sea, use the Herb in Sallets, in Broths, in bread, and in Table-Beer; and apply it outwardly in Fomentations, and other External medicines for the Eyes.'

Although eyebright had been used in this way at least since the fourteenth century, by the eighteenth century medical men had begun to cast doubt upon its safety; this was a time when the medical fraternity was attempting to rationalize medicine and wanted to distance themselves from 'old wives' tales'.

Lightfoot, however, in his *Flora Scotica* (1777) ignores official disapproval and remarks that 'The Highlanders do however still retain the practice of it, by making an infusion of it in milk, and anointing the patient's eyes with a feather dipped in it.' His defiance was not without good cause. In modern-day medical herbalism, the plant is still used for conjunctivitis as well as inflamed eyelids. And, just as in the Isle of Lewis, it is used to counteract catarrh.

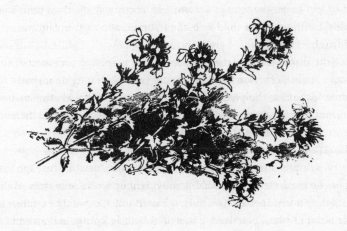

Fairy Flax
(*Linum catharticum*)

The tiny, star-like, white flowers of this delicate plant are to be found in summer in mountains, moorland and grassland throughout Britain. It has been said that it got its name because the fairies used it to make their diminutive clothes of linen. It is a plant that has been specially valued in the Celtic areas of Britain.

In folk medicine, fairy flax has featured strongly in the highly secretive areas of pregnancy and menstruation; clues to this use lie in several of its Gaelic names, which mean 'menstrual plant' or simply 'monthly'. Alexander Carmichael in his collection of songs and ballads tells us that in Barra, fairy flax was put under the soles of a woman in labour and 'the child came into the world without toil or trouble to its mother'. However, the plant was also used to terminate unwanted pregnancies. In the western Highlands, this was one of the plants used for the euphemistically named 'suppression of the menses'; James Robertson recorded its use in 1768. Fear of disapproval by society and the Church, as well as natural reticence on such a sensitive matter, has meant that few folk remedies (or indeed official ones) for abortifacients were ever mentioned in the literature (see also CLUBMOSSES, PENNYROYAL, MUGWORT).

Fairy flax was also well-known as a purge, and was still used for that purpose on the Scottish island of Colonsay right up to the early years of the twentieth century. In the Highlands, a handful of flax would be taken in either water or whey. In Ireland, it was used both as a purge and an emetic; Michael F. Moloney recorded in 1919: 'It is said that when boiled with the flower end uppermost the infusion prepared will promote vomiting ... with stem uppermost purging is produced by the infusion.' It was as a purge that the plant appears in the herbals, and in 1694 Pechey tells us: 'The whole Herb, infus'd in Whitewine, for a whole Night, over hot Ashes, purges strongly Watery Humours.'

Fairy flax was also used in official medicine for the treatment of rheumatism. The butler to a Norfolk gentleman, S. Hoare, Esq., wrote down this recipe in 1801 (now kept in Cromer Museum). It refers to flax by one of its alternative names. Whether the remedy was for himself or his master, we do not know.

> Mountain Flax made into strong Tea for the Rheumitizm [sic] $\frac{1}{2}$ pint to be taken for 9 Mornings & 9 Evenings then miss for a Time.

Nowadays the plant is little used by herbalists. Its cousin, the much larger blue-flowered flax, linseed (*Linum usitatissimum*), which is grown commercially for its oil and fibre, is used instead. Linseed seeds, invaluable in poultices, are also used as a bulk laxative.

Fat Hen
(*Chenopodium album*)

Good King Henry
(*Chenopodium bonus-henricus*)

These common weeds of dung-hills and wasteland have grown in Britain since prehistoric times, but may not strictly be native. They are closely related members of the plant family Chenopodiaceae, which includes many of our modern vegetables such as beetroot, sugar beet and spinach. The generic name *Chenopodium* is derived from the Greek *chen*, meaning 'goose', and *pous*, meaning 'foot', and refers to the shape of the leaves. The name 'Good King Henry' is thought to refer to a sixteenth-century German elf called Heinrich, renowned for his healing powers. The 'King' crept into the English name, but the reasons for this are not known. These plants both have a large number of country names, some of which they share. Probably the two plants were used more or less interchangeably in the past.

In folk medicine, there are only a few records of their use. In Isleham in the Cambridgeshire fens, a cure was recorded of a man's weeping eczema (there called scurvy) by using these plants. A local woman instructed the man to grind up the plant 'in water and drink it. That cured the scurvy and cured my sweaty feet too.' In Ireland, a similar infusion was drunk for rheumatism. Other ailments treated have included 'sore fingers' and wounds. Bryant in 1783 says of Good King Henry, 'The country people call the plant All-good, from a conceit that it will cure all hurts.'

Official medicine confirms the plants' efficacy against chronic sores and adds gout and colic to the list. By the eighteenth century, both plants were little used in official medicine.

Over the centuries, the primary use of both fat hen and Good King Henry has been as a nutritious ingredient in cooking, and an important source of food for animals too. People have been eating these plants since ancient times, and perhaps are still doing so – as recently as the early twentieth century, people in Ayrshire were still adding fat hen to their soup. The Anglo-Saxons called fat hen *melde* and there are still places that preserve the name, such as Melbourn in Cambridgeshire ('Meldeburna', the stream where *melde* grew). Traditionally, the leaves were boiled and pounded with butter, but other parts of the plant could be used too. The young tips were eaten as salad, and the extremely nutritious seeds were used in gruel and even dried and ground into flour for breadmaking.

The last meal of the 2,000-year-old Tollund Man included seeds of fat hen. He was excavated from a raised bog in Finland in the 1950s and was so well-preserved that it was possible to identify his stomach contents, which included many other wild plants as well as barley and linseed.

Good King Henry was cultivated in Lincolnshire where it was known as Lincolnshire Spinach, but 'true' spinach, introduced from Asia in the sixteenth century, swept in and replaced fat hen and its cousin.

We may no longer cultivate these plants for the dinner table but gardeners may like to know that they are still well worth planting among more favoured plants. Their deep roots bring up valuable minerals from lower down in the soil and make them available for more shallow-rooted species.

FERNS

I had no medicine, sir, to go invisible
No fern seed in my pocket.

Ben Jonson, *The New Inn*, I, vi, 18–19

These primitive, varied and beautiful plants usually grow in damp woodland areas and this has added to their mystery as well as their aesthetic appeal. The word 'fern' is thought to be shortened from the Anglo-Saxon *fepern*, meaning 'feather', and many ferns do indeed have feathery fronds. The Victorians were fascinated by the plants, and collecting, growing and pressing them became a popular pastime. Some of the elaborate greenhouses built to house them still remain. Magical powers are often attributed to ferns; their spores were said to make a man invisible, an idea celebrated by Jonson (see above), and also by Shakespeare:

... we have the receipt of fern-seed, we walk invisible.

Shakespeare, *Henry IV*, II, i, 83–84

For invisibility to be conferred on a person, the fern 'seed' must be collected at midnight, on the eve of St John the Baptist; the seed had to fall of its own accord, rather than being shaken onto a plate. This rather difficult method of collection might go some way to explaining the fern's lack of success but, nevertheless, the belief lingered at least into the nineteenth century.

There was also a belief that cutting or burning ferns brought rain, and when Charles I visited Staffordshire his chamberlain wrote to the local sheriff asking him to ensure that no fern should be burnt or cut during the king's visit, so that the weather would be fine.

Ferns have been widely used in folk medicine, and records show that they have been used to treat a variety of ills, from toothache in the nineteenth century (you had to nibble the first frond that appeared in the spring) to the chilblains of a twentieth-century Essex bus driver. This fascinating story from 1965 concerns a hermit-like character called Dido who lived in Hainault Forest.

'He was a very adroit man at making herbal medicine and ointments which cured whooping cough, measles, backache, liver trouble, burns etc ... From a fern, Dido made a green ointment which was highly spoken of.

With this ointment, he cured the chilblains of the bus driver on the Lambourne to Woodford route. Dido said the fern was getting very scarce – the only place where he could find it was Loughton.'

Adder's Tongue Fern
(*Ophioglossum vulgatum*)

This little fern is widespread throughout Britain especially in the lowlands, in grassland and open woodland. It differs in appearance from all the other British ferns. The plant is small and bears an undivided, oval frond that encloses a single spike bearing two rows of spore-cases. The spike is said to resemble the tongue of a snake, which may have given rise to its English and its botanical names. It was, however, also used to treat adder bites, another possible explanation. Other names for this fern include 'serpent's tongue' and 'Christ's spear'.

For many centuries, this fern has been used as a wound-healer for man and beast alike. As recently as the 1930s, a so-called Green Oil of Charity was prepared from its leaves and was commercially available. Some herbal practitioners still recommend this fern today, and often make their own ointments from the leaves. A suggested remedy for bruises, chilblains, sores and ulcers, as well as wounds, is to coat a leaf with the ointment and then bandage the entire leaf in place over the afflicted part.

This fern was also said to be effective against tumours, but the plant had to be gathered when the moon was waning for the treatment to be successful.

Bracken
(*Pteridium aquilinum*)

Get home with the brake,

To brue with and bake,

To cover the shed,

Drie over the hed,

To lie under cow,

To rot under mow,

To serve a burn,

For many a turn.

Thomas Tusser, *Five Hundred Pointes of Good Husbandrie* (1557)

Bracken, or brake, is so widespread in many upland heaths as to be a pest, and this, combined with the recent scares about the toxicity of its spores (it has been suggested that inhaling them could cause cancer) have combined to give the plant a very bad image indeed. But it has proved extremely useful in the past in many ways: as bedding for man and animals; in the Scottish Highlands, for roofing; and as kindling (in Lincolnshire, bracken is called 'light-fire'). Bracken does burn very fiercely and in Sussex was at one time used to burn lime. Even the ash had its uses and was often mixed with tallow to make soap balls, and sometimes used in glassmaking.

It was discovered that if you sliced the rhizome (the underground stem) of bracken, the cross-section would give the appearance of a Greek χ, the initial of Christos. From this emerged the belief that witches hated the plant, and so bracken was used as protection from their powers. Whatever the truth of that, intestinal worms certainly hate it, and a valuable remedy for man and beast alike has been derived from the rhizome.

Both bracken and MALE FERN are toxic, and ingesting them can cause blindness. Could this be related to the idea that their spores confer invisibility?

Male Fern
(*Dryopteris filix-mas*)

Like bracken, this has proved to be invaluable in the war against the dreaded intestinal worm. Pechey tells us that in the seventeenth century 'mounte-banks keep this as a great Secret, and use it to kill Worms.' Nearly two centuries later, Kemsey tells us that 'it is said that the King of France paid a large sum of money for the secret.' There was no quack medicine afoot here: it has been shown that the oleo-resin this fern yields paralyses the muscles of the tapeworm, making it release its hold on the gut wall. Medical herbalists still use male fern today, with caution given the plant's toxicity (SEE BRACKEN), for the same purpose.

Male fern had other applications in official medicine. Pechey in 1694 records its efficacy for burns, while in 1693 Salmon describes it as a purge and adds that it is useful for treating sores. By the nineteenth century, only its worm-killing properties were still valued.

Royal Fern
(*Osmunda regalis*)

This fern has a lovely and intriguing country name: 'Osmund the Waterman'. Royal fern is a tall plant, often reaching several feet in height, and it is said that a waterman of Loch Tyne named Osmund hid his family among a patch of it when the Danes invaded. It is a plant of wet places, common in Ireland and parts of Scotland, and it is in these countries that it is valued most highly in folk medicine.

Such was the faith in the healing power of the royal fern in the Scottish Highlands that even the liquid in which its roots had been boiled was said to cure a dislocated kneecap. According to one witness, when the liquid was applied to the knee, 'forthwith the pain stopped, all swelling disappeared and the kneecap went back to its original place'. On Colonsay and in Cumbria, the mucilaginous roots were chopped and steeped in water to treat sprains. In Cumbria, the plant was also called 'bog onion' and was used as a remedy for rickets. It has been found to have had a very ancient use indeed; in prehistoric times, its spores were added to mead to halt its fermentation.

The royal fern was not only employed in folk medicine. In official medicine, it was recommended in the seventeenth century for ulcers, colic, bruises and wounds, according to Pechey in 1694. These remedies subsequently died out and today the plant is little-used in medical herbalism in this country.

Like many other ferns, this one had a magical aura and was used in love charms. One particular charm requires nine stalks of royal fern:

> A love charm for thee, water through a straw, the warmth of him [her] thou
> lovest, with love to draw on thee, Arise betimes on Lord's day, to the flat rock on
> the shore, Take with thee the butterbur and the foxglove. A small quantity of
> embers, in the skirt of thy kirtle, a special handful of sea-weed in a wooden shovel.
> Three bones of an old man, newly torn from the grave, Nine stalks of Royal fern,
> newly trimmed with an axe. Burn them on a fire of faggots, and make them into
> ashes; sprinkle in the fleshy breast of thy lover, against the venom of the north
> wind. Go round the rath of procreation, The circuit of five turns, And I will vow
> and warrant thee that man [woman] shall never leave thee.

Feverfew
(*Tanacetum parthenium*)

Feverfew is not a native plant but a common, naturalized weed of gardens and waste ground. Its leaves are a characteristic yellowish-green, shaped like those of a garden chrysanthemum. The plant is bushy and upright and its numerous, neat, daisy-like flowers are held upright too, making it easy to distinguish from the mayweeds (*Matricaria* and *Tripleurospermum* species). The flowers are longlasting and the generic name *Tanacetum* is said to be derived from the Greek word *athanato*, meaning 'immortal'. It is thought that the plant was introduced in the Middle Ages, perhaps for medicinal uses. Feverfew can often be found growing in country churchyards, for a very melancholy reason, as this Norfolk man, Wigby (1990), recounts:

'As there were no chapels of rest, the corpse was placed in a coffin, placed on trestles and left there until the funeral. In summertime feverfew was placed around it and also on the lid as it was taken to the place of burial. Many seeds of the feverfew fell off en route and that is why the plant is or was frequently found in many village churchyards, mainly on the north side where paupers, or those who had committed suicide, were buried.'

Feverfew is perhaps more famous as a rare example of a plant remedy that has been investigated scientifically and shown to be effective in a clinical trial. It has proved to be of great help in the treatment of migraines, and many sufferers find relief by taking the herb in tablet form or by eating the fresh leaves in bread and butter (however, this can result in inflammation of the mouth). The plant does, indeed, taste extremely bitter. It was Pechey back in 1694 who recommended it for headaches: 'Take of Feverfew one handful, warm it in a Frying-pan, apply it twice or thrice hot; this cures an

Hemicrania'. Hemicrania, meaning literally 'half-head', was the word from which migraine was derived.

In official medicine, feverfew was also recommended for slightly unusual ailments such as melancholy, vertigo and 'against opium taken too liberally'. A good many gynaecological complaints, such as irregular menstruation, were also helped by feverfew. It was still being recommended, rather delicately, in the 1838 *The British Herbal* 'for the diseases of women who have children. A decoction, or a tea made of it is an emmenagogue, and being sweetened with honey may be used with good success to ease a cough'.

There are very few records of feverfew in folk medicine in the past – a situation common with non-native plants – but its popularity now for treating migraine probably will result in it having a folk role in future. Within living memory, the herb has been used to allay pain and as a cough treatment.

We should look even more favourably on this plant in the summer when insects are numerous. It has been used in Scotland for repelling those that bite, and Pechey has this piece of advice: 'Bees cannot endure it; wherefore those that abound with good Humours in the body, and are most apt to be stung with Bees, may secure themselves, when they walk in Gardens where Bees are, by carrying Feverfew in their Hands.'

Figwort

(*Scrophularia nodosa, Scrophularia auriculata*)

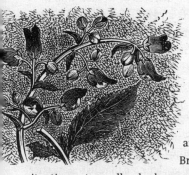

This is a distinctive plant with a tall, upright, emphatically square stem, pairs of large, oval leaves and terminal spikes of odd-looking, reddish-brown flowers. The upper part of the flower is two-lobed and projects like a little roof above the rest. When crushed, the plant has a pungent and unpleasant scent. It is native throughout Britain and grows particularly in damp situations at woodland edges and beside streams and rivers. Anglers find the plant a nuisance because it frequently gets tangled up in their rods.

In folk medicine, figwort has been famed as a wound-healer. In Ireland, it was particularly highly prized; there it was called the Queen of Herbs and was used to treat everything from piles (formerly known as 'figs', hence the name 'figwort'), skin conditions, wounds and liver, kidney and stomach complaints. It was advisable to quote this charm while gathering figwort:

> I will pluck the figwort,
> With the frutage of sea and land,
> The plant of joy and gladness,
> The plant of rich milk.

Alexander Carmichael, *Carmina Gadelica* (1900–1971)

The plant also had a firm reputation as a painkiller, and young mothers must have found figwort quite indispensable; they would take dried pieces of the stem and thread them together to make teething necklaces for children. The child would chew on it and find some respite from a sore mouth. For the remedy to work, a man should pick figwort for a girl child, and a woman for a boy. Figwort's painkilling properties were known countrywide:

in Devon, where it was known as 'poor man's salve', a poultice of it was used to relieve skin conditions and aches and pains; in the fens of Cambridgeshire, leaves were gathered from the dykes and used to treat sore heels and chapped toes. 'They soon relieved the pain.'

In official medicine, it had one clear use above all – for treating scrofula, in modern terms glandular tuberculosis. It was believed that kings of England had the power to cure this disease simply by touching the sufferer, hence the name of 'King's evil'. Culpeper recommends figwort in 1653 for the King's evil, for wounds and 'knobs, kernels, bunches or wens', as well as for piles.

Pechey in 1694 says of figwort that 'this and some other herbs, do good in the King's Evil; but nothing has been found so effectual, as Touching.' He goes on to say that anyone trying to treat the disease 'will find Reason of Acknowledging the Goodness of God, who has dealt so bountifully with this Nation, in giving the Kings of it, at least, from *Edward the Confessor*, downwards, if not for a longer Time, an extraordinary Power in the miraculous Cures thereof'. Figwort was so closely identified with scrofula that it sometimes goes by the name 'rose-noble', the royal golden coin that, in the absence of the King himself, was reckoned to be the next best thing for curing scrofula.

By the nineteenth century, scrofula began to disappear, replaced by the more deadly pulmonary tuberculosis that is still all too common in the poorest and most overcrowded countries today. Why the even more virulent form of tuberculosis should have taken over from scrofula is not clear.

However, the use of figwort for other ailments has continued: present-day medical herbalists prescribe figwort for a variety of skin conditions and for the healing of burns, haemorrhoids, ulcers and wounds.

Forget-me-not
(*Myosotis* species)

Nor can I find, amid my lonely walk
By rivulet, or spring, or wet roadside
That blue and bright-eyed flowerlet of the brook,
Hope's gentle gem, the sweet Forget-me-not!

Samuel Taylor Coleridge, *The Keepsake* (1802)

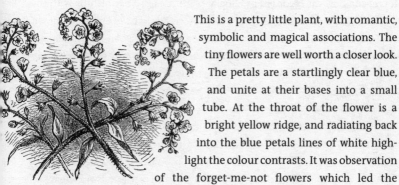

This is a pretty little plant, with romantic, symbolic and magical associations. The tiny flowers are well worth a closer look. The petals are a startlingly clear blue, and unite at their bases into a small tube. At the throat of the flower is a bright yellow ridge, and radiating back into the blue petals lines of white highlight the colour contrasts. It was observation of the forget-me-not flowers which led the eighteenth-century German botanist Sprengel to formulate the idea of 'honey guides' – patterns on the flower which direct the pollinating insect to the nectar, ensuring pollination occurs in the process.

Forget-me-not was adored by the Victorians who, in the language of flowers, regarded it as a symbol of love. Its name was said to be derived from a German legend, of a knight who picked a bunch of the flowers for his sweetheart, slipped and fell into the river, and threw the flowers to his love as he was swept away, calling, 'Forget me not.'

Another theory states that Henry of Lancaster was responsible for the flower's symbolism: 'the royal adventurer, Henry of Lancaster ... appears to have been the person who gave *Myosotis arvensis*, or forget-me-not, its emblematical and poetical meaning'. During his exile in France he gave a piece of the plant, along with the message *Souveigne vous de moy*, to his hostess, at that time the wife of the Duke de Bretagne. Later, as dowager Duchess of Brittany, she became Henry's second wife, so she clearly did remember him. More simply, forget-me-not in Yorkshire is sometimes called 'love-me'.

Tracing the history of this plant is made difficult by the confusion over its English name. Gerard was the first in 1597 to record the plant in Britain, but he knew of no English names for it, and called it 'scorpion grass', because of a slight resemblance of the coiled flowering stem to a scorpion's tail. In official medicine, it was taken to be the plant named by Dioscorides as scorpion grass and used for treating snakebites.

The plant has been little-used in folk medicine; made into a decoction or a poultice, it was used to treat sore eyes. On the island of Colonsay, the forget-me-not was regarded as a lucky plant.

Foxglove
(*Digitalis purpurea*)

The Foxglove's leaves, with caution giv'n,
Another proof of favouring Heav'n,
Will happily display;
The rapid pulse it can abate:
The hectic flush can moderate;
And, blest by Him whose will is fate,
May give a lengthen'd day.

Eighteenth-century rhyme

The foxglove must surely be one of our most stately wild flowers, as well as one of the easiest to recognize. It grows in damp woodland and is especially common on acid soils in the north and west of Britain. The plant's tall spire is much visited by bees; its rosy-pink flowers are held at an angle to the stem, and each provides a conveniently jutting-out lobe which acts as a doorstep on which the bee can alight.

The story of how a modern heart drug was developed from the use of foxglove in country herbal medicine is world-famous and must be the best-known example of the overlap between folk and official medicine. The man behind it was William Withering, a mid-eighteenth-century physician. While he was practising in Stafford, an interest in wild flowers was sparked by his courtship of a girl who enjoyed painting them. In 1775, he encountered a Shropshire family recipe for dropsy and realized that an important ingredient of it was the foxglove. He knew that dropsy was often caused by heart failure and his thorough investigation of this ultimately led to the discovery of digoxin, still one of the mainline drugs in heart treatment. His patient years of experiment and observation on the effects of foxglove infusion have led to his being honoured as the father of modern clinical pharmacology.

Ironically, the effect of foxglove on the heart was almost forgotten by orthodox medicine, and was only revived thanks to the work of two London physicians, Mackenzie and Lewis, in the early years of the twentieth century.

Prior to Withering's time, the foxglove had had a chequered history in official medicine. Gerard in 1597 was dismissive, saying that foxgloves 'are of no use, neither have they any place amongst medicines, according to the Antients'. A century later, Salmon reported that foxglove was being employed in official medicine for a diverse range of ailments including sores, the King's evil (scrofula) and epilepsy. By the nineteenth century, Kemsey was advising handling foxglove with caution, but did recommend it for dropsy.

In addition to dropsy, folk practitioners used the plant for a variety of other ailments, from eczema in animals and humans, to treating infected sores. In the Scottish Highlands, foxglove leaves were chopped, mixed with butter and onion, and applied as a warm poultice for diphtheria and 'bad knees'. No doubt all treatments were applied with great caution. In the folk museum at Kingussie in Scotland, there is a handwritten note giving instructions and wholehearted approval for a very different remedy:

> For a man in great pain from an internal growth or swelling, a pulp was made from squashed foxglove roots, then applied inside flannel, after the pulp had been heated, as a poultice to the swelling. The man received immediate relief, and continued to do so until the cure was completed.

In medical herbalism, the foxglove provided a heart tonic in the nineteenth and early twentieth centuries, but nowadays its use is restricted by law, and it can be prescribed only by a physician. Currently, a related species (*Digitalis lanata*) is the main source of the glycoside digoxin for the pharmaceutical industry.

The plant is, of course, quite deadly. Its numerous country names, such as 'fairy's thimbles' and 'dead men's thimbles', imply an element of magic, as is so often the case with plants that are poisonous. In the Scottish Borders, foxglove leaves were placed in babies' cradles to prevent them from being bewitched and, in seventeenth-century Ireland and Wales, children suspected of being changelings were rubbed all over with the juice.

Although the flowers are very easily recognized, the leaves have sometimes been confused with those of comfrey, with fatal results. Birds and animals will not go anywhere near it; humans are often tempted. The magical legends surrounding the plant may have been intended as a deterrent, especially to children, who were warned not even to pick foxglove let alone eat it. Children would often be told that if they ate foxglove flowers, they would be carried away by the fairies. However, it seems that children have always liked to play dangerous games. The Reverend MacFarlane relates that in the 1920s in Scotland children 'have the habit of sucking the honey-bags of the foxglove flowers. Wonderful is their immunity.' Children also enjoyed popping the unopened buds, which are beautifully sealed, like little parcels – another game parents must have warned against time and time again.

Despite its known dangers, the foxglove remained in use in folk medicine right into the early decades of the twentieth century:

'My mother had eleven children and I was the eldest girl. Mother breastfed us all and when she weaned the baby we went into the woods to gather the largest leaves of the foxgloves. These she [mother] put on her breasts like plasters. They dried her milk with no ill effects.'

Mrs E. D—, Somerset (1985)

The list of animal complaints for which foxglove has been used includes eczema, mange, red-water fever, sheep scab and strangles. In Limerick, pieces of foxglove were strewn around to kill rats and mice. Even the well-researched foxglove may not yet have yielded up all its secrets to science.

Fumitory
(*Fumaria* species)

Fumiter is erbe, I say,
That springyth in April and in May,
In field, in town, in yerd and gate
There land is fat and good in state

Stockholm medical manuscript (*c*.1400)

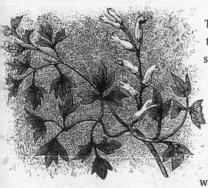

The name fumitory means 'smoke', and the plant is sometimes called 'earth-smoke', but the link between smoke and fumitory remains as elusive today as it ever was. Some have suggested that the very fine leaves are a reminder of smoke; others that the tiny, purple-edged, tubular flowers look like the lighted ends of matches. To muddy the waters even further, there is a legend suggesting that the plant arises mysteriously from the earth in the form of smoke. In ancient times, exorcists claimed that the smoke from the burnt herb had the power to expel evil spirits.

Despite these dark origins, in both folk and official medicine, fumitory has been valued mainly as a cosmetic, an enhancer of young women. An infusion of the flowers was meant to make the face more beautiful and remove spots and freckles.

In official medicine, the plant was recommended to treat jaundice as well as skin conditions:

Get water of fumiter liver to cool
And other the like, or go die like a fool.

The juice dropped into eyes was claimed to clear the eyesight, although

Culpeper warned in 1653 that 'it procure some pain for the present and cause tears'. In the eighteenth century, Sir John Hill related that 'Some smoke the dried leaves in the manner of tobacco for disorders of the head with success.' *The British Herbal* of 1838 gives uses of the plant very similar to Culpeper's: 'It is good for obstructions in the viscera and jaundice. The juice of fumitory and dock, mingled with vinegar, cures scabs, pimples, wheals, or pushes.'

As well as a cosmetic, there were a few additional roles for fumitory in folk medicine. Fumitory in whey provided a healthy tonic drink until the twentieth century, and a preparation of the plant was used to treat cradle cap in infants. It was also used to treat worms in humans and in animals. In parts of Ireland, the plant was dried and burnt and the smoke inhaled as a remedy for stomach trouble.

Garlic
(*Allium sativum*)

'When the medicine of Dr Cullen failed, I shall give him garlic in brandy ... I shall engage it will free him from worms, and it is attended with no inconvenience, but his breath will perfume the air.'

Eighteenth-century letter

Garlic is thought to have originated in Asia, and was a great delicacy of the ancient Egyptians. The date of its introduction to Britain is not known but it has been grown here at least since the fourteenth century. For the countryfolk, RAMSONS, or wild garlic, probably often took the place of cultivated garlic.

Its virtues, medicinal and culinary, have perhaps not been appreciated quite as much as in continental Europe, and yet its reputation has never faltered over the centuries. Even today, it is still considered in many households to be not just a food but a health-giver, a good guard against many ailments.

A few folk remedies used garlic rather than ramsons – in Ireland, for ringworm and jaundice. A twentieth-century treatment for whooping cough in England was to rub the child's hands and feet with garlic. This same remedy is described by one who remembers it vividly:

> I was born in 1910, and when I was a child at the age of four years I was put to bed unwell by my mother who told me I had whooping cough ... My mother looked up the remedy book called *Common Ailments* to see what to use; it said Garlic Pods to be crushed to a pulp and put on lint then apply to the soles of the feet; it was *not* to touch the skin. Lots of folk refused to believe this cure and laughed about it but she had the last laugh when a peaceful night was had and the next morning there was no sign of the whoop.

Mrs E. M—, Essex Age Concern essay (1991)

In official medicine, Culpeper lists innumerable ailments in 1653 for which garlic can be used, including the treatment of the bites of 'venomous creatures', dropsy, jaundice and the treatment of worms. For this latter ailment, garlic was favoured throughout the centuries. Pechey in 1694 recommended it, as did the writer of the eighteenth-century letter quoted above and Kemsey in 1838; in the 1930s, it was still in use for treating worms in children. It was also found to keep cats and dogs worm-free if added to their food.

The scientific underpinnings behind the power of garlic began during the First World War when it was used, literally by the ton, in first-aid treatment of wounds. The government offered growers one shilling per pound of bulbs, and were willing to buy all that could be produced. In those pre-antibiotic days, it was the most effective antiseptic available. Since then garlic has been subjected to extensive scientific research which has 'justified' many of its uses. A substance named allicin, released when the clove is crushed, has a strongly antiseptic and antibiotic action that is effective against a number of bacteria, viruses and fungi. We are also beginning to understand the complex biochemistry behind its observed effects in lowering blood pressure and reducing cholesterol levels.

Modern-day herbalists recommend garlic for treating infections of all kinds and also value it for lowering cholesterol levels and blood pressure. It has been shown to be effective in some cases of diabetes too. The more we discover about garlic, the more remarkable its powers seem to be.

Goat's Beard
(*Tragopogon pratensis*)

And goodly now the noon-tide hour,
When from his high meridian tower
The sun looks down in majesty,
What time about, the grassy lea.
The goat's beard, prompt his rise to hail,
With broad expanded disk, in veil
Close mantling wraps its yellow head,
And goes, as peasants say, to bed.

Bishop Mant (1776–1846)

Goat's beard is a plant of rough grassland and roadside verges. In midsummer, its yellow flowerheads close up tightly in the middle of the day, giving rise to the country name of 'Jack-go-to-bed-at-noon'. The flowers are succeeded by a large, spherical seedhead like a giant dandelion clock, but it is the long silky hairs on the seed that have given rise to the name of goat's beard, a literal translation of the generic name of *Tragopogon*.

The plant is closely related to salsify (*Tragopogon porrifolius*), a root vegetable once popular but now less so. Like salsify, the long taproots may be eaten raw in salads, or cooked and served like parsnips. This of course was a simple way of ingesting the plant's goodness.

In official medicine, Gerard recommends in 1597 this method: 'The same boiled in water until they be tender, and buttered as parsneps and carrots, are a most pleasant and wholesome meate, in delicate taste far surpassing either Parsenep or Carrot: which meat procures appetite, warmeth the stomacke, and strengthneth those that have been sicke of a long lingring disease.' The root could also be boiled in wine for pain and stitches in the side. Respiratory and urinary complaints were also treated with goat's beard.

Folk medicine in Britain does not seem to have used this plant very much at all (with the one exception of the Scottish Highlands, where it was used for stomach troubles). Official medicine perhaps did not value goat's beard quite as much as it should, for it is now known to contain a substance called inulin, which is broken down in the body to fructose, rather than glucose. This makes it a useful food for diabetics.

Present-day medical herbalists in this country use it for liver and gallbladder problems.

Goldenrod
(*Solidago virgaurea*)

Reaching up through bush and briar
Sumptuous brow and heart of fire,
Flaunting high its wind-rocked plume,
Brave with wealth of native bloom, –
Golden rod!

Elaine Goodale Eastman (1863–1953), *Golden Rod*

We are more familiar with goldenrod as a garden plant than as a wild plant, but in its native state it grows in open woodland, grassland, cliffs and hedgerows. As its name suggests, it has a wand-like form with a flexible, very upright stem bearing neatly arranged leaves. In late summer, the stem bears a cluster of tiny gold stars, each a minute daisy in form. Bees love the flowers and it has been said that an acre of land planted with goldenrod would supply a hundred hives with their winter stores. Traditionally it was said to be useful as a divining rod: 'the golden rod has long had the reputation in England of pointing to hidden springs of water, as well as to treasures of gold and silver.' Yet in some parts of the country it is considered unlucky to bring it into the house or even to have it growing in the garden.

In folk and in official medicine, the plant was renowned as a wound-healer and for treating broken bones. Its generic name, *Solidago*, means to 'make whole'. For generations, goldenrod has been used in this way, often in the form of an ointment.

Doris E. Coates's book about country life in the early years of the twentieth century records how goldenrod was always grown in the herb patch and used for wound-healing, as well as a variety of other complaints. An infusion of the leaves was used for scratches, or the fresh leaf could be pressed on the injury 'as it was thought to be antiseptic. The infusion could also be drunk for indigestion.' In Derbyshire, goldenrod alleviated backache; in Yorkshire, it was applied to 'sore infected places'. In Irish folk medicine, goldenrod was used to treat colds, indigestion, kidney trouble and even heart conditions. It was known there as the 'herb of the Palsy' and 'is said to have worked wonders in cases of general apathy and depression'.

In official medicine, the plant was also used primarily as a wound-healer and no doubt was much in demand, but was subject to the vagaries of commerce, as Gerard in 1597 comments: 'I have known the dry herbe which came from beyond the sea sold in Bucklersbury in London for half a crowne an ounce. But since it was found in Hamstead wood, even as it were at our townes end, no man will give halfe a crowne for an hundred weight of it.' And yet, as he goes on to say, the plant 'no doubt have the same vertue now that then it had, although it growes so neere our owne homes in never so great quantity'.

Culpeper in 1653 and Pechey in 1694 praise it as a wound herb and Pechey also suggests its usefulness for treating kidney stones, as does Kemsey in 1838. So it is perhaps no surprise that although the plant's use as a wound-healer has largely discontinued, its value as a remedy for various urinary disorders continues in modern herbalism.

Goosegrass
(*Galium aparine*)

Our grandmother wearing what must have been the last of the proper sunbonnets (I have never seen another) gathered goosegrass which she cooked and fed to the goslings, hence the name, but a pad soaked in the liquid and bandaged over a wound was supposed to help the tissue to knit quickly. Goosegrass is the weed that children call Sweethearts probably because of its propensity to cling. We were asked not to gather it as the seeds were too tiresome to remove from our clothing.

Mrs E. M—, Essex Age Concern essay (1991)

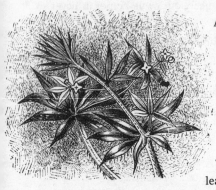

Although it is known as a troublesome, sprawling weed to most gardeners, this plant deserves a better press. Children are familiar with it, as are dog-walkers; the entire plant is covered with barbed bristles which cause it to stick to anything it comes into contact with. In parts of Scotland, it has been called 'bluid-tongue' because 'children with the leaves practise phlebotomy upon the tongue of those playmates who are simple enough to endure it.' The small, round fruits are likewise bristly and easily dispersed, a factor that must in part account for the plant's commonness, especially by footpaths and field margins. The minute, white flowers are borne in the axils of the whorls of leaves.

The main uses of goosegrass seem to have been culinary although, of course, anything made from it was considered health-giving. The whole plant is nutritious, and as its name suggests, it was fed to poultry to fatten them. It was a constituent of many country tonics for humans too, including in East Anglia a fizzy, beer-like drink made in the springtime from NETTLES and goosegrass. The tiny fruits were also roasted to make a coffee substitute (although unfortunately not a very pleasant one).

Practical uses are very varied. Dairy farmers used the juice as a vegetable rennet for making cheese and junket. The generic name of *Galium* is derived from the Greek word for milk, *gala*. On Colonsay in the Hebrides, goosegrass shoots were bunched together and used as a sieve and, in Ireland, even the water in which goosegrass had been boiled was considered valuable as 'a marvellous hair tonic'. Birds however must beware; the root yields a red dye and it is claimed that if they eat the root their bones will be stained red.

The medicinal role of goosegrass has been varied but all three strands (folk, official, modern herbalist) include its role as a springtime tonic. In addition, in official medicine it was used to treat a wide variety of illnesses, among them burns and bites, dropsy, gravel and stone (urinary stones) and scrofula (glandular tuberculosis). Gerard in 1597 recommended eating goosegrass if you wanted to lose weight, and yet poultry farmers fattened up their geese on it. The plant is strongly diuretic, which might in part account for its claimed slimming properties.

In folk medicine the plant was associated with completely different ailments: it was a first-aid treatment for cuts and scratches and, in particular, leg ulcers. It was also widely used to treat coughs, colds, wounds and occasionally tumours. Goosegrass's role in folk medicine is a strictly seasonal one; the plant has to be used fresh and in the springtime: this is probably why official medicine and herbalism have not in recent times exploited it to the same extent.

Nineteenth- and twentieth-century medical herbalists have used goosegrass in a similar way to its cousin LADY'S BEDSTRAW, mainly to treat urinary complaints, swollen lymph glands and skin conditions such as psoriasis.

Gorse

(*Ulex europaeus*)

Love is out of fashion
When the gorse is out of bloom.

Proverb

As the saying implies, gorse flowers all year round, and it is not unusual to find some bushes in flower outside its normal flowering season. It is a prickly and very abundant plant, widespread in heathland throughout Britain, and so much a part of the landscape that it features in many poems and paintings. Anyone who has smelt the sweet, coconut-like smell of the vivid yellow flowers on a sunny day will find it a quite unforgettable fragrance.

In British rural life, gorse has been indispensable. It was an important source of fuel where trees were few and far between, and provided good fodder for cattle when grass was scarce. When the young green leaves were available, livestock would graze on them; at other times of the year, the gorse was cut, pounded and chopped for feeding to the livestock. In Scotland, it was believed that butter from gorse-fed cattle had a better colour. Other practical uses included using the branches to make fishermen's creels; making wine from the blossoms; and extracting a dark green and yellow dye, used in Morayshire, for example to colour Easter eggs. In the wool-dyeing process, gorse bark would be boiled with other dye plants to deepen and fix their colours.

Gorse was shrouded in superstition and tradition. In Ireland, it was 'considered lucky, and was generally grown close to the house because of its value as a clothes dryer', a nice mix of magic and practicality. In fact it was a washday bonus, because its ashes could be mixed with clay to make soap.

In Devon the gorse, sometimes known as the furze bush, was considered an emblem of constancy – in some places, a sprig was included in the bridal bouquet. In this same county, it was used as a 'kissing bush' at Christmas in much the same way as mistletoe, a practice still current in the 1950s. It was often dusted with flour to resemble snow, decorated and planted indoors in a tub. But although it could be brought into the house for Christmas, it was considered unlucky to bring it indoors during May; such action could bring about the death of a family member. In parts of Scotland, it was considered an unlucky flower that should never be given to anyone. Conversely, in Ireland a bunch of gorse was brought into the house by the youngest family member on a May morning; this was called 'bringing in the summer'.

Its applications in folk medicine are several. In nineteenth-century Suffolk, it was an emmenagogue (menstruation stimulant). Perhaps it was used in this way as contraception, giving a less lighthearted meaning to the saying quoted at the top of this entry. Gorse seems to have been especially effective when made into an ointment. In Wales, an ointment made from crushed gorse was used to treat sores while, in Whitby in Yorkshire, fishermen soothed their chapped hands with a salve made from gorse flowers and lard.

Ireland had so many practical uses for gorse that a whole book has been written about them. Other medicinal uses there include the treatment of coughs and colds, indigestion, intestinal worms, jaundice, heart trouble and skin conditions. The Irish probably used the only truly native gorse *Ulex gallii*, which is found only in the west of the British Isles. The now far commoner *Ulex europaeus* was introduced for fencing and foraging.

In official medicine, gorse has been little used. It was recommended for gravel (small urinary stones), stone and jaundice from Gerard's time but its decline was absolute; it is not used at all in modern-day medical herbalism.

Greater Celandine
(*Chelidonium majus*)

The celandine ain't such a very common plant to meet with, and I can tell you a queer thing about it. You'll never find it growing far from houses. Often enough it will be under a garden hedge close against the road, or in among nettles on a rubbish heap. It have something of the look on a small yellow poppy ...

'My gipsy friend', quoted Mary Thorne Quelch,
Herbs for Daily Use (1941)

Despite its name, this plant is not related to the spring-flowering lesser celandine; instead it is a member of the poppy family. It is not strictly native to Britain, but was introduced by the Romans and is now widely naturalized. In the seventeenth century, Pechey commented: 'Celendine [sic] grows in shady and rough Places and amongst Rubbish', a description which still holds good today. The plant flowers in early summer, its bright yellow, four-petalled flowers dropping their sepals as soon as the flower opens (just like the field poppy). The flower can be a useful weather forecaster, because it closes up when the weather is deteriorating and opens again in the sunshine. The whole plant has a striking, bright orange sap.

In folk medicine, the plant has been used above all to remove warts and corns, but among its subsidiary uses has been the removal of whitish opaque spots on the eye that people once called 'kennings'; this has given rise to its country name of 'kenning-wort'. The juice of the plant is rather caustic and this treatment would have been painful. In a Devonian folk cure for a sore eye, the sufferer is advised to place the crushed plant on the wrist: the right-hand wrist for a right sore eye, and vice versa.

Despite its acrid juice, the plant has also been used internally as a kidney stimulant and (in Suffolk) for treating cancer of the liver. It was still in use for treating jaundice in the early decades of the twentieth century. A lady now living in Norfolk recalls how, as a young girl of twelve in 1929, she was treated for jaundice by her grandmother, at Denver Mill in Cambridgeshire. After the medicine the doctor had given her did little good, her granny treated her with a celandine concoction of which she had to drink an eggcupful each day for several days. She remembers it tasted dreadful, but it did the trick and her jaundice vanished.

In official medicine, as in folk medicine, the plant had been recommended since Classical times for improving the eyesight. Gerard in 1597 claims that 'it cleanseth and consumeth awaie slimie things that cleave about the ball of the eye'. He recommends it too for improving the eyesight of hawks; hawking was a favourite sport at that time.

Culpeper, in similar vein, once experimented on the eyesight of swallows. His reason for doing so sprang from an old and fascinating story that the greater celandine was so named (*chelidon* is Greek for 'swallow') because swallows use the plant to restore the sight of their young. Culpeper, the empiricist, put the idea to the test: 'They say, that if you put out the eyes of young swallows when they are in the nest, the old ones will recover their eyes again with this herb. This I am confident, for I have tried it, that if we mar the very apple of their eyes with a needle, she will recover them again; but whether with this herb or not, I know not.' An alarming experiment, but it would seem that no harm was done. Salmon in 1693 also recommends the juice for clearing the eyesight but advises 'it is best to allay it with Brest milk and so drop it in'. He recommended it too for jaundice as well as for removal of sores, ulcers, warts, 'Ring-worms, spreading Cankers &c'. A very similar list of uses is named by Kemsey in 1838.

Present-day medical herbalists use the plant, with care, to treat asthma, gallstones, whooping cough and a variety of skin conditions, including eczema, malignant skin tumours and warts. Its acrid nature means that greater celandine is no longer recommended for treating eyes.

Modern pharmacological studies of this plant are revealing a wealth of alkaloids which have a variety of physiological effects on the body. Some are antibacterial and antiviral, others affect blood pressure and muscle contraction. Studies of their effectiveness against certain cancers are looking hopeful, and clearly, much of the story of this plant remains to be told.

Greater Plantain
(*Plantago major*)

And you, Waybread, mother of worts,
Open from eastward, powerful within,
Over you chariots rolled, over you queens road,
Over you brides cried, over you bulls belled;
All these you withstood, and these you confounded,
So withstand now the venom that flies through the air,
And the loathed thing which through the land roves

Lay of the Nine Healing Herbs

This is from the Lay of the Nine Healing Herbs, a poem celebrating the herbs most valued by the Anglo-Saxons. It occurs in the famous early medical manuscript known as the 'Lacnunga', and was originally written in the Wessex dialect. It shows just how highly respected this lowly plant was.

As the poem (above) implies, this tough plant withstands trampling, and so is often to be found colonizing otherwise bare ground in field entrances and along pathways. Its country name of 'waybread' refers to this habit of growing along paths trodden by man. The native Americans call it 'white man's footsteps', since it was introduced by white settlers to North America and followed in their tracks. Part of the reason it can withstand trampling so well is the toughness of its leaves, which can flatten against the earth and take the weight of a person with no ill effect. In addition, the growing point of the plant is sheltered well, right at ground level.

This plantain does not lend itself to children's games in the same way as its close relative, RIBWORT PLANTAIN, because its stems are so tough and very hard to break, but nevertheless children have always, and still do, amuse themselves by scraping the greater plantain's leaf-stalk to reveal the very elastic veins, which when stretched become the strings of a toy violin or banjo.

Aside from children's games, the greater plantain has been a celebrated wound-healer, used in folk medicine to treat cuts, insect bites, stings, wounds and even broken bones. One Norfolk lady currently forbids her family to remove any greater plantains from her lawn, because she uses them to treat varicose ulcers on her legs.

In official medicine, greater plantain was used in similar ways. Gerard, writing in the sixteenth century, although he recommends the juice for sore eyes and ears, is strangely dismissive of the plant and all the magic associated with it:

> I find in antient writers many goodmorrowes, which I think not meete to bring into your memorie againe; as That three roots will cure one griefe, four another disease, six hanged about the neck are good for another malady, &c. all which are but ridiculous toyes.

Yet Shakespeare, writing at the same time, has Costard in *Love's Labour's Lost* (III, i, 68–69) calling 'O, sir, plantain, a plain plantain; no l'envoy, no l'envoy; no salve, sir, but a plantain!' to mend his broken shin. In 1693, Salmon confirms the use of 'Broad Plantane or Way bred' as a wound-healer, also for spitting of blood and for scurvy, as does his contemporary John Pechey. By the nineteenth century, plantain was still officially recommended by Kemsey for treating sore eyes and ears, as well as dropsy and jaundice. In modern medical herbalism in this country the plant continues to be used to treat cuts, wounds, inflammation, sprains and fractures. What is known so far about the plant's chemistry endorses many of these uses.

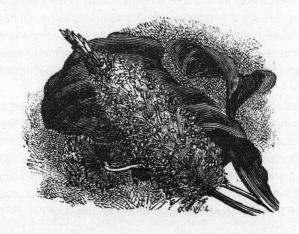

Ground Elder
(*Aegopodium podagraria*)

Ground elder was introduced in the Middle Ages as a vegetable, and ever since, it has made itself perfectly at home throughout Britain – much to the gardener's dismay. By Gerard's time, it 'groweth of it selfe in gardens without setting or sowing, and is so fruitfull in his increase that where it hath once taken roote, it will hardly be gotten out again, spoiling and getting every yeare more ground, to the annoying of better herbes'. The plant spreads by seed and by underground stems, and even one small piece can quickly regenerate. In some areas, ground elder is called 'jump-about' and in Ireland it has earned itself the name of 'farmer's plague'.

Ground elder's reputation as an ineradicable nuisance sadly obscures its good qualities, medicinal and otherwise. It is actually an attractive plant; its pinkish flowerheads gradually fade to white as they mature and can look very beautiful, like old, handmade lace. The boiled shoots make an addition to the dinner table, tasting like a spicy version of spinach.

In official medicine, the plant was used primarily for the treatment of gout and other 'joint-ache': both its common name of 'goutweed' and its specific name, *podagraria*, reflect this use. Gout was usually a disease of the more monied classes and this is reflected in another of the plant's country names, 'bishop's weed'. Kemsey in 1838 still advocated its use for 'the cold gout and sciatica' and added that 'carrying it about the person eases the pains of gout, and prevents the disease'. But Kemsey's recommendation was not enough and the plant is seldom used today by medical herbalists in this country.

Folk medicine, however, harnessed the plant in treating a wider variety of conditions, including arthritis (in Orkney a decoction of ground elder was taken for this complaint). And unlike official medicine, folk medicine has continued to find a place for ground elder. Mixed with comfrey, it has formed a first-aid ointment – the inventor of this ointment uses it on her family to this day. It is known simply as 'green stuff'. In Essex, this conversation was recorded in the early decades of the twentieth century:

'That's a terrible useless plant, Fred! Serves no useful purpose I know of!'
Fred then told me 'I only know one thing it is good for and that is to boil some
of it up, and then when cold, use the solution on piles – it will cure them.'

Essex Age Concern essay (1991)

Ground Ivy
(*Glechoma hederacea*)

This little creeping plant carpets the floor of open woodland sites and hedgerows with its neat, dark-green, scalloped leaves, and then in spring-time produces spikes of blue (or occasionally pink) flowers. Chaucer described it as 'ground ivy that makes our yard so merry' in the *Nun's Priest's Tale*. When fully open, the leaves are slightly convex, catching the light so that they appear shiny, even though the entire plant is covered with hairs. The young growing tips are often tinged with purple, which dramatically shows off the small, bluish flowers.

When crushed, the plant has a very strong smell, and was used as a bitter in ale before the introduction of hops in the sixteenth century – hence the alternative names of 'alehoof' and 'gill-go-by-the-ground' (from the French verb *guiller*, 'to ferment'). Ground ivy not only added a tang to the flavour of the ale, it also clarified and preserved it. Its leaves were used to adorn the stake that marked an alehouse, and alehouses were sometimes known as 'gill houses'. It was one of the herbs sold by 'criers' in the London markets of the past:

Here's fine rosemary, sage and thyme.
Come, buy my Ground Ivy.
Here's featherfew, gillyflowers and rue.
Come, buy my knotted marjoram, too!

Roxburghe Ballads, collected by the Third Duke of Roxburghe
(1740–1804)

Magical properties were ascribed to ground ivy. Its long runners would be wound with a combination of other flowers into a garland that was said to endow its wearer with the ability to distinguish witches from other folk. Margaret Plues (1828–1901), one of eight children of a Yorkshire clergyman, remembers that: 'We used to dislike it as children, because when we were seeking Sweet Violets we were often misled by the blossoms of Ground Ivy, and so we called it "the Deceiver". But its introduction into fairy tales, where it is mentioned as both knowing and showing the way to the enchanted well, completely reconciled us to it.'

In folk medicine, ground ivy had a number of applications. Gathered in the spring and made into an infusion, it eased coughs and colds throughout the year in 'gill tea' and was still in use in the 1930s in England, as a spring-time tonic and for relief of colds. It was recommended for headaches too. In the Scottish Highlands, the dried leaves were made into snuff for this purpose.

The fresh leaves have also been used to heal minor cuts and wounds and the plant combined with YARROW in a poultice to treat abscesses. According to Mrs Daisy P— of Little Totham, an infusion of ground ivy was used in East Anglia to treat 'bad eyes'.

Ground ivy in official medicine was used in mediaeval times to treat fevers and coughs. Gerard in the sixteenth century recommended it for tinnitus as well as eye ailments. It was a remedy for kidney stones and jaundice as well. Salmon in 1693 quotes the Classical sage Hollerius as saying 'The juice of this herb has cured many at the point of death, being drunk'. By the nineteenth century, the plant was still officially approved, as Kemsey states: 'The juice of it, with a little fine powdered sugar, is good for the eyes and for films growing over the sight; also, boiled with a little honey and verdigris, cleanses fistulas, ulcers, and cancers. It heals green [fresh] wounds upon being bruised and bound thereto.'

Nineteenth- and twentieth-century herbalists used the plant as a treatment for kidney complaints and indigestion as well as abscesses. Medical herbalists in this country today employ it mainly to clear catarrh and ease indigestion.

Groundsel
(*Senecio vulgaris*)

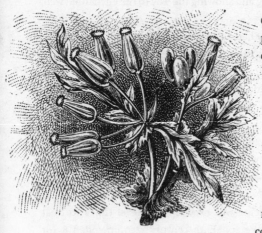

Groundsel is familiar to most people as a garden weed and an edible treat for cagebirds. It is a small and unimposing plant, with yellow, composite flowers that lack ray florets (petals) and divided leaves like a miniature RAGWORT, to which it is closely related. Groundsel was once grown as a crop, for animal fodder, is rich in minerals and makes a useful contribution to compost. The plant produces an enormous amount of downy seed and is a very successful colonizer of bare ground. In Culpeper's words, 'it will spring and seed twice in a year at least if it be suffered in a garden.'

The plant was widely appreciated in folk medicine for its ability to raise and absorb pus – it has been made into a poultice to bring boils to a head and to treat infected cuts. Rolf, the self-styled King of the Norfolk Poachers, left a fascinating memoir early in the twentieth century, of his life as a poacher turned gamekeeper. He was raised largely by his grandmother, to whom he remained very close. Rolf recalls some of the herbal remedies that she used: 'Secenction [a corruption of its botanical name] was a good thing for boils . . . .' Groundsel was valued in particular for cuts made with an iron implement and so the instructions for gathering groundsel were specific: the plant should not be gathered by cutting it with a metal implement, but by hand-pulling.

The plant had a bewilderingly wide range of other uses. In Devon, the leaves were plucked 'downwards for a purge, and upwards for a vomit'. Culpeper in 1653 tells us that it was used in Lincolnshire for pains and swelling. An infusion of the whole herb in boiling water is good for treating chapped hands and, made into a poultice, it was applied in a poultice to the stomach to treat fevers. It could help with the pain of rheumatism, teething and toothache, and could even staunch nosebleeds. With such a wide range of healing properties, it is no wonder that one of its Gaelic names was simply *am bualan*, 'the remedy'.

The uses of groundsel were similar in official medicine. Gerard in 1597, for example, mentions its use as an emetic and that 'the leaves stamped and strained in to Milke and drunke, helpe the red gums and frets in Children'. A century later in 1693, Salmon recommends it as an emetic and for treating a variety of illnesses including epilepsy, gout, jaundice and the stone (large urinary stones).

Groundsel is now known to contain substances toxic to the liver, and its internal application is no longer advised. In modern medical herbalism in Britain, it is little used. However, it continues to be utilized as a poultice to treat infected sores and boils. In the 1940s, this recipe was given by a gypsy to a man suffering from a bad outbreak of boils:

> Wash groundsel, remove just the leaves, make them into a flat parcel in a piece
> of linen, old sheet, etc. Pour on boiling water, squeeze out the parcel and put
> it on the boil.

The man's boils were cured and never returned and his family were so impressed that they subsequently used the same remedy very successfully for treating sore and inflamed skin.

Harebell
(*Campanula rotundifolia*)

E'en the slight harebell raised its head,
Elastic from her airy tread:

Sir Walter Scott, *The Lady of the Lake* (1810), XVIII, 14–15

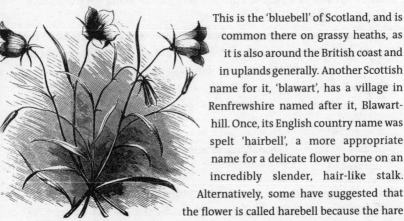

This is the 'bluebell' of Scotland, and is common there on grassy heaths, as it is also around the British coast and in uplands generally. Another Scottish name for it, 'blawart', has a village in Renfrewshire named after it, Blawarthill. Once, its English country name was spelt 'hairbell', a more appropriate name for a delicate flower borne on an incredibly slender, hair-like stalk. Alternatively, some have suggested that the flower is called harebell because the hare frequents the same places, and the hare is associated with magic and witches. There are various legends associated with this flower; some say that the bells 'ring' to warn the hare of approaching danger; others that the fairies ring the bells to warn of the approaching hare. Many of the flower's country names have magical overtones, such as 'fairy bells' and 'witches' thimbles'. In the nineteenth century, children played a game with the papery flowerbells: a blossom was inverted on the back of the hand and smacked sharply to produce a popping noise.

In some areas, the flower was considered unlucky and there was a danger associated with picking it, although the white-flowered variant was considered lucky. In the northeast of Scotland, it was 'regarded with a sort of dread, and commonly left unpulled'; there it went by the name of 'Aul'man's bell' (devil's bell). The colour blue is often associated with true love in folklore, so that one poet suggested:

> The harebell, for her stainless, azured blue,
> Claims to be worn of none but those are true.

Certainly cattle and sheep seem to avoid it, but there is no mystery in this – the entire plant tastes acrid. Its specific name of *rotundifolia* refers to the round basal leaves, which wither away before the plant flowers. More usually noticed are the fine, grass-like leaves on the flowering stems.

There are no known medicinal or practical uses for this plant, but for sheer beauty the harebell deserves our wholehearted appreciation.

Hawthorn
(*Crataegus* species)

By the craggy hill-side,
Through the mosses bare,
They have planted thorn trees
For pleasure here and there.
If any man so daring
As dig them up in spite,
He shall find their sharpest thorns
In his bed at night.

William Allingham (1824–1889), *The Fairies*

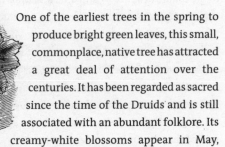

One of the earliest trees in the spring to produce bright green leaves, this small, commonplace, native tree has attracted a great deal of attention over the centuries. It has been regarded as sacred since the time of the Druids and is still associated with an abundant folklore. Its creamy-white blossoms appear in May, straddling spring and summer, and hawthorn is often simply referred to as 'may'. In England on May Day, that celebration of the onset of summer, the hawthorn, which was believed to have protective powers, was brought from the woods to decorate the maypole. Perhaps on account of its magical associations as well as its toughness, it is a favourite wood for carving walking sticks.

Along with summer comes fecundity, and hawthorn was often planted in hedges around pastures as a symbol of fertility. At lambing and calving time, the afterbirth was tossed onto a hawthorn to ensure the reproductive prowess of the next generation of animals, a practice that continued at least in East Anglia up to the twentieth century. The hawthorn played a role in human courtship too. It was said that if a girl wished to be married she should pick some may blossom and walk home in silence. In addition, if she washed her face in dew from the hawthorn tree, she would always be beautiful.

Prohibitions and warnings about the hawthorn are many and varied. It could not be cut down or damaged because it was said to be the trysting place for fairies. In Ireland, a 'fairy bush' or maybush could be grown close to the front door, to bring good luck and to serve (like gorse) as a clothes dryer. Yet it is generally regarded as being extremely unlucky to bring its flowers into the house. Some have attributed this to the flowers' characteristic smell. 'The hawthorn hath a deathly smell' was the title of one of Walter de la Mare's poems – and he was correct. The flowers contain trimethylamine, one of the first products of putrefaction.

The symbolism of the hawthorn was later Christianized – Christ's crown of thorns was believed to be made from the tree. In homage to this, many of the foliate heads carved in our cathedrals depict hawthorn leaves. Perhaps the most celebrated hawthorn tree – many individual thorn trees were revered – is the famous Glastonbury thorn, growing in the grounds of Glastonbury Abbey. This is a variety of hawthorn which flowers during the winter and, according to one legend, it sprouted from the staff of Joseph of Arimathea when he arrived in Glastonbury.

There is documentary evidence to suggest that there was indeed a holy thorn growing at Glastonbury as early as the twelfth century. It became part of the Glastonbury legend and cuttings of it were sold during the reign of James I but, in the mid-seventeenth century, it was cut down by a zealous Roundhead. However, descendants of the original tree were by then growing elsewhere in gardens all over the country, and these continued to be venerated. It is possible that the original holy thorn really was brought from Palestine, since some populations of hawthorn there flower in the winter.

In contrast to the near-cult worship of this tree, the attitude of children towards the hawthorn is simple – it's a source of food. In many country areas, the leaves and young buds – often called 'bread and cheese' – are nibbled as a snack by children.

'Happy memories they are of eating "bread and cheese" on the way to school in the spring. As the hawthorn hedge broke into tiny delicious leaves, we picked them gently not to get pricked by the thorns and enjoyed a second breakfast all the way to school.'

Mrs A. B—, Cheshire (2002)

The haws (berries) are not sweet enough to appeal to young tastebuds, although they can be eaten raw, but in excess can result in poisoning. Children do like the round stones within them however and find them good ammunition for popguns.

As with several other berry-bearing trees, a good crop of haws indicated a hard winter ahead: 'Mony haws, mony snaws' is a Scottish proverb. In Scotland, they were considered at their best after Hallowe'en, when the witches had flown over them. Like sloes, their flavour and texture are improved by the first frosts, and they can then be made into delicious wine and jam.

In folk medicine, hawthorn was used in a number of ways, some symbolic and some purely practical. A very widespread folk cure for warts involved passing a snail or slug over the wart and then impaling it on a thorn of either hawthorn or BLACKTHORN; as the mollusc died, so the wart would wither and disappear. In the Scottish Highlands, both the flowers and leaves were used as infusions to treat sore throats and, in Ireland, the bark was chewed for toothache. Both the flowers and berries have been used as a heart tonic in places as far apart as the Isle of Man and Devon, while in the Scottish Highlands it was used to 'balance' blood pressure.

In official medicine, Culpeper in 1653 suggests that it is useful in dropsy and stone (large urinary stones), and that an infusion of the leaves helps to remove thorns; 'the thorn gives a medicine for its own pricking'. Salmon in 1693 recommends use of the berries to cure 'fluxes' and haemorrhage as well. The seventeenth- and eighteenth-century Gunton Household Book gives a recipe for a conserve prepared from haws, skinned and stoned, which was used to treat diabetes, and also a thick paste made from the haws mixed with cider or wine for the easing of kidney stones.

Several generations later, a nineteenth-century Irish physician called Dr Green found that hawthorn was very effective in treating heart conditions. Modern medical herbalists continue to reap benefits from this rediscovery and prescribe hawthorn for the treatment of angina, coronary heart disease and both high and low blood pressure. In official medicine in this country it is not used at present, although recent pharmacological studies have confirmed that it is effective in treating congestive heart failure.

Like many other herbs, this plant is an example of the phenomenon known as 'synergism', where the properties of various substances that are present in the plant combine to produce the observed effect. An extract of the whole plant therefore has effects that are different from those produced by any one isolated compound. This in turn means that such a plant does not lend itself to exploitation by a drug company wanting to produce a single, quantifiable, known active principle. It is to be hoped that somehow this gulf between herbalism and the modern pharmaceutical industry can be bridged so that in future some of our most effective plant remedies may be re-introduced into mainstream medicine.

Hazel
(*Corylus avellana*)

Choose the willow of the streams,
Choose the hazel of the rocks,
Choose the alder of the marshes,
Choose the birch of the waterfalls.

Alexander Carmichael, *Carmina Gadelica* (1900–1971)

Hazel was one of the first trees to colonize the land after the end of the last Ice Age and for a great period of time it would have been one of the most abundant tree species. It is still widespread, but no longer dominates the landscape. With such an ancient history, it is no surprise to learn that hazel has been one of the most important sources of wood since early times; over the centuries, it has gathered around it a great deal of folklore and superstition.

When man first settled in Britain the forests were full of hazel: its flexible but strong branches made it highly suitable for making wattle in house walls, as well as for fencing and the manufacture of baskets and tools. Ancient trackways on the Somerset Levels were built with foundations of hazel wattles and it is likely that the growing and coppicing of hazel as an industry had already begun. Coppicing is the practice of cutting back the tree to the stump, to stimulate it into sending up fresh shoots; a succession of crops of sturdy poles can then be cut and used in building and fencing.

In some parts of Scotland, it was believed that the hazel was best cut when the moon was waxing; during the waning moon, the sap 'retreated' to the roots and the wood was dry and brittle. Hazelwood charcoal was an important sideline. Pechey in 1694 states that 'painters use the Coal of it, to delineate. Gunpowder was made of the Coals, before the Coals of Alder were found more commodious for that Use.' Thin poles of hazel wood were used for making switches and, in some parts of the country, the verb 'hazeling' was synonymous with flogging. In Scotland, the traditional game of shinty used a ball made from a lump of hazel root that had been boiled in a pot of water over the fire to toughen it.

The hazel was used on several occasions in official medicine. Gerard in 1597 tells us that 'The kernels of Nuts made into Milk like Almonds, doth mightily binde the belly, and is good for the laske and the bloody fluxe. The same doth coole exceedingly in hot fevers, and burning agues.' People made hazelnut 'milk' for years and it was believed to be highly nutritious; it was often given to small or sickly children, especially in Scotland, and was sometimes mixed with honey. An oil derived from the wood of wild hazel was 'reported to be very good against the Epilepsie and other Disease of the Head and Brain'. Hazel is rarely used in modern medical herbalism in this country.

There are only a few records of the use of hazel in practical folk medicine; in Ireland, the bark was used to treat boils and cuts and the ashes of burnt hazel to assuage burns. However, hazel was regarded as a magical tree and so has frequently served as a talisman, believed to protect people from misfortune and illness. For example, hazelnuts were carried in pockets in Ireland to ward off rheumatism and lumbago and, in Devon, to prevent toothache. A double hazelnut was a useful amulet to protect against the evil eye. In common with the ash tree, the hazel was thought to have power against snakes and, in Wales, a cure for snakebite was made from hazel leaves, together with TANSY and ground ash.

Other ways of calling upon the power of hazel included bringing in small bunches of hazel twigs to protect a house from thunder and lightning and bringing in catkins at lambing time to protect the sheep. In Cambridgeshire, it was believed that hazel twigs brought into the nursery would ensure that a baby's eyes would turn brown. Hazel was one of the first woods to be used in kindling ceremonial fires in pagan festivals such as Beltane – a May Day festival – in Scotland. Also in Scotland, children born in autumn who were fed the 'milk' from unripe hazelnuts were said to develop the power of prophecy. The proper source of water-divining rods is also hazel.

Hazel has long been associated with fertility and childbirth. A good hazelnut crop was thought to foretell a large number of babies born in the locality. There is a West-Country saying: 'Plenty of Catkins, Plenty of Prams'. A twentieth-century story concerns a Somerset girl returning from London to be married: she announced her intention of not having children for a while because it would interfere with her freedom. But locals all contributed to a present for her of a large bag of hazelnuts and four children soon followed. 'Hazel-nutting' was a euphemism for courtship and lovemaking, and the nuts were sometimes used in love divination. A double nut shared with a loved one was sure to make the relationship last.

Hazel provided important food sources too. The leaves were eaten by domestic animals, and the nuts were an important, if seasonal, source of protein for humans. In eighteenth-century Scotland, they were ground into flour to make biscuits and bread. Apart from their nutritional value, hazel-nuts were an important commercial crop for the dye industry. Some families living in Dorset at the beginning of the twentieth century were able to make enough money from the proceeds to pay their annual rents.

At the present time, the hazel is under threat. Grey squirrels consume most of our hazelnuts, a process that is accelerating the decline of hazel tree numbers in Britain.

Heartsease
(*Viola tricolor*)

Yet mark'd I where the bolt of Cupid fell.
It fell upon a little western flower,
Before milk-white, now purple with love's wound,
And maidens call it love-in-idleness.
Fetch me that flow'r; the herb I showed thee once.
The juice of it on sleeping eyelids laid
Will make or man or woman madly dote
Upon the next live creature that it sees.

Shakespeare, *A Midsummer Night's Dream*, II, i, 167–172

This miniature pansy, a common weed of arable land and one of the ancestors of the garden pansy, is so small that it is easily overlooked, and yet it must be among the daintiest and prettiest of our wild flowers. As *tricolor* implies, the flower is three-coloured: gold heart, delicate, creamy lower petals, and the upper pair of petals a faint shade of purple. In the words of poet Abraham Cowley (1618–1667) in his poem *Of Plants*:

Gold, silver, purple are thy ornament:
Thy rivals thou mightst scorn hadst thou but scent.

Although the flowers are tiny, as Darwin noted they are visited by bees, as well as smaller insects. When fertilized, the seed capsule splits into three parts, and as the capsule wall dries out the seeds are expelled with some force – a very efficient way of self-seeding: 'the roote perisheth every yeare, and raiseth itselfe up plentifully by its owne sowing, if it be suffered.'

Most of the plant's country names, including heartsease, refer to the use

of the plant as a love potion. One of the longest of its country names is '
Meet her i' the entry, kiss her i' the buttery'. Sometimes the name is
shortened to 'buttery entry'.

The plant does not seem to have had a significant role in folk medicine,
but in official medicine it was used, according to Gerard in 1597, for treating
fevers, convulsions and skin conditions. John Moncrief in his *Poor Man's
Physician* of 1731 states that 'Pansies, or Heart's-ease taken in Meat or Drink,
for the Space of nine Days, perfectly cureth a Rupture, which I have often
tried. You may also apply a Plaister of these Herbs.'

In modern medical herbalism, the plant is used to treat skin conditions
including eczema, as well as bronchitis, cystitis, rheumatism and whooping
cough.

Heaths and Heathers
(*Erica* species and *Calluna vulgaris*)

... Those wastes of heath,
Stretching for miles to lure the bee,
Where the wild bird, on pinions strong,
Wheels round, and pours his piping song,
And timid creatures wander free.

Mary Howitt (1799–1888)

The purpling of moors and heaths with heather flowers in late summer is a dramatic sight, just as spectacular on lowland heath as on the sweeping expanses of the northern uplands, where the plant is conserved for sheep and grouse. An abundant flowering of the heather is thought to foretell a harsh winter. No doubt those who made their living from the surrounding land appreciated its beauty, but day-to-day living in a harsh rural economy probably made them value its practical uses a great deal more.

Heather has provided bedding for man and beast, thatch for roofs and much-needed woody stems for hedging and kindling. It burns very efficiently and, in the days of clan warfare in the Scottish Highlands, beacons of blazing heather were used to summon soldiers to battle. (The colours of their clan tartans owed much to heather too: yellow, orange and green dyes could be obtained from the flowers.) In more recent times, heather was lit as a torch to lure fish to the surface of the water at night.

Domestic uses for heather are endless: tough, burnt roots were fashioned into nails and pegs; clumps of it were used in drainage layers underneath the gravel of tracks, and as filters at the entrances to drains; mats and baskets were woven from it; and its branches were turned into besoms to sweep floors and chimneys and to groom horses. The tough, wiry stems were also woven into rope, a centuries-old tradition – heather rope was found during the excavation of a 4,000-year-old village in Orkney. Heather rope was still being made in more recent times in the Scottish Highlands. Often two people collaborated; a stick was passed through the end of a loop of heather stem, then one person fed in new pieces of heather while the other walked slowly backwards, using the stick as a handle to twist the stems clockwise.

Heather has played several roles in folk medicine. Records do not distinguish between the more common heather (*Calluna vulgaris*) and heath (*Erica tetralix*) or bell heather (*Erica cinerea*); presumably they were employed interchangeably. (The illustration on the previous page is of a heath.) A heather infusion was used for insomnia in the Scottish Highlands and was given to tuberculosis sufferers as a tonic. Coughs and colds were also treated with heather in parts of Scotland and, in Cumbria, rheumatism as well as stomach upsets were found to benefit from it.

Official medicine seems to have largely ignored the plant, although in modern-day herbalism heather is a urinary antiseptic and a treatment for rheumatism.

We do continue to use heather in some of its many traditional ways. White heather is still seen as a symbol of good luck, frequently worn at weddings, and sprigs of it are still slipped into a pocket or tucked into a buttonhole. Presumably the white version was prized simply because it is relatively rare. In Scottish folklore, it was said to grow where fairies rested, and various victories in battle were attributed to it.

Heather honey is still rightly celebrated today, for its delicate and unusual taste. The honey may be made into mead, and of course the traditional heather ale is still brewed and has been since the times of the Vikings. Robert Louis Stevenson (1850–1894) celebrated this in a famous poem, *Heather Ale*:

> From the bonny bells of heather,
> They brewed a drink long syne,
> Was sweeter far than honey,
> Was stronger far than wine.

Even after a law was passed in the eighteenth century prohibiting brewers from using anything other than hops to ferment ale, heather continued as an ingredient in domestic brewing. Not only did it aid fermentation, it also imparted a lovely mead-like flavour. A Glasgow firm revived the brewing of heather ale on a commercial scale in the 1980s, and it is now brewed in Argyll. The recipe is based on an old Gaelic one and includes heather flowers and leaves of BOG MYRTLE. It is marketed under the name of *Fraoch*.

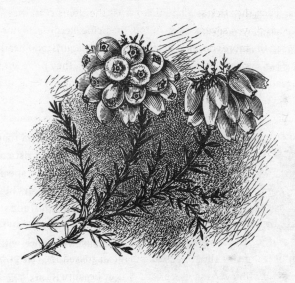

Hellebore
(*Helleborus* species)

Borage and hellebore fill two scenes,
Sovereign plants to purge the veins
Of melancholy, and cheer the heart
Of those black fumes which make it smart;

Robert Burton (1577–1640), *Anatomy of Melancholy*

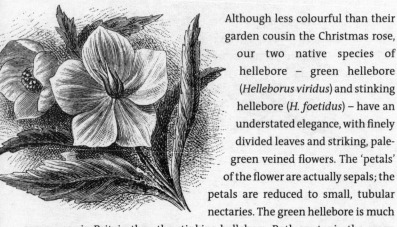

Although less colourful than their garden cousin the Christmas rose, our two native species of hellebore – green hellebore (*Helleborus viridus*) and stinking hellebore (*H. foetidus*) – have an understated elegance, with finely divided leaves and striking, pale-green veined flowers. The 'petals' of the flower are actually sepals; the petals are reduced to small, tubular nectaries. The green hellebore is much commoner in Britain than the stinking hellebore. Both are toxic, the green less so than the stinking. Arrow poison was once made from this plant. The plants were violent purges and were used to get rid of intestinal worms, but their action was so fierce and sometimes even fatal that, unsurprisingly, this practice was eventually discontinued. In Gilbert White's words: 'Where it killed not the patient it would certainly kill the worms; but the worst of it is, it will sometimes kill both.'

In official medicine. a related species, the Christmas rose (*H. niger*), was used a great deal more for treating gout, jaundice, sciatica, and leprosy even, but wild species were also prescribed, mainly for killing worms in children. Obviously familiar with the difficulties of getting children to take medicine,

Gerard in 1597 recommended drying and crushing the leaves, then folding the resulting powder into a raisin or fig to sweeten the pill; or even mixing the powder with honey and spreading it onto a slice of bread. However, he warns that 'This strong medicine made of white Hellebor, ought not to bee given inwardly unto delicate bodies without great correction; but it may be more safely given unto countrey people which feed grosly, and have hard tough and strong bodies.' Should a dose of hellebore be too high, Culpeper in 1653 tells us that the antidote for poisoning is to take goat's milk.

We know that hellebores were gathered in the wild for use in official medicine. Curtis in his *Flora Londinensis* in the eighteenth century described how a large quantity of wild hellebore root was collected and sent up to Guy's Hospital. Doubtless, this large-scale gathering contributed to the plant's increasing scarcity.

In the twentieth century, hellebore leaves were found to contain cardiac glycosides and for a while it was employed in small doses as a heart stimulant for the elderly, but its toxicity caused it to fall out of favour – a familiar story with this plant.

Hellebores were widely used in animal medicine, in both official and country practice, particularly for treating various kinds of swelling. Dried and beaten with cumin, it also produced a remedy for fleas, ticks and lice in dogs. Some of the plant's country names, such as 'oxheal', reflect this association with animal medicine. In the process known as 'settering', a piece of the plant was inserted into a slit made in the animal's ear or dewlap; this was thought to drain away 'bad humours'. Hellebore was also used to predict if a sick animal would recover.

> For a pig that has anything wrong with its wind pass a bit of the leaf stem of Hellabor [sic] under the skin of the ear ... If the part swells up ... the pig will live.

Occasionally, those who worked with animals would administer the same medical treatment to themselves. Here is an eighteenth-century remedy taken from a horseman's notebook:

> For the Itch in a Christain take 2 peneworth of Black Elebore Powder and 4 peneworth of red Precipitate powder mixed with Pork Lard and rub your joints with the same.

Within living memory, horse remedies were often used by farm labourers on themselves and on their families because they were free, unlike a visit from a doctor. Even after the advent of the National Health Service, the scarcity of doctors in many rural areas meant that many were self-dependent in times of illness. A natural 'perk' of the poorly paid farm labourer was access to animal medicines: one elderly lady recalled using 'hoss oils' for her rheumatism, arguing that if it worked for the horses it would probably help her too.

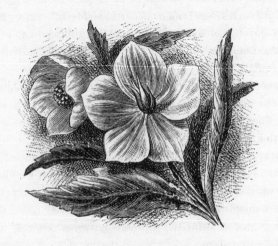

Henbane
(*Hyoscyamus niger*)

Henbane has a very dark and sinister history indeed and has been described as one of the oldest narcotics in the world. It was harvested at the waxing of the moon by the root-gatherers of ancient Greece. Poisoners from the last King of Pergamos (who died 134 BC) to the infamous Dr Crippen have used it to kill their enemies. In 1910, Crippen murdered his wife with henbane and fled to Canada with his lover: the evidence presented at his trial is now considered to be the basis of our modern forensic medicine.

Henbane is a strange-looking plant, with an unpleasant smell that has been likened to dead rats. Its repellant appearance seems to give the game away. The entire plant is hairy and slightly sticky; its leaves are large, soft and toothed or lobed. The flowers have a funnel-shaped corolla that is pale yellow with a net-like pattern of purple lines; the throat of the corolla itself is deep purple. The fruits, which are spherical, release their ripe seeds by opening small 'lids'.

Henbane has been present in Britain at least since Neolithic times, and its unusual properties have been well recorded. When ingested, it gives a sensation of flying, and was one of the constituents of the 'flying ointments' given to women accused of witchcraft. Their accusers would administer a good dose of henbane as well as other hallucinogenic herbs; these unfortunate women were then so convinced that they had been flying that it was child's play to convict them. A fortunate few were reprieved, like Jane Wenham whose trial in 1712 was presided over by a Mr Justice Powell. He is claimed to have stated at her trial that there was no law against flying and her case was dismissed.

More recently, in the nineteenth century, an incident was recorded in which henbane roots were mistakenly eaten for chicory:

> A rather amusing instance of partial poisoning by this plant is related by Dr Houlton, in which the inmates of a monastery eat the roots for supper. They were all attacked by a sort of delirious frenzy, more or less violent, but in some accompanied by the most strange delusions. One got up at midnight and tolled

the bell for matins; the rest attended at the summons, but some could not read, others fancied the letters were running around like ants, and some read what they did not find in their books.

Sowerby and Johnson, *The Useful Plants of Great Britain* (1862)

In folk and official medicine, the plant's more constructive properties were exploited. There is some evidence, from an archaeological find of henbane and hemlock seeds at the site of a mediaeval hospital in Scotland, to suggest that henbane may have been used as an anaesthetic during surgery. Gerard in 1597 says that 'To wash the feet in the decoction of Henbane causeth sleepe; and also the often smelling to the floures', and that henbane 'mitigateth all kinde of paine'.

Culpeper in 1653 lists numerous uses for the plant, including for deafness, gout, headache and swellings, but he warns against taking it internally and gives instructions on how to prepare an antidote. John Pechey in 1694 gives similar uses for the plant. Writing in the nineteenth century, Kemsey recommends a fomentation of the leaves for treating painful ulcers and swellings. Internally, he says, it is given for rheumatism and 'spasmodic affections'. He stresses its dangers and states that the best antidote is vinegar.

Animals too could be sedated with henbane. It was one of the plants used in controlling shire horses; simply the smell of a mixture of potent herbs including henbane could render them biddable. One eighteenth-century recipe to 'make a gelding quiet' suggests using henbane leaf mixed with aromatic oils:'Mix the oils with the leaf and ware it in your Pockett Let him smell of that.'

As a painkiller, the herb was particularly good for toothache. Centuries ago, toothache was often ascribed to a worm in the tooth, and some claimed that after treatment with henbane, the worm would emerge and could be clearly seen. Gerard in 1597 dismisses this as nonsense, but nevertheless still recommends henbane root for this ailment. Folk medicine also exploited henbane in treating toothache; here is a record from twentieth-century Suffolk:

Toothache caused a lot of distress before dentistry became more common or human [sic]. Poultices of hot salt, or sand, were applied to the side of the face. Another, and to me rather strange and even dangerous, remedy was to get the

flowers of the deadly poisonous henbane. These were placed in a hot tin and
the person held his mouth open over the fumes.

Mr C—, English Folklore Survey, University College London (1960s)

Folk medicine had other applications for the plant including treatment
for earache, headache and the measles. In Ireland, the juice was apparently
given for 'the nerves' and an infusion of the leaves for whooping cough.
Necklaces were made for teething infants of dried henbane stems cut into
short pieces; it was believed that the fumes given off by the henbane had a
sedative effect and protected against the convulsions thought sometimes to
accompany teething. And in Wiltshire, and probably elsewhere in Britain,
henbane was used to induce a 'twilight sleep' during labour; the patient
remained awake, but was unaware of what was going on.

Henbane's extracts were listed in the British Pharmaceutical Codex until
well into the twentieth century. It was cultivated for medicinal purposes
during the First World War and was still in use, combined with morphine,
for procuring twilight sleep in the 1930s. One of its constituents is hyoscine
(also present, although in smaller quantities, in DEADLY NIGHTSHADE); this
is still in use as a pre-operative sedative.

In modern medical herbalism the plant is employed, with caution, as a
painkiller and sedative. Ongoing research suggests that the plant could be
useful in the treatment of Parkinson's disease.

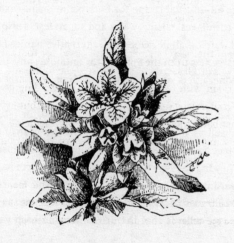

Herb Bennet or Wood Avens

(*Geum urbanum*)

Where the root is in the house the devil can do nothing, and flies from it;
wherefore it is blessed above all other herbs.

Anon., *Ortus Sanitatis* (1491)

This bristly little plant of woodland edges has small, five-petalled, yellow
flowers, which have earned it the country name of 'gold star'. The seedheads
are spherical, spiky, brown balls, ready to catch on passers-by, whether animal
or human. The name herb bennet seems to have come from the mediaeval
Latin *Herba benedicta* meaning 'blessed herb', and it is said that the devil
shuns the plant. The roots are aromatic and spicy-smelling, which may
account for the devil's aversion. In the kitchen, however, it is warmly
welcomed and can be used in place of cloves, in apple pies for example.

Herb bennet was once employed to flavour ale and prevent it from souring.
Peggy Hutchinson's book of homemade wines, *More Home-made Wine
Secrets*, includes an unusual recipe for herb bennet wine, made from herb
bennet, barley, cornflakes, raisins, water and sugar. It was also believed that
the plant could ward off all ills. One of its alternative names is 'wood avens'
(the word 'avens' comes from the Spanish for 'antidote') and, in the fifteenth
century, the stonecarvers of our great cathedrals regularly chose it as a
subject.

In official medicine, the plant was recommended for bites, fevers and
indigestion, as well as for internal wounds. The powder of the root was
deemed to protect against the plague, perhaps again because of its sweet
smell; John Pechey in 1694 says that 'Wine wherein the Root has been infus'd
has a fine pleasant Taste and Smell: It chears the Heart, and opens
Obstructions.' In Elizabethan England, herb bennet was used as a moth repellent. Gerard in 1597 tells us that the dried roots 'do keep garments from

being eaten with Mothes, and make them to have an excellent good odour'.

John Moncrief in 1731 includes in his *Poor Man's Physician* the following remedy: 'For Inward Wounds; Drink the Decoction of Avens-roots. It prevails also for Pains in the Breast and Sides, and to dispel internal crudities.'

Strangely, this plant has not figured much in British folk medicine. Such records as have been traced are all of gypsy origin. It was stewed in vinegar, for treating sore eyes, and the roots were taken for diarrhoea and sore throats. In modern-day herbalism, the plant is used for mouth and throat infections and gut irritations.

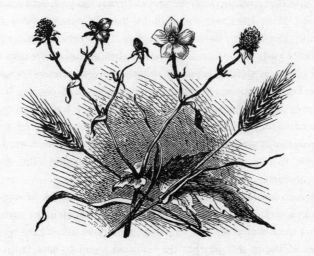

Herb Robert
(*Geranium robertianum*)

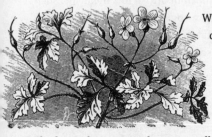

With soft ferny leaves, red-tinged stems and dainty, purplish flowers, herb Robert is a most attractive wildflower, found in abundance in hedgerows and around the edges of woodlands. Its flowers droop in dull weather, proving to be very useful for rural weather forecasting.

The leaves have an unpleasant smell when crushed, and the plant often goes by the unlovely names of 'stinking Roger' or 'foetid cranesbill'. Its acrid scent repels insects and within living memory in Orkney has been used against the dreaded midges. The name cranesbill, for this and related species, derives from the characteristic, beaked seed capsule. This explodes when ripe and propels the seeds for a distance of several metres, ensuring wide dispersal.

The plant was apparently named after the eleventh-century French Saint Robert, but it has been given an enormous number of country names – perhaps because it was found all over the land and each community developed a name for it. Some of the names are rather sinister for such a simple and unassuming plant, for example 'death-come-quickly'. In Somerset, there is a belief that 'If 'ee pick'n someone'll take 'ee', implying a link with the fairies, or worse.

However, some country names such as 'red Roger' and 'bloodwort' are to the point and clearly indicate the plant's main application in the past, which was as a blood-stauncher. Within living memory in Ireland, the plant has been employed in this way but the tradition seems to have faded much earlier in Britain, although there are relatively recent records of garden-grown geranium leaves being used to treat cuts. In Ireland, the plant was recommended also for coughs, kidney troubles and sore throats, and elsewhere for a wide variety of skin conditions.

In official medicine, the herb's role has been – as in folk medicine – mainly as a treatment for bleeding, both internal and external, and for a wide variety of skin conditions. Pechey in 1694 describes herb Robert as 'Vulnerary ... It cleanses Wounds and Ulcers', and Kemsey in 1838 tells us that the plant 'speedily heals all green wounds, and is an effectual cure for old ulcers'.

Modern-day medical herbalists in this country continue the tradition and use herb Robert, although only occasionally, as a wound-healer.

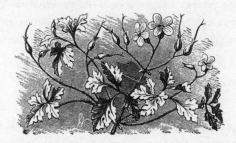

Hogweed
(*Heracleum sphondylium*)

'I have just been cutting … hogweed shoots for an invalid ewe … hogweed shoots and leaves seem to go down stalk first. Their flowers too are a delicacy, especially when just open, they have a faint fragrance, somewhat like elderflower.'

Mrs M. P—, Somerset (2002)

This tough, large member of the umbellifer family (Apiaceae) is a common hedgerow plant, abundant too in grassland and waste ground. Its flowers are attractive to insects, so much so that at least one hundred and eighteen different insect species visit them. As its name suggests, the plant has been a food for livestock. The farmer quoted above discovered that sickly sheep enjoyed hogweed shoots, which 'were gobbled up in preference to grass'. In the Statistical Account of Scotland, there is this impressive testimony from Aberdeenshire: 'An old woman in the parish gives her cow a creel-full of this plant in season for supper, and she says that the milk-pail next morning bears testimony to its virtues.'

In folk medicine, hogweed has been used to treat jaundice and its juice applied to warts. An unusual remedy for sores, within living memory in Essex, was to dust them with hogweed pollen. A similar remedy was recorded in Ireland, where the plant was also used to treat rheumatism in cows.

Hogweed has been exploited in very different ways in official medicine. Gerard in 1597 claims that:

If a phrenetick or melancholicke mans head bee anointed with oile wherein the leaves and roots have been sodden, it helpeth him very much, and such as be troubled with the head-ache and the lethargie, or sickness called the forget-full evill [sic].

Culpeper in 1653 likewise recommends it for 'drowsy evil' as well as for shortness of breath, falling sickness and jaundice. John Pechey in 1694 reports that 'The Seed is excellent for Hysterick Fits'.

However, despite these successes, hogweed has not stood up to the test of time and is not utilized in modern-day medical herbalism in Britain. Perhaps we should appreciate hogweed a great deal more. The young stems taste just like asparagus, and were once eaten as a digestive in eighteenth-century Mull.

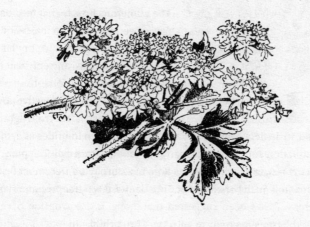

Holly
(*Ilex aquifolium*)

Holly and Hazel went to the wood
Holly took hazel home by the lug.

Irish saying

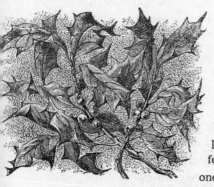

This is a much-loved evergreen tree, with highly distinctive, glossy, prickle-fringed leaves and bright scarlet berries. The sweetly scented flowers go largely unnoticed, except by the numerous insects that feed on the nectar secreted at the bases of the petals. Holly is immensely popular as a festive plant, but its ancient history is one of superstition and folklore.

Since Classical times, holly has been endowed with great protective powers and influence. It would be planted near a house to keep it free from lightning strikes and, in ancient Rome, holly wreaths were given to brides as symbols of congratulation and to protect marrying couples from evil. The plant was part of many festivals, including the Roman Saturnalia, a December festival of merrymaking. With the advent of Christianity, it was adopted as a symbol of Christmas; it has been suggested that 'holly' is a corruption of 'holy', indicating the tree's association with the Christ child.

Hollies were often planted at the boundaries of property as markers, and it was considered bad luck to cut them down – a prohibition which still lingers in some parts of the country, especially East Anglia.

Bringing holly into the house was also fraught with superstition. Sometimes the plant has leaves without prickles; such a plant was often referred to as 'he-holly' and the more usual, prickled kind as 'she-holly'. In Derbyshire, it was said that if prickled holly was incorporated in the

Christmas decorations the man would be master for the following year; if smooth holly was used, then the wife would reign instead. The belief in Somerset was that berried holly should be brought into the house only by a man. Sterile holly in the same county was viewed with fear and, if no berried holly was available, a sprig of box should be included in a holly wreath to cancel the resulting ill luck. In Scotland, holly branches were sometimes brought into the house and laid against the doors to protect the house from evil. The proverb 'He lies never but when the Hollen is green' was once common in the Scottish Borders.

Once Christmas was over, great care still had to be taken with holly. It was considered unlucky to burn holly, and so it was important to remember to throw it out rather than cast it on the fire. Come New Year's Day in Scotland, there was a tradition that one boy should thrash another with holly; every drop of blood spilt added a year to the victim's life.

Holly thrashing also played a role in folk medicine. Sprigs of holly were used to thrash chilblains, a brutal-sounding remedy that was widespread throughout England. Sometimes it was specified that the beating should continue until the skin bled. The same method was applied in Somerset to arthritis and in Ireland for a stiff neck. Gentler treatments for chilblains included an ointment prepared from holly berries and, for rheumatism, an infusion of the leaves. Holly leaves were also applied to burns. In Hampshire, whooping cough was treated by giving the child milk to drink in a cup made from the wood of a variegated holly.

In official medicine, the uses of holly were different. Culpeper in 1653 suggests the fresh berries as a purge; the dried ones, on the other hand, are binding. Holly bark he claims is useful as a 'fomentation for broken bones'. Pechey in 1694 states that:

> The prickles of the Leaves boyl'd in Posset drink, wonderfully ease the Cholick, and Pains in the Bowels. With this a Gentlewoman cured her self, and many others, when other Medicines would do no good.

In the nineteenth century, holly continued to be utilized – the bark only – for treating fevers, and today's medical herbalists use holly very little.

Holly wood has found plenty of applications in modern times, though. The wood takes up stain readily and can be used as an ebony-substitute; it has been made into veneers and knife handles. There is a fan-maker in

Norfolk who uses only holly wood because it is strong, and light in weight and in colour.

Holly is nature's barbed wire and makes an excellent stock-proof hedge; because it is slow-growing, it needs little trimming. The shrub may be pruned like box into topiary and ornamental hedges and its innumerable horticultural variants provide a range of colours throughout the year.

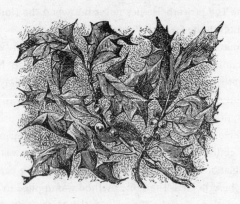

Honeysuckle or Woodbine

(*Lonicera periclymenum*)

Sleep thou, and I will wind thee in my arms ...
So doth the woodbine the sweet honeysuckle
Gently entwist;

Shakespeare, *A Midsummer Night's Dream*, IV, i, 37–40

The rich scent of honeysuckle flowers on a summer evening is deeply evocative; it would seem that nature invented aromatherapy long before we did. Parkinson in the seventeenth century was obviously an admirer of the plant and, very unselfishly, wanted everyone to be able to enjoy it. In 1629, he wrote: 'The Honisuckle that growth wilde in every hedge, although it be very sweete, yet doe I not bring into my garden, but let it rest in his owne place, to serve their senses that travel by it, or have no garden.'

More recently the botanist and author Phebe Lankester (1825–1900) recalled, 'Well do I remember ... becoming almost overpowered with the perfume, as bough after bough was pulled from its native Suffolk hedge, and piled up, so as to make a floral couch in a carriage in which I sat one still warm summer evening in July.'

The honeysuckle is unusual among our wild flowers in being a woody, semi-evergreen climber, and the height to which it can scramble up a tree, on the edge of woodland, is surprising. The botanical family to which it belongs, Caprifoliaceae, includes cousins such as ELDER and viburnum. Each honeysuckle flower opens for the first time in the evening, just after the pollen-bearing anthers have ripened; the tall stamens provide a convenient landing stage for pollinating moths.

Countless children have enjoyed the drops of nectar at the bases of each flower, by biting off the end of each flower tube – hence the name honeysuckle. Chaucer called the plant 'wodebyne' (woodbine) and portrayed it as a symbol of steadfastness in love; 'bine' is the same word as 'vine', denoting a climber. The stems are surprisingly tough and have been used for centuries to make rope. (Recognizable pieces of honeysuckle rope were found in an excavation of the recently discovered Bronze Age 'Wood-Henge' in Norfolk.) In much more recent times in the Outer Hebrides, honeysuckle stems were formed into bridles for pack ponies.

In folk medicine, the plant has been used for one condition above all others, namely asthma. An infusion of the flowers was used to treat this, as well as other respiratory complaints. Honeysuckle tea was also used to treat nervous headaches, and to remove skin blemishes. Jaundice was treated in Ireland with honeysuckle bark and a lotion for mouth and throat infections was prepared from the leaves and flowers.

Honeysuckle was used for asthma also in official medicine. Pechey in 1694 tells us that: "Tis chiefly used in an Asthma, and for a Cough. It helps Difficulty of Breathing, and hastens Delivery, and expels Gravel [small urinary stones]'. A century and a half later, Kemsey wrote, 'It has been observed that it is fitting that a conserve made of the flowers of it were kept in every gentlewoman's house as a cure for asthma.'

In the early part of the twentieth century, herbalists still used syrup of honeysuckle flowers for asthma and an infusion of the leaves as a laxative, but today the plant is little-used in modern medical herbalism in this country.

Horsetail
(*Equisetum arvense*)

The Root is small, black, jointed, and creeping, and has many small Fibres arising
from the joints. It springs up with heads somewhat like Asparagus, which grow
into hard, rough, hollow Stalks, jointed at many places, one within another. At
every Joint grows a Bush of rusty, hard Leaves, resembling an Horse-tail.

John Pechey, *The Compleat Herbal of Physical Plants* (1694)

The primitive, spore-bearing horsetail is directly descended from a giant of
the Palaeozoic period, when dinosaurs roamed the land, and the basic struc-
ture of the plant has changed little since then. It has characteristic jointed
stems, with a whorl of brownish scales at intervals. In the axils of these
scale-like leaves are whorls of brittle branches, which are still a feature of
children's games. Pull the stem upwards and it will break neatly at a node;
the broken stem may then be replaced, like a candle in a candlestick. This
pleasing aspect of the plant has earned it the modern and very appropriate
name of 'Lego plant'.

The horsetail has been known by many country names, of which one of
the most evocative is the Anglo-Saxon *dysshwasshynges*, recorded in the
sixteenth century – surely a much nicer word than pan-scourer. The plant
contains scratchy silica crystals that make it ideal for cleaning, for polishing
pewter and sanding timber.

Horsetails have a unique ability to concentrate gold in their tissues, so
they have been used as indicators by gold prospectors. Horsetail's high
mineral content can compensate for its reputation as a troublesome garden
weed by providing a good fungicide against black spot and mildew. Other
practical uses have included tying the plant onto the tails of livestock to
keep flies away, as a dyestuff and as a vegetable – it is said to taste a little
like asparagus.

In folk medicine, the plant has been utilized to staunch bleeding and in
an infusion for indigestion. In the nineteenth century, Barton and Castle

record that 'an infusion of the dried herb is frequently used as a tea by poor people for diarrhoea'.

The plant was also used to remedy bleeding in Classical medicine, and this is the way in which Culpeper recommended it in 1653. In addition, he claimed it was useful for all types of flux, for skin eruptions, for swellings, for stone (large urinary stones) and that it would 'solder together the tops of green wounds'. Pechey in 1694 confirmed that it was good for wounds, 'even when the nerves are cut'. In the nineteenth century, it was still being used in similar ways, for treating bloody urine, fluxes and inflammations.

Today's medical herbalists continue to value horsetail, for staunching bleeding both external and internal, and for aiding healing. They also recommend it for treating emphysema and swollen legs.

As with all herbal medicine it is important to be sure of the plant's identification. The marsh horsetail (*Equisetum palustre*), larger but similar in appearance, is toxic and should not be used. Cases of poisoning of horses with this plant have been reported. Perhaps the giant ancestors of our present-day horsetails were toxic to the creatures of the Palaeozoic era and therefore survived their attention to become the ancestors of our Lego plant.

Houseleek

(*Sempervivum tectorum*)

An ancient author recited (among divers other experiments of Nature) that if
this herb, houseleek or sygreen, do grow on a house-top, the same house will
never be stricken by lightning or thunder.

Thomas Hill, *Natural and Artificial Conclusions* (1670)

Most of the plants that have been widely used in folk medicine in Britain
are native ones: the reasons for this are various. Wild plants are freely available, and in the past only the relatively wealthy had gardens. The 'learned'
classes had access to books of remedies as well as to plants grown in their
gardens; they could also import herbal plants from abroad or buy them
from apothecaries. However, the majority of people had to look to wild plants
as the only material available for the common person's do-it-yourself medicine. Houseleek is one plant that breaks the mould.

This plant is not a British native, but has been widely used in folk and
official medicine. Its country of origin is unknown; however, all over Europe
its characteristic succulent rosettes were often deliberately planted on
rooftops and outhouses, where they served the dual function of keeping
away lightning and providing a store for first-aid material. On slate roofs,
they had the added bonus of binding the slates together and on thatched
roofs they provided protection against fire. On any house, they keep witches
away. In Suffolk, it was said that if a houseleek grew on your house you
would never be penniless. It was considered unlucky to uproot houseleek, a
superstition that probably grew from the simple fact that it was of great
practical value.

The plant has innumerable country names, of which the longest and best
is certainly 'welcome-home-husband-however-drunk-you-be'. How it got this
particular name is unclear; it may be because the offshoots, which bear small
rosettes, are sometimes dislodged by the wind and roll drunkenly down the
roof slope. The houseleek was dedicated in Classical times to a rather more

distinguished figure, Jupiter the Roman god of thunder and lightning, which explains the plant's supposed protective role against lightning strikes and fire.

In folk medicine, houseleek's uses mirror those of its cousin NAVELWORT. In extensive areas of Britain where navelwort does not occur, houseleek seems to have played a similar role. It has been used as a poultice to treat abscesses, wounds and skin conditions, ranging from burns and eczema to ringworm and shingles. Its juice was dropped into sore eyes and ears (in the Middle Ages it was called 'erewort'). The plant also treated asthma, croup and fevers.

In official medicine, the plant was regarded as 'cooling', and from Classical times onwards was used to treat inflammations. Gerard in 1597 recommended the plant for burns, corns and sore eyes, and Pechey added fevers to this list in 1694. In the nineteenth century, it was still being recommended for the same ailments and Kemsey describes it as 'easing all inward and outward heats'. He also includes 'immoderate courses' (heavy periods), nosebleeds and bee and nettle stings. Kemsey's recommendations closely resemble those of Culpeper, from two centuries earlier. This early nineteenth-century recipe taken from the diary of Maryanne Weston of Thorpe, Norwich, wholeheartedly endorses another use:

To cure the coming-off of children's hair attended with a dry humour, and scurfiness.

Slightly bruise the full grown but tender leaves of House leek, strain the juice and add to it a little cream. Moisten a piece of soft old Irish linen several times double with it, till wet through put it on the affected part when the child goes to bed at night keeping it as moist as you can all night and wash it well off in the morning with soft soap and water. This I found a perfect cure.

Today's medical herbalists use houseleek primarily in the treatment of skin conditions, and advise its use externally, but not internally because it can cause vomiting.

Ivy
(*Hedera helix*)

Love the strong and weak doth yoke,
And makes the ivy climb the oak

Giles Fletcher (d. 1623), *Wooing Song*

This evergreen climber is a familiar sight, scrambling over the ground and up trees in woodlands throughout Britain. Ivy often grows over dead tree stumps, suggesting that the ivy is harmful, but whether or not it does any damage to live trees is still a controversial matter among botanists. Ivy takes only water from the trunk through its clinging roots, and many have claimed that it does the host tree no harm at all. Certainly, attitudes towards ivy are ambivalent, and its long-held image as a plant of ancient ruins and melancholy places does not help. In some areas, it was considered unlucky to bring it into the house. But on the whole the image of ivy is as beneficial and protective.

Ivy's evergreen nature symbolizes immortality and it has been made into wreaths and crowns for centuries, not just at Christmas-time but in the pre-Christian era too. Together with BRAMBLE and ROWAN, ivy was twined into wreaths in the Scottish Highlands and worn for protection against evil. It was similarly included in wreaths hung above the lintels of cow byres to defend the cattle against the evil eye and infection.

Ivy was used in love divination and to foretell health in the coming year. In a twentieth-century collection of country remedies from schoolchildren in Norfolk, one child recorded the following from her grandparents:

Find a green ivy leaf on New Year's Eve and put it in a dish in water. Cover the dish. Leave it covered until the sixth of January, then take the leaf out ... If the leaf is still green and healthy you will have a year's good health.

In folk medicine, the use of ivy has been a mixture of the symbolic and practical. An ivy leaf dipped in vinegar provided a cure for a corn; an ivy tree growing on an ash has particular value. Warts were similarly treated. In Wales, it was considered important to start this cure when the moon was waning.

Ivy leaves had applications for other skin conditions. A recent report from 2002 describes the wearing of a cap made from ivy leaves to cure a scabby head in a child. The cap of leaves was bandaged in place and, within a month, the sores had disappeared.

Another remarkable first-hand account of an ivy cure comes from Ayrshire in Scotland. A man now in his seventies remembers as a child playing with a friend who had an accident and was badly burned on his face. His grandmother sent him to collect ivy from the wall of the byre. She pounded the leaves in olive oil, laid them all over the injured boy's face, and covered the whole with a brown paper mask. By the time the doctor had arrived, the boy was in much less pain, so the doctor decided to do nothing further. The lad's burns healed without any scar.

Folk medicine used ivy for other ailments too. Twigs boiled in butter helped the discomfort of sunburn in the Scottish Highlands (a remedy probably not called upon very often). Sore eyes and swellings were eased with ivy lotions and ointments and the berries were eaten for aches and pains. A cure for whooping cough in Cheshire was to make a cup from ivy wood, from which the child had to take all its drinks.

In official medicine, Gerard in 1597 recommends an infusion of ivy leaves for eye troubles. Culpeper suggests in 1653 the use of the same for washing foul ulcers and soothing headaches. The berries, he tells us, were good against the plague as well as heavy periods, kidney stones and worms, and the leaves were included in an unusual hangover cure:

> There seems to be a very great antipathy between wine and Ivy; for if one hath got a surfeit by drinking of wine, his speediest cure is to drink a draught of the same wine wherein a handful of Ivy leaves, being first bruised, have been boiled.

This association between ivy and drink goes back to Classical times when it was a symbol of Bacchus. The idea was preserved for many centuries in the custom of marking a tavern with a 'bush' of ivy. This is the origin of the phrase 'a good wine needs no bush'. There is a saying in Somerset: 'Put a trail of ivy across a drunkard's path and he will become a sober citizen.'

Salmon in 1693 states that ivy berries can help to expel a dead child and cleanse the afterbirth. By the nineteenth century, Kemsey describes ivy berries as 'diuretic and emmenagogue' and the leaves as useful in cleansing sores and burns and scalds, and easing pains and stitches. Thereafter, official medical use of ivy died out and today the plant is little exploited in medical herbalism in Britain, although its application persists in continental Europe.

Ivy's value as a skin-soother, for sores, burns and scalds, continued in folk medicine right through the nineteenth and into the twentieth century. Farmers still occasionally feed ivy to their livestock. Sheep and cows will not normally eat the plant, but when they are sick they often will, and find benefit from it. One shepherd went so far as to say that if a sheep won't eat ivy you might as well give up on it. Other applications are varied. The plant is given to cattle, goats and sheep to help expel afterbirths; chewed ivy leaves were applied to cataracts in cows and sheep and given to those suspected of mineral deficiency. Sick goats were sometimes given ivy leaves, but care had to be taken – if given to nanny goats, the ivy tainted the milk.

Household servants found good use for ivy too. It could revive the colour of black silk and would remove the shine from serge. For these purposes, ivy leaves were boiled until the water turned dark, and the material was rinsed in the resulting liquid.

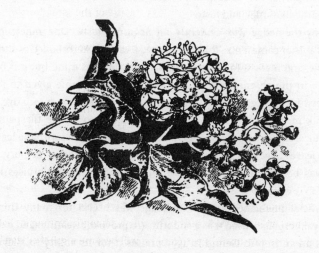

Jack-by-the-hedge
(*Alliaria petiolata*)

> The poor people in the country eat the leaves of this plant with their bread, and on account of the relish they give, call them sauce-alone. They also mix them with Lettuce, use them as a stuffing herb to pork, and eat them with salt fish.
>
> Charles Bryant, *Flora Dietetica* (1783)

This member of the cress family grows in hedgerows, on the edges of woodland and on wasteland. The very bright green leaves form a starched ruff for the cluster of dazzlingly white flowers at the top of the unbranched stem. The leaves smell of garlic when crushed, and the smell is attractive to midges, which pollinate the flowers. It has long been used as a flavouring on account of its garlicky taste; 'garlic mustard' is one of its common names. The shoots were usually eaten as a vegetable or made into sauce to accompany meat. Gerard in 1597 recommended it with fish as well. Some called it 'sauce-alone': the 'alone' part of the name derived from 'ail', meaning garlic and referring to the garlic-like smell and taste.

Jack-by-the-hedge was evidently an acquired taste. One nineteenth-century author comments: 'It has been used as a salad herb, boiled as a table vegetable, and made into sauce in the same manner as mint; but it is only tolerable in the absence of all other vegetables.' The name given to it in Leicestershire of 'beggar-man's-oatmeal' sounds equally unappreciative.

In folk medicine, the fresh leaves were chewed to relieve the pain of mouth ulcers. A Somerset cure for cramp was to rub the feet with the leaves, and the leaves have also been applied to wounds. Within living memory, the plant was boiled and made into an ointment for treating bruises and sores.

In official medicine, Jack-by-the-hedge was useful for many things. Mediaeval herbalists used it as a sudorific (to provoke sweating) and externally as an antiseptic. Gerard in 1597 praises it for its ability to alleviate colic and kidney stones and, a century later, Salmon also advocates it for indigestion and colic. A syrup with honey is 'good against Coughs, Colds, Horsness, Weesings, &c.' and the 'essence' of the plant is, he tells us, an 'Antidote against the Plague and all pestiliential Fevers'. The seeds rubbed and put up the nose provoke sneezing and clear the head, according to Pechey in 1694. Culpeper in 1653 recommends it in addition for leg ulcers, a use mentioned again in *The British Herbal* of 1838. This was its last recommendation and official herbalism in this country seems to have forgotten the plant after this.

Jack-by-the-hedge is still gathered in season, when fresh, and added to salads to lend them a lovely, mild garlic flavour.

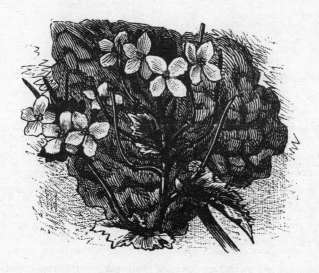

Juniper
(*Juniperus communis*)

Marie Hamilton's to the kirk gane,
Wi' ribbons in her hair;
And the King thought mair o' Marie Hamilton,
Than ony that was there.

She hadna been about the King's Court
A month, but barely ane,

When frae' the King's Court Marie Hamilton,
Marie Hamilton durstna' be

The King is to the Abbey gane,
To pu' the savin tree,
But for a' that he could do or say,
The babe it wadna dee.

Traditional ballad, 'The Queen's Maries'

Juniper's fragrant, evergreen needles and dark blue berries are a common sight in the Mediterranean; in Britain, our native juniper is confined to areas of heath and mountain, mostly in the highlands of Scotland and Wales. It was once, of course, far more abundant. The common name 'savin' is probably derived from the botanical name *Juniperus sabinus*, the species most widely used in official medicine. The name has been further corrupted to 'saffen' and even 'saffron', as in this letter from W. Wallace in the *East Anglian Magazine* of December 1975:

> I remarked on a small shrub that stood in the middle plot and asked him what it was. Bill, an ex-horseman, replied: 'That's saffron. You must have seen it growing round churchyards many a time and there's no harm now in telling you what we used to use it for. If you had a good working mare in your stable and the gaffer wanted her in foal and you didn't, you'd mix some dried saffron

leaves in her grub and the stallion could keep coming round all he liked but she'd never click for a foal. Not only that, it made her coat shine.'

In some parts of East Anglia, juniper was known as the 'threepenny bit herb', because the dose for a horse was no more than would cover a silver three-penny piece.

Juniper had an underground reputation as an abortifacient. In southwest England, it went by the uncompromising name of 'bastard killer'. Naturally, there are few written records kept on this delicate subject, but it is known that juniper has been used for hundreds of years to get rid of unwanted babies. In Oxford's Pitt Rivers Museum, there are sprigs of juniper that a woman once wore in her boots for nine days with the aim of producing an abortion; we do not know if it worked. If fresh juniper could not be found, gin – which is flavoured with its berries – would be tried instead.

The herbalists were well aware of juniper's powers: Pechey in 1694 tells us that 'it forces the Courses and causes Miscarriage: Upon which Account they are too well known, and too much used by Wenches.' In Scotland, 'giving birth under the savin tree' was once a euphemism for an abortion. The extract above from the ballad 'The Queen's Maries' indicates that its use was commonly known. The 'Abbey' in the ballad is Holyrood House in Edinburgh. Alas for Marie Hamilton, the juniper did not work and she was executed in the Tolbooth.

The uses of juniper in folk medicine have not all been controversial and other juniper remedies are many and varied. An infusion of its leaves has been used to treat jaundice, its berries for kidney ailments, rheumatism, toothache and, in Scotland, to poultice snakebites. In Achill Island, off the coast of County Mayo in Ireland, the gathering of the unripe berries was ceremonially performed on the last Sunday in July. The berries were then preserved in whisky for 'ailments' unspecified. A recent first-hand account states that 'juniper berry gin is excellent for backache (6 berries to one gill)'.

In official medicine, Salmon follows the Classical tradition and in 1693 recommends juniper wood, as an infusion or as smoke. It will, he says, 'comfort the Viscera, strengthen the nerves, and help Palsies', while the berries are suitable for a whole host of conditions, including 'sharpness and heat of Urine'. Oil of juniper was in official use as a carminative (a relief for flatulence) up to the 1940s. Juniper is still used in modern medical herbalism in this country, to treat rheumatic conditions, colic and cystitis. Although the continental species *Juniperus sabinus* is more powerful as an abortifacient, all types of juniper should be avoided during pregnancy.

Like many other evergreens, juniper has been regarded as having special protective powers. Sprigs of juniper were hung in cows' byres to protect them from the evil eye in the Scottish Highlands. Teething rings of juniper wood were used in Scotland for the same reason: a child when teething was thought to be vulnerable to all kinds of ills, natural and supernatural. A nineteenth-century botanist states that 'In former times a few sprigs of Juniper flung into the fire were thought very efficacious in protecting the bystanders and their property from evil spirits and witchcraft.'

Juniper was also brought into the home for another reason: its fragrance was effective in fumigating byres and houses, especially at times of infection. As recently as the twentieth century, juniper leaves and berries were put on the open fire to remove the smell of new paint after decorating.

The plant's wood was used as fuel, especially valued for illicit stills because it burns with very little betraying smoke. In Ellis' eighteenth-century work, *Modern Husbandman*, we read:

> When women chide their husbands for a long while together, it is commonly said they give them a juniper lecture; which, I am informed, is a comparison taken from the long lasting of the live-coals of that wood, not from its sweet smell.

Twigs of juniper were used to smoke hams and were woven into baskets; when mixed with oil of linseed, juniper made a useful varnish for pictures, tables and to protect iron from rust. And was it an accidental discovery? – eating and drinking utensils made from juniper wood were said to give a 'grateful relish' to their contents.

Kingcup or Marsh Marigold
(*Caltha palustris*)

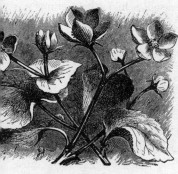

The name kingcup is easy to understand; its flowers light up bogs and marshes like the world's biggest buttercups. Its generic name *Caltha* is derived from the Greek *kalatho*, meaning 'a goblet'. The flower's striking beauty has earned it what is possibly a record-breaking number of country names: Geoffrey Grigson lists more than eighty. One very common alternative name is marsh marigold.

Emphatically a plant of springtime, kingcup is associated with the advent of the cuckoo and of emergence of the growing season; perhaps they are Shakespeare's 'cuckoo buds of yellow hue' (*Love's Labour's Lost*, V, ii, 883). In the Isle of Man and in Ireland, the plant was used in the May Eve rites to protect the households from fairies. It was one of several flowers made into garlands in Scotland to protect milk.

Like many other members of the buttercup family, the plant has very acrid juice, and this might explain the relative scarcity of its use in folk medicine. In Ireland, boils were poulticed with its leaves and a drink prepared from the flowers was employed for heart conditions.

Official medicine largely neglected this plant, although Turner in the sixteenth century recommended it for toothache. Withering, of FOXGLOVE fame, made an unusual observation regarding kingcups: 'on a large quantity of the flowers . . . .being put into the bedroom of a girl who had been subject to fits, the fits ceased'. This success was to be repeated over the years, with an infusion of the flowers sometimes utilized to treat fits.

In the kitchen, kingcup had its uses too. The buds were at one time pickled in vinegar as a caper substitute; the leaves may be cooked and eaten like spinach. In the dairy, kingcups were added to milk in lieu of rennet, especially in Fife.

A most intriguing property of kingcup is its 'alleged power to save the wearer of it from making unkind remarks himself, or from suffering such remarks from others'. Essential, then, to carry it at all times.

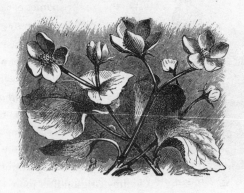

Knapweed
(*Centaurea nigra*)

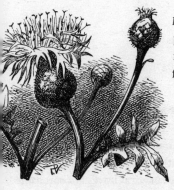

Most of the country names of this common plant of grassland and wayside refer to its most striking feature: its hard, dark brown flowerheads. The name 'loggerheads' is used in Northamptonshire; a loggerhead was a vicious weapon – a spherical iron ball at the end of a wooden stick. When the flowerhead opens, the numerous purple florets give a thistle-like appearance to the plant, but the leaves and stems, although tough, are soft and devoid of prickles.

In folk medicine, the plant seems to have played a minor role, although an infusion was used in Essex for indigestion, in Sussex as a bitter tonic and in Wales for treating boils. It has been more widely used in Ireland, again as a tonic and also for treating jaundice and respiratory complaints.

In official medicine, knapweed seems to have lived up to its generic name of *Centaurea*; it was named after the Centaur, famous for his gift of healing. Wounds, whitlows and felons [inflamed and infected sores, usually on a finger] were treated with knapweed, and Culpeper in 1653 recommends it for fluxes, for 'those that are bursten [have hernias]', for running sores, green wounds and sore throats. In the mid-nineteenth century, the herb was still being prescribed for 'green wounds, bruises, sores, cancers, scabby head, and fistulas', but medical herbalists in this country no longer use the plant.

Knapweed plays a well-known role in love divination, where the plant foretells whether a girl's affections will be returned: any open florets are plucked off a flowerhead and it is placed inside the girl's blouse; if after an hour more florets have opened, then her love will be returned.

Knotgrass
(*Polygonum aviculare*)

Knotgrass, a diminutive member of the dock family, is a common weed of arable land. It has smooth, wiry, green stems with swollen 'joints' at each node, where the tiny oval leaves are borne and shelter in their axils minute, pinkish flowers. When gathered, the stem normally breaks at a joint, a characteristic that has given rise to such names as 'ninety-knot' and 'centinode'.

The plant's black, three-angled seeds are eaten by many of our small birds, and cattle and pigs eat the plant readily. Gerard in 1597 tells us that 'It is given to swine with good successe when they are sicke and will not eat their meate, whereupon the country people so call it Swine's Grass.' Yet, oddly, there was a belief that eating knotgrass stunted growth in humans, as referred to in the verse above. Shakespeare also refers to its stunting properties in *A Midsummer Night's Dream* (III, ii, 327): 'Get you gone, you dwarf; you minimus, of hindering knot-grass made.'

Although very common throughout Britain, surprisingly, knotweed does not feature prominently in our folk medicine. In Somerset, it was sometimes harnessed to treat nosebleeds – the plant would be rubbed into the nostrils – and, in Ireland where the plant is called 'pigroot', it was used for treating swine fever. No other uses are recorded.

In complete contrast, the plant was exploited in official medicine for a bewildering assortment of conditions. Culpeper's list in 1653 is long: for bleeding of all kinds, for kidney conditions including gravel and stone (small and large urinary stones), for inflammations, to kill worms, to treat bites, broken joints and ruptures. Salmon in 1693 adds the 'comforting' of 'nerves and tendons'. The seventeenth- and eighteenth-century Gunton Household Book suggests knotgrass and plantain applied hot 'to put up the fundament being out'; this presumably refers to some kind of prolapse. Kemsey in 1838 also recommends it for 'ulcers, old sores, fistulas, and cancers'.

And so it goes on. Modern-day medical herbalists use it for an impressive range of complaints including bleeding of all kinds, diarrhoea, lung complaints, piles and worms. Recent research in China has shown the plant to be effective in treating dysentery.

Lady's Bedstraw
(*Galium verum*)

This plant is as soft as its cousin the GOOSEGRASS is rough. Its leaves are fine and delicate and its flowers smell of honey. As it dries, the whole plant gives off the scent of new-mown hay; the Manx name for it translates as 'herb of the sweet smell', and it would often be placed among clothes to sweeten them and to repel moths. It is also known as 'fleaweed', perhaps because it was once used to repel these unwanted bedfellows. All these properties make it ideal as bedding for man or beast. Chaucer refers to it in connection with illicit love: 'O perilous fyr, that in the bedstraw bredeth.' A German tradition suggests that the plant got its name because the newborn Christ was placed on a bed of bracken and bedstraw; the bedstraw alone acknowledged the Christ child, and was rewarded by having its flowers turned to gold; other related bedstraws have white flowers. In Scotland, the plant is sometimes called 'a-hundred-fald', after the vast numbers of its tiny flowers.

Lady's bedstraw does not seem to have been used in British folk medicine. In official medicine though the plant was used to staunch bleeding, an application that was reported in the seventeenth century by Pechey and continued right into the early nineteenth century. The herb also had a role in easing sore feet. Gerard in 1597 tells us that 'An ointment is prepared which is good for anointing the weary traveller.' In the eighteenth century, Miller's *Botanicum Officinale* reports that 'a bath made of it is very refreshing to wash the feet of persons tired with overwalking' and it is good for gout too.

Modern herbalists in this country use it for urinary complaints, including kidney and bladder stones, and also for skin conditions.

Like GOOSEGRASS, the plant has also been used to curdle milk, hence the name 'cheese rennet', given to it in some parts of Britain. Gerard mentions this and, loyal to his own county, he remarks that 'The people in Cheshire, especially about Namptwich where the best Cheese is made, do use it in their Rennet, esteeming greatly of that Cheese above other made without it.' He adds that the milk from goats fed on lady's bedstraw is 'sweeter and more pleasant in taste, and also more holsome, especially to break the stone [large urinary stones]'. Within living memory, the plant was still in occasional country use as a rennet substitute: if the whole aerial shoots are used the resulting cheese is green while using just the flowering tops gives a yellow cheese.

Clearly, there were many reasons why lady's bedstraw was a plant worth gathering. In some parts of the country, the entire plant, roots and all, would be picked to extract the dye from its roots and shoots. Yellow dye was obtained from the flowering shoots and red from the roots, and the tweed industry in the Hebrides and in other parts of Scotland employed it a great deal. In the Scottish Highlands, its flowers were used to colour butter. Because the roots are so fine, it was necessary to collect large quantities of the plant; in coastal regions, the consequent erosion became such a problem that the eighteenth-century landowners had to prohibit gathering of the plant. As synthetic dyes have largely taken over from plant pigments commercially, there is no longer any demand for large quantities of lady's bedstraw.

Lady's Mantle
(*Alchemilla vulgaris*)

This plant grows on grassland throughout Britain but is more commonly found in the north of the country. It has tiny, greenish-yellow, inconspicuous flowers but its leaves are uniquely beautiful. Their shape and the way in which they are folded in the bud suggest the form of a Tudor mantle, a cloak, and this accounts for the plant's common name. To modern eyes, the leaves resemble inverted, half-opened umbrellas. They often have trapped dewdrops nestling in them first thing in the morning; one of the Gaelic names given to this plant translates as 'dew-cup'. It is easy to understand why this dew should have magical associations, because it appears overnight and looks so enchanting.

It has been suggested that the generic name *Alchemilla* is derived from the Arabic word *alkemelych*, meaning 'alchemy', and is a reference to former uses of the plant in magical potions. The dew shaken from the leaves was said to restore feminine beauty, however faded. In Ireland, the plant's magic also extended to livestock. The juice squeezed from its leaves and shoots was added to a cow's drinking water and sprinkled over its ears to cure it from 'elf-shot', a disease thought to be caused by supernatural beings.

In folk medicine, the plant was used in the Scottish Highlands to treat wounds and sores. In Ireland, it has been utilized for a wider selection of ailments, including burns, kidney trouble and nosebleeds. Its names of 'colickwort' and 'bowel-hive grass' both suggest that in the past the herb was used against intestinal pain and flatulence.

In official medicine, lady's mantle had a reputation as a wound-healer. Culpeper in 1653 proclaimed it to be 'one of the most singular wound herbs that is'. John Pechey echoes that in 1694 and recommends the plant for treating heavy periods as well as wounds and ruptures. Its official use as a wound-healer continued well into the nineteenth century. The plant had another subsidiary use. Gerard in 1597 tells us that 'it keepeth downe maidens paps or dugs, and when they be too great and flaggie, it maketh them lesser and harder'. A hundred years later, Pechey recommends the plant for 'lax breasts'. It was still in favour in the nineteenth century: 'The good women in the north of England apply the leaves to their breasts, to make them recover their form, after they have been swelled with milk. Hence it has got the name of ladies' mantle.' It has even been claimed that an infusion of the plant is so effective in contracting tissue that it has been used to shrink the female genitalia to give the appearance of virginity.

Lady's mantle is still used today by medical herbalists to treat heavy periods, fibroids and endometriosis.

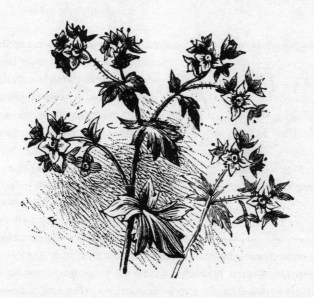

Lady's Smock
(*Cardamine pratensis*)

When daisies pied and violets blue
And lady-smocks all silver white
And cuckoo-buds of yellow hue
Do paint the meadows with delight,
The cuckoo then, on every tree,
Mocks married men ...

Shakespeare, *Love's Labour's Lost*, V, ii, 881–886

This cousin of the watercress is a springtime flower of damp places, water meadows and riverbanks throughout Britain. Its dainty, pink or white flowers have four overlapping petals and its leaflets are long and narrow, giving the plant a delicate appearance. Its leaves have the unusual ability to root at the point where they touch the earth and produce new plantlets. Like watercress, the leaves have a peppery taste and can be added to salads and sandwiches.

The plant seems to have had amorous associations, 'smock' being a derogatory word for women, in much the same way as we refer today to 'a piece of skirt'. Shakespeare implies similar associations in the song quoted above. The common names of 'cuckoo flower' and 'cuckoo spit' have been attributed either to the association of the cuckoo with unfaithfulness, or to a more prosaic fact – that there is often 'cuckoo spit', the froth formed by a small bug, present on the plant.

In folk medicine, the plant has been used in the Scottish Highlands to treat scurvy and fevers and in England to treat persistent headaches.

In official medicine, Culpeper in 1653 also recommended it for scurvy, as well as a diuretic and for treating kidney stone, restoring appetite and soothing indigestion. From the seventeenth century onwards, lady's smock was described as 'antispasmodic' and was used to treat fits, St Vitus's dance and hysteria.

For a while the herb came into vogue as a treatment for epilepsy. Sir George Baker in 1767 read a paper before the College of Physicians that was entirely about the medicinal value of this plant. According to him, the flowers had to be toasted in pewter dishes, then powdered and boiled in bottles that were covered not with cork but with leather. The flowers' application for epilepsy later seemed to fall out of favour. By 1862, when C. Pierpoint Johnson wrote his treatise on the *Useful Plants of Great Britain*, he mentions that lady's smock was formerly used for epilepsy, but in his day was utilized only by the peasantry. Epilepsy was often attributed to supernatural causes and folk treatments for it were often magical, rather than herbal. It is interesting that lady's smock is also called 'cuckoo flower'; several of the charms used against epilepsy have cuckoo associations.

The plant is now known to have a high vitamin C content, which explains its usefulness in fighting scurvy and makes it a good addition to salads. It is little used today by medical herbalists in this country, although elsewhere in Europe it is still employed as a tonic and an antispasmodic for coughs.

Lesser Celandine
(*Ranunculus ficaria*)

The bright yellow, starry flowers of lesser celandine are one of the first flowers of early spring, bringing a little brightness to damp riverbanks and shady hedgerows in the last gasp of winter. Burgess in 1868 refers to these 'golden varnished flowers' so loved by Wordsworth, who expressed it perfectly in his poem *To the Small Celandine*, when he referred to the flowers:

Telling tales about the sun,
When we've little warmth, or none.

In Wales, the appearance of the lesser celandine was a sign that it was time to sow crops. The celandine's petals are green on their undersides, so when they close up, as they do before rain, the flower becomes almost invisible among the leaves. Bunches of the roots and bulbils (small bulbs formed in the leaf axils) were hung in cowsheds in Devon and in the Scottish Highlands, to increase the cream content of the milk.

Lesser celandine has whitish roots and bulbils – these parts have mainly been utilized in medicine. In folk medicine, an ointment prepared from the bulbils has been applied not only to piles (which were known in the past as 'figs') but also to other swellings, including corns and warts. The English names of 'figwort' and 'pilewort' spring from this use. The entire plant, like many members of the buttercup family, contains an irritant juice, which was exploited by beggars in order to produce sympathy-evoking sores. The caustic juice was also applied to corns and warts to burn them off. Both the petals and the leaves helped to clean teeth. Within living memory, an infusion made by pouring boiling water on the leaves served as a skin cleanser.

In official medicine, the plant was also used to alleviate piles. Gerard in 1597 recommended the plant for this, as did later herbalists. Culpeper in 1653 commends it too for treating the swellings of the King's evil (scrofula): 'with this I cured my own Daughter of King's evil, broke the Sore, drew out a quarter of a pound of Corruption, cured it without any scar at all, and all in one week's time'. Pechey in 1694 found it useful not only for piles but also for cleaning teeth, jaundice and scurvy. Like many plants, it was dropped from official medicine in Britain in the nineteenth century.

Present-day medical herbalists still recommend ointment or suppositories prepared from lesser celandine to treat piles. Modern studies suggest that compounds called saponins in the plant are, at least in part, the reason the plant is so effective in treating haemorrhoids. The herb has also been shown to have antifungal and antibacterial properties.

LICHENS

These strange plants, biologically a combination of an alga and a fungus, are good indicators of air pollution: where roof tiles and tree bark are covered with lichen, the air is clean. In the past, they were a source of occasional food and medicine – the different types often were only vaguely distinguished – but, perhaps just as importantly, lichens were a crucial source of material for the dye industry. In Wales and Scotland, a large number of different lichens, in particular *Parmelia* species, were collectively called crotal and used to dye wool. Crotal gave Harris tweed its characteristic smell.

The lichen would be scraped off the rocks and steeped in urine for three months before use; doubtless this too contributed to the smell of the tweed. The lichen was then layered with the wool in a cauldron and boiled until it was a deep red. Red and purple dyes came from a lichen called 'cudbear' (*Ochrolechia tartarea*) and yellow and green from species of 'hairmoss' (*Usnea*). Brown shades could also be obtained. Cudbear is said to be named after Dr Cuthbert Gordon who helped set up a dye-works at Leith in the eighteenth century that exploited this lichen. Incidentally, crotal was never used to dye fishermen's jerseys because of the superstition that the lichen would cause its wearer to return to the rocks and be shipwrecked.

It was still possible in the early nineteenth century to make a living by gathering lichen and selling it at the Glasgow markets. However, commercial development of the lichen industry was unsustainable because lichens are extremely slow-growing.

Folk uses for lichens were very varied. In the Scottish Highlands, crotal was dried and powdered and sprinkled on the feet to prevent them from getting sore and inflamed and, in Ireland, it was applied to burns, cuts and sores.

Sea-green lichen (*Peltigera aphthosa*) was employed both in folk medicine and in official medicine, for treating thrush in children, a condition that used to be described in medical circles as aphthous ulcers (hence the specific name *aphthosa*). Withering, of FOXGLOVE fame, reported in the eighteenth century that this lichen was boiled in milk and given to children for thrush; that in larger doses it caused vomiting and purging; and was also effective against intestinal worms.

Dog Lichen
(*Peltigera canina*)

Dog lichen became famous in the eighteenth century for the treatment of mad-dog bites and was still in use in official medicine in the nineteenth century. This lichen is also confusingly known as 'ash-coloured liverwort', although it does not belong to the true liverworts, which are themselves closely related to the mosses. As that name suggests, the lichen was used to treat liver complaints. Salmon in 1693 describes its application for jaundice, rickets, wounds and sores and Culpeper in 1653 claimed that 'it fortifies the liver exceedingly, and makes it impregnable', but as a dog-bite antidote it reigned supreme.

The Only receipt against the bite of a mad dog which never yet failed:

Take dwarf-box, ash-coloured liverwort, wild periwinkle, and wild trefoil (the best time for laying in a stock of the latter is in June), of each an equal quantity. When they have lain by to be sufficiently dried, rub them, and sift them into a fine powder. Then give three quarters of an ounce in a pint of new milk fasting to either man or dog; let it be repeated for three mornings; the sooner the better after the bite.

Scots Magazine, February 1751

Tree Lungwort
(*Lobaria pulmonaria*)

This grey lichen grows mainly on trees and has been used for centuries in official medicine to treat lung complaints. Culpeper in 1653 recommends it for coughs, wheezings, shortness of breath, and ulcers. Pechey gives a vivid description of it in 1694: 'It grows on old Oaks and beeches, in dark, shady, old Woods. It has broad, greyish, rough Leaves, variously folded, crumpl'd and gash'd on the edges, and sometimes spotted on the upper side. It bears no Stalk, nor Flower ... It stops Bleeding, and cures fresh Wounds. It stops the Courses, and the Flux of the Belly. The Powder, the Syrup, and the distill'd Water of it are commonly used for Diseases of the Lungs.' Kemsey in 1838 echoes Culpeper from two centuries earlier when he tells us that 'It cures coughs, wheezings and shortness of breath, in man or beast. It is an excellent wash for ulcers.'

Folk medicine too utilized this lichen. In the nineteenth century, it was still collected in the New Forest and an infusion in milk used to treat consumption.

Herbalists still advise it for lung complaints, as well as various gastro-intestinal problems, and one eminent medical herbalist in this country describes it as 'a beneficial but under-used remedy'.

Lily of the Valley
(*Convallaria majalis*)

The Conval-lily is esteemed to have of all others, the sweetest and most agree-able perfume; not offensive or overbearing, even to those who are made uneasy with the perfumes of other sweet-scented flowers

John Lawrence, *The Flower Garden* (1726)

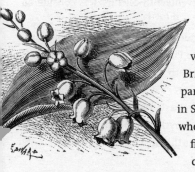

Surely one of the most delightfully fragrant of our wild flowers, lily of the valley is native in woodland throughout Britain, although it is not common. It is particularly abundant in St Leonard's Forest in Sussex and, according to legend, it grows where St Leonard's blood was spilt during a fight with a dragon. The only other fable connected with this plant is considerably less violent; it is said that the nightingale is lured into woodland by the scent of the flowers to find a mate. The aromatic oil farnesol, which gives the flowers their wonderful scent, was once a constituent of snuff. Although lily of the valley has had good and holy associations in many places, it is never-theless considered by some to be unlucky to bring it into the house; in Devon, it was unwise even to plant it in the garden.

The plant's broad green, cooling leaves lend themselves to first aid, but their use in folk medicine in Britain has been minimal, probably because of the relative scarcity of the plant. In Gloucestershire and in East Anglia, within living memory, the leaves were bound onto cuts and, in Hampshire, they were infused in boiling water, wrapped in muslin and applied as a poultice to abscesses.

In official medicine, the plant has been employed since the time of the ancient Greeks to treat heart conditions and dropsy. We now know that the plant contains cardiac glycosides, which, while making the plant poisonous and dangerous to use, are responsible for its action on the heart.

Other applications of this plant were many and varied. One of the most unexpected came from Gerard, in the days when the plant was abundant on Hampstead Heath. He suggests in 1597 depositing the flowers in a glass vessel, placing it in an anthill for a month, and using the resultant liquid to treat gout. Culpeper in 1653 says of lily of the valley that 'it strengthens the brain, recruits a weak memory, and makes it strong again'. He recommends the flowers for eye conditions and also the distilled spirit of the flowers, because they restore 'lost speech, help the palsy, and is excellently good in the apoplexy'. The distilled water from the blossoms used to be known as *aqua aurea* (golden water) and in the seventeenth century was considered a good preservative against infections.

Lily of the valley continued to be included in official medicine right up to the mid-twentieth century. During the First World War, the after-effects of poison gas were treated with it. The herb was still listed in the *British Pharmacopoeia* of 1949.

Today's medical herbalists use the plant as a heart tonic, administering it in small doses to regulate heart rate and rhythm. It is better tolerated than foxglove but its poisonous nature requires that it should be prescribed only by professionals.

Lousewort
(*Pedicularis* species)

There be two kinds of rattle grasse, one which beareth redde floures and leaves finely jagged or snipt ... The stalkes be weake and small, whereof some lye along trayling upon the ground and do beare the little leaves, the rest do growe upright as high as a man's hand, and upon them grow the floures from the middle of the stemme round about even up to the top, somewhat like to ye floure of the red nettle. The which being falle away there grow in their place little flat powches or huskes wherein the seede is contained.

Rembert Dodoens, *A Niewe Herball, or Historie of Plantes*, trans. Henry Lyte (1578)

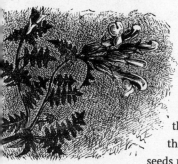

Lousewort can be found on peaty heathland throughout Britain. In the same family as FIGWORT, it is a low-growing plant with attractive, hooked, pink flowers, which grow in a dense spike. The flowers are followed by papery, brown calyces, which puff up after the seed is set. This characteristic has earned the plant the name of 'rattle' since the ripe seeds really do rattle in the bladder-like calyx.

For such a pretty plant, the name 'lousewort' seems unjustifiably insulting, but people thought there was good reason for it. Some believed, as Gerard in 1597, that the plant 'filleth sheepe and other cattle that feede in medowes where this groweth full of lice', an idea which probably arose because the poorly-drained soils on which it grows are likely to harbour parasites such as liver fluke. There is confusion surrounding the name lousewort. Before the nineteenth century, we are told that people wore a sprig around their necks; the perfume of this attracted fleas and lice from other parts of the body, which could then be destroyed. On the other hand, we now know that lousewort contains an insecticidal compound called aucubin, so another explanation of the name may be that it was found to destroy these pests.

In folk medicine, the plant was little used, but lousewort poultices were made by the inhabitants of Jura in the Hebrides to cure a painful disease known there in the eighteenth century as 'fillan'. The disease was thought to be caused by a thread-like worm and left many of the inhabitants crippled for life. This was chronicled by a distinguished botanist and visitor to the island, Dr John Walker; he recognized the plant that they used to treat the disease as lousewort. It is impossible to know in modern terms what the disease 'fillan' referred to, and equally impossible to identify its cause.

In official medicine, the applications of lousewort were few in number. Gerard in 1597 suggested that the plant was useful for bloody fluxes and Culpeper in 1653 recommended lousewort for healing ulcers and fistulas, as well as for bleeding. These remedies continued into the nineteenth century, but gradually declined. Lousewort is not much utilized by present-day medical herbalists in this country.

Mallow
(*Malva* species)

The uses of mallow are infinite.

J. T. Burgess, *Old English Wild Flowers* (1868)

The commonest type of mallow grows as a wayside weed, but it is one of great beauty and usefulness. Its lobed leaves resemble umbrellas in various stages of opening and its tall, hairy stems bear striking, pale purple flowers. Each flower is twisted neatly in the bud and, when open, has five petals that are shaped like elongated hearts and individually striped with darker veins. In rural areas, the flowers would be strewn in front of houses on May Day, and there is a saying that marsh mallow grows only near a happy home.

The flowers are followed by round, flattened fruits and country people still remember nibbling them: they are called 'biscuities' in Scotland, 'cheeses' in England. The fruit is actually a mild laxative; it tastes pleasant, slightly sweet and nutty, and was regarded as a desirable alternative to a weekly dosing with sulphur and molasses – something that many elderly people recall vividly from their childhoods. The dried fruits were strung on necklaces too as a game.

The main function of mallow in folk medicine was as a healer of sore and inflamed skin. The plant contains abundant, soothing mucilage, and was crushed and applied as a poultice to sores and boils, insect bites and stings, cuts and grazes. It was used for swellings and sores on animals as well. In a book on farriery published in 1842 (A. Lawson, *The Modern Farrier*), there is this remarkable testimony to the plant's powers:

A neighbouring farmer had cut his thumb in a very dangerous manner, and, after a great deal of doctoring, it was got to such a pitch that his hand was swelled to twice its natural size. I recommended the use of mallows to him: gave him a little bunch out of my store, it being winter time, and his hand was well in four days ...

The other instance was this: I had a pig: indeed it was a large and valuable hog, that had been gored by the sharp horn of a cow. My men had given it up for lost. I had the hog caught and held down. The gore was in the side, and so large and deep that I could run my finger in beyond the ribs. I poured in the liquor in which the mallows had been stewed, and rubbed the side well with it besides. The next day the hog got up and began to eat ... upon examining the wound I found it so far closed up that I did not think it right to disturb it. I bathed the side over again; and in two days the hog was turned out and running about along with the rest.

In official medicine, mallow was used in some similar ways, also to 'ripen Tumours, and to ease Pain' and mallow juice was prescribed for consumption and shortness of breath. Folk medicine does not always distinguish between the true marsh mallow (*Althaea officinalis*) and the much more common mallow (*Malva sylvestris*), but in official medicine preference was given to the former. (This preference is likely to be due to the fact that the Classical authors favoured it). Kemsey in 1838 states that mallow 'is in every respect inferior to that of marshmallow'.

Modern-day herbalists, too, use the marsh mallow most, but the common mallow is still utilized to soothe skin conditions and as a laxative. The sweets that bear their name were once made from the roots of the marsh mallow; nowadays they contain no mallow at all.

Marjoram
(*Origanum vulgare*)

With margerain gentle,
The flower of goodlihead,
Embroidered the mantle
Is of your maidenhead.

John Skelton (1460–1529), *To Mistress Margery Wentworth*

Marjoram is a delicately beautiful plant, with slender stems and purple bracts surrounding clusters of pink flowers. The generic name *Origanum* means 'joy of the mountains'. In ancient Greece and Rome, brides wore a garland of marjoram. This may be because the plant had been recommended in the fourth century BC by Theophrastus for childbirth, so wearing the garland could have symbolized successful childbearing. There was a tradition of planting marjoram on the grave of a loved one; it was said that if the marjoram grew there it meant that the dead person was happy.

In rural areas, the herb was picked and dried in bunches for winter use. One country writer, Doris E. Coates, recollects that because of its sweet smell it was a favourite to gather in the wild while nibbling the leaves. 'Marjoram tea was a fragrant drink and was a relief for headaches. It was also thought to drive out the poisons which caused outbreaks of spots or boils.'

In official medicine, Gerard in 1597 advocated wild marjoram for a long list of ailments, including seasickness: 'It is very good against the warmbling [sic] of the stomach, and stayeth the desire to vomit, especially at sea.' Culpeper in 1653 describes wild marjoram as valuable in the treatment of indigestion, consumption, dropsy, jaundice, and says that the juice dropped in the ears 'helps deafness, pain and noise in the ears'.

Modern medical herbalists use the plant for indigestion (again, the calming of the stomach) and coughs, and prescribe the oil rubbed onto aching teeth or joints.

In the days when it was a constant battle to keep a home smelling agreeable, marjoram had a major role to play. As a fragrant herb, in the sixteenth century it was strewn on floors, and in dairies too where, together with wild thyme, it was thought to prevent milk from curdling during a thunderstorm. Until recent times the herb was used, like lavender, to freshen clothes and linen. Other practical uses are fascinating. It dyed wool purple and linen red and preserved beer while lending it an aromatic flavour. Various herbal mixtures were used by horsemen as a means of controlling and calming horses, and marjoram oil would be a vital constituent, as recorded in this eighteenth-century horseman's notebook:

The Art of Catching a Vicious horse or wild Colt in Any Field,

Take ginger bread and swett it under your arm or elsewhear and scent it with the Oil of Origanum and the Oil of Cinnamon and the Oil of Fennel, and the Oil of Rosemary you must get the windy side of him.

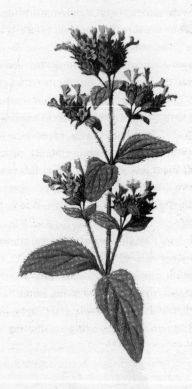

Meadowsweet
(*Filipendula ulmaria*)

Meadowsweet is a member of the rose family, and grows in damp meadows throughout Britain. Its rough, tough leaves and red-tinged stems are followed in early summer by a surprising mass of soft, creamy, fragrant flowers that smell of the very essence of summer. The petals drop very readily, their points of attachment to the flower being very narrow. The scent of the flowers attracts insects, but the flowers have no nectar. However, the pollen is so abundant that it is still worthwhile for bees to visit and collect the pollen, fertilizing the flowers in the process.

Meadowsweet has an abundance of pretty names, including 'bridewort' and 'queen of the meadow', but its former generic name of *Spiraea* has the most interest. In 1835, biochemists isolated a substance from meadowsweet called salicylic acid; at the end of the nineteenth century, this was synthesized and used to make aspirin, named after *Spiraea*. In contrast with aspirin, an infusion of meadowsweet does not produce stomach upsets or ulceration; it seems to have a built-in protective agent, which is not yet fully understood, and can actually relieve heartburn and indigestion.

In folk medicine, the plant has been used for a wide variety of ailments, including coughs, colds, sore throats, headache and fevers – many of the complaints for which today we take aspirin. It was reported by Aubrey in the seventeenth century that 'There is a woman in Bedfordshire who doth great cures for fevers with meadowsweet, to which she adds some green wheat'. In addition, sore eyes, diarrhoea, stomach-ache, sunburn were all treated with this plant, as well as in Ireland jaundice and dropsy. Doris E. Coates, in her book *Tuppeny Rice and Treacle: Cottage Housekeeping* (1900–1920), quotes the saying that meadowsweet 'makes old men young and young men strong'.

In official medicine, the root was used to treat gravel and stone (small and large urinary stones), coughs and colds and the leaves treated colic and piles. Pechey in 1694 recommended the plant in particular for treating fluxes and, in the early twentieth century, herbalists still prescribed it particularly for treating diarrhoea in children.

Medical herbalists today employ meadowsweet for treating diarrhoea, indigestion and some arthritic complaints. It is particularly used as a safe remedy for diarrhoea in children.

People have found many other applications for meadowsweet. The leaves when crushed are sharply fragrant and have been used to flavour claret. The difference in scent between the flowers (sweet) and the crushed leaves (aromatic and sharp) gave rise to the country name of 'courtship and marriage'. When infused in water, they yield a liquid that tastes like orange water. Such an infusion was used in the Scottish Highlands as a cosmetic to improve the complexion. A more common use of meadowsweet was to lend flavour to mead, and it is from this, rather than the word 'meadow', that the name of meadowsweet is thought to be derived. In the Scottish Highlands, the whole plant has been added to soups and stews for extra flavour.

The plant's fragrance made it of immense value as a strewing herb for the house and Elizabeth I would have nothing but meadowsweet in her chambers. Gerard in 1597 was full of praise for it:

> The leaves and flowers excel all other strowing herbes for to deck up houses, to straw [sic] in chambers, halls and banqueting houses in the summer time, for the smell thereof makes the heart merrie, delighting the senses; and neither does it cause headache, or lothsomenesse to meat, as some other sweet smelling herbes do.

Some people believed that the flowers should not be brought into the house since they could bring bad luck – an idea associated with many white flowers – but certainly this belief could not have been prevalent in Gerard's time when the plant was used liberally to rid the house of bad odours.

Milkwort
(*Polygala vulgaris*)

This tiny plant grows in short turf and grassland throughout Britain. Its flowers are deep blue, or sometimes pink or white. In Donegal, it is called 'fairy soap', and it is said that the fairies make a lather with its roots and leaves.

In the north of England, milkwort is called 'gang flower' and was a favourite plant for Rogation Week, a festivity also known as Gang Week, from the Saxon word *gang*, 'to go'. The purpose of Rogation Week was to give a blessing to the surrounding fields and livestock, and often involved a day when parishioners would walk ('go') around the edge of the parish, confirming the boundaries. This of course was in the days before maps. As part of the procession, children would carry a long pole decked with a profusion of flowers, among which milkwort was especially prominent. Records of these Rogation processions occur as early as AD 550 and the practice continued until the eighteenth century.

As the name milkwort implies, this plant was thought to increase milk production. Early mediaeval herbalists identified it as the *polygala* (much-milk) of Classical tradition. In later official medicine, Gerard in 1597 speaks of milkwort's 'virtues in procuring milke in the brests of nurses'. Pechey in 1694 mentions its purgative properties. In the nineteenth century, Johnson and Sowerby refer to the root being utilized in treating pleurisy and coughs.

There is no evidence to support the idea that milkwort actually increases milk production, and its reputation may well rest on misidentification by mediaeval herbalists. Its other main role, in assuaging coughs, seems to be better established. However, modern herbalists in this country use the non-native species *Polygala senega* and our native milkwort is now rarely used.

There are few records of milkwort in folk medicine, and those that we do have seem likely to have been 'borrowed' from written official medicine, rather than preserved as an oral tradition. There were magical uses for the plant though. In the Scottish Highlands, it would be bound together with several other plants into a magic hoop and placed under the milk vessel to prevent 'the substance of the milk from being spirited away'. Alternatively, the plant could be placed in the milk to reverse the effect of bewitchment. This was always feared because, once bewitched, the milk would not turn into butter and cheese.

Mint
(*Mentha* species)

> The savour or smell of the water Mint rejoiceth the heart of man for which
> cause they strowe it in chambers and places of recreation, pleasur, and repose,
> and where feasts and banquets are made.
>
> John Gerard, *The Herball; or, Generall Historie of Plantes* (1597)

Mint is native throughout Britain with many species cultivated for domestic use. It is perhaps best known as mint sauce – an accompaniment to lamb – and children are still sent out to the garden to pick a few sprigs for Sunday lunch. The origin of this practice makes perfect sense; mint is an aid to digestion.

Most mints in the wild grow in damp places, and water mint likes it even damper still – anyone who has walked through boggy heathland will be familiar with its pungent smell. There are a great number of different mints because the plant hybridizes readily, and the resulting group of mints is complex. Peppermint, for example, is a hybrid between *Mentha aquatica* and *M. spicata* and was first discovered in the late seventeenth century in Hertfordshire. Its flavour soon became so popular that it was widely grown and cultivated. An eighteenth-century Scottish newspaper, the *Edinburgh Evening Courant*, carried an advertisement for peppermint water 'distill'd neat and fine, as they do in London'.

Mint was a superb treatment for digestive complaints of all kinds: 'it is marvellous wholsome for the stomacke,' Gerard reported in 1597, and Culpeper in 1653 says that bites, sores, headaches and heavy periods were all greatly eased by mint. By the nineteenth century, only peppermint was still listed in the 1838 *British Herbal*, as a digestive. Modern medical herbalists use peppermint mainly to soothe wind and colic; it is a constituent in many proprietary treatments for indigestion.

In folk medicine, the plant has a long list of applications in addition to its commonly known reputation as a digestive aid. Its leaves have been

rubbed on insect bites and stings; it has been drunk hot or cold for a headache; and an infusion of water mint has been recommended for heavy colds
and flu. Athlete's foot, sore gums and hayfever have all been alleviated by it
– hayfever was eased with a sprig of mint under the pillow. Nursing mothers
relieved the pain of congested breasts by applying a hot mint poultice and,
in Yorkshire, women who experienced 'difficult monthlies' were given scalded
POPPY seeds and peppermint. Even appendicitis was treated in the early
twentieth century with a compress of ELDER and peppermint, applied externally and then injected internally into the bowel.

At home, mint has many uses. Before tea was introduced, a mint infusion
was commonly drunk in Scotland, and was a mediaeval flavouring for whisky,
too. A jar of mint kept in the house freshens the air and keeps flies and mice
away. A sprig of mint worn about the person was believed to ward off infection or if placed in milk was said to prevent it souring. If mint is rubbed
over a new beehive, it will stop the bees from deserting.

It has been suggested that when growing mint in the garden one must
not look at it for a month after planting because it is shy: 'It needs time to
settle down.'

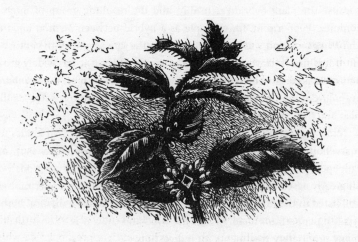

Mistletoe
(*Viscum album*)

It is easy to see why people have been fascinated by this plant. It is parasitic, growing on apple trees and occasionally on other host trees. Birds love to eat the berries and, in the process, they rub the sticky seeds off their beaks to lodge in cracks on the tree, there to germinate and form new plants. Mistletoe therefore never touches the ground, and this has lent it great symbolic significance. Its appearance is strikingly different from any other in our flora; its rounded mass of stems and paired leaves are a pale olive green, and bear the familiar white berries. Also, it is evergreen – a symbol of immortality.

Mistletoe has been revered at least since the time of the druids. It is the famous Golden Bough of legend, cut at the winter and summer solstices by Celtic druids. In Norse mythology, it was the plant accused of killing Baldur the Sun God, after all plants and animals in heaven and earth had sworn not to harm him. The mistletoe, growing as it does neither in heaven nor on earth, but in-between, was not included in this oath and the evil Norse deity Loki used the mistletoe to slay Baldur.

Within the house, mistletoe was believed to protect the inhabitants from harm and bring them good luck and fertility. In Dorset, the plant has the name 'kiss-and-go'. The familiar practice of kissing under the mistletoe at Christmas is all that remains of a much more complicated symbolism that was once attached to the plant. Even today it is considered unlucky to allow the mistletoe to touch the ground; in some areas, the Christmas mistletoe is pushed up the chimney after the festivities have ended, where it will eventually be burnt. Many churches still exclude mistletoe from their Christmas decorations because of its pagan associations.

Cutting down a tree that bears mistletoe is believed to bring catastrophe, as a famous Scottish story bears witness. The Hay family of Errol in Perthshire believed that they would flourish only as long as their great oak tree, which bore mistletoe, survived. They adopted the mistletoe as their badge, and pieces of it would be cut with great ceremony on All Hallow's Eve (the old

Celtic New Year's Eve), having walked three times round the tree sun-wise. They believed that the mistletoe could provide protection in battle, and that a sprig in a baby's cradle prevented fairies from stealing it and replacing it with a changeling. The family has scattered now, the estate is broken up and the oak no longer exists, but history does not record the order in which these events occurred!

Mistletoe was regarded in ancient Britain as a heal-all, an antidote to poison, even a resolver of conflicts. One of its Gaelic names translates as 'all-heal'. Folk medicine employed the plant in various ways. It was used in eighteenth-century Scotland for treating fevers and elsewhere for epilepsy, St Vitus's dance (a disorder of the central nervous system) and hysteria. Cut small and crushed, in the nineteenth century, it staunched bleeding. In the same century, a lady in Inverness drank an infusion of mistletoe to cure her heart palpitations; she was indeed giving herself the best cure. It is now known that mistletoe does have an action on the heart, lowering blood pressure and correcting heart rhythm. One Suffolk family with a history of strokes currently grows mistletoe for self-medication:

'We use mistletoe from our apple tree, spring and autumn, to prevent strokes – soak a leaf overnight and gently warm the next day and drink.'

Mrs D. W—, Colchester (1990)

In official medicine, the plant was recommended for epilepsy and to relieve 'hard knots, tumour and imposthumes'. Pechey in 1694 tells us that 'The Wood is chiefly used for the Falling-sickness, and is counted a specifick for it. 'Tis also used for Apoplexies and Giddiness.' Mistletoe had fallen from use in official medicine by the nineteenth century.

Today medical herbalists in this country use the plant chiefly to lower blood pressure and heart rate and as a treatment for anxiety. It is also sometimes used to treat epilepsy. The plant and particularly the berries are toxic, so mistletoe should be used only with professional guidance.

The beneficial action of mistletoe on the heart is now beginning to be understood. Current research is also lending support to its use against certain cancers: it has the surprising, dual effect of destroying some cancer cells and stimulating the body's immune system. There are clearly chapters still to be told in the story of mankind's use of mistletoe.

Monkshood
(*Aconitum napellus*)

> ... I have heard that Aconite,
> Being timely taken, hath a healing might
> Against the scorpion's stroke.

Ben Jonson, *Sejanus*, III, iii, 30–32

This is a highly poisonous member of the buttercup family, once used for putting criminals to death. On the Aegean island of Chios, it was used in ancient times for euthanasia. Much later, in a sixteenth-century experiment, two criminals were given an extract of it and both died quickly. Monkshood is native to Britain, growing locally in shady places. The deep purple-blue flowers are very beautiful and it is often cultivated as a garden plant. The intriguing shape of the flowers has led to a great variety of country names, including 'wolfsbane', 'old woman in her bed', 'three faces in one hood' and, more sinisterly, 'old woman's nightcap'.

Monkshood was probably exploited by hunters as a poison for killing prey. The generic name *Aconitum* is thought to derive from the Greek *akos*, meaning 'dart'; the implication is that darts were once made poisonous with the juice of this plant. It is not surprising to find that there are no records of its use in folk medicine. Official medical practitioners also approached the plant with great caution on account of its toxic nature and there are countless warning tales against its use.

It was thought that monkshood could counteract the effect of other poisons, a belief that Jonson referred to in his play *Sejanus* (see above). Gerard in 1597 wrote about the attempts of physicians to make counterpoisons from flies that feed on the plant. He paints a dramatic picture of the symptoms of the original poisoning: 'Their lipps and tongue swell forthwith, their eyes hang out, their thighs are stiffe, and their wits are taken from them.' An unfortunate, early-eighteenth-century incident sounds equally appalling:

A person having eaten some of the leaves of the *Aconitum napellus*, became maniacal and the surgeon who was called to his assistance declared that the plant was not the cause of his disorder; and to convince the company that it was perfectly innocent, he ate freely of its leaves, and soon after died in great agony.

Despite such disasters, monkshood was sometimes utilized by later practitioners. One nineteenth-century surgeon, Kemsey, states in 1838: 'it requires to be used cautiously. It has been advantageously employed in chronic rheumatism, gout, paralysis, schirrhus, scrofula, cancer, and intermittants [sic].'

A liniment, an ointment and a tincture of aconite are all included in the *British Pharmacopoeia* for 1914. The plant was still in use in the 1930s, but by then mainly as a liniment for relieving the pain of neuralgia and rheumatism. It was finally dropped from the official Pharmacopoeia in the 1950s.

Nowadays, monkshood is occasionally applied externally by British medical herbalists to treat neuralgia. Investigations have shown that it contains the alkaloid aconitine, which does have a pain-relieving effect but in higher doses can lead to cardiac arrest. It is clearly a plant to be used, if at all, only under professional advice.

Mugwort
(*Artemisia vulgaris*)

If they would eat nettles in March
And Mugwort in May
So many young maidens
Would not turn to clay.

Proverb

Mugwort is a very common plant, usually found growing on waste ground. It has tiny, greenish flowers borne on a tall, tough stalk, and dark green leaves with silvery undersides. When crushed, it gives off an aromatic scent reminiscent of autumn apples and chrysanthemums. It is an inconspicuous, modest plant and yet was the subject in the past of much human attention.

The clue to its value lies in the generic name of the plant; *Artemisia* is named for the goddess Artemis, famous for aiding women in childbirth. Various species of *Artemisia* have been used for treating infertility, irregular menstruation, pregnancy, labour, and possibly as contraceptives.

An Essex man recalls: 'In our garden, my father grew a clump of mugwort and I think my mother used this for irregularities peculiar to women.' This is the tail end of a tradition reaching back at least to the time of the ancient Greeks. The sensitivity surrounding gynaecology and childbirth is reflected in the fact that there are relatively few records of the folk use of mugwort in this country. What knowledge we do have has largely to be inferred, for example from old names for the plant such as 'moderwort' and 'maidenswort'. Various writers have suggested that the young maidens of the poem quoted above were suffering from consumption, but it seems more likely that they were in danger from difficult childbirth.

In thirteenth-century Wales, there was a famous family of 'hereditary' doctors who based their practice on a blend of official and folk medicine. They were known as the Physicians of Myddfai after the village they lived in and numerous legends grew up around them. They left written records of many of their remedies, including one for a difficult delivery: 'let the mugwort be bound to her left thigh'. The seventeenth- and eighteenth-century Gunton Household Book, written by successive generations of a landed family, includes a recipe for 'a poor country woman in labor': it consists simply of mugwort.

In official medicine, Pechey in 1694 tells us that: ''Tis frequently used by Women, inwardly and outwardly, in all the diseases peculiar to them.' He adds that it is also useful for 'hip-Gout' (sciatica). Salmon in 1693 states that the herb 'is specificated to the Womb' and that it provokes menstruation and facilitates birth and delivery of the afterbirth. He also refers to its role in treating jaundice, sciatica and the King's evil (scrofula).

Medical herbalists in the twentieth century have used mugwort in the treatment of amenorrhoea, anorexia and indigestion, and occasionally for roundworm infestation. Mugwort should never be taken during pregnancy because of its known action on the womb. Today its main use is as a digestive tonic.

There was a widespread belief that the plant could give strength and protection, especially to travellers. It had an aura of magic about it. The lucky charm effect was first described by Pliny the Elder (AD 23–79) and recorded in greater detail in the *Herbarium Apuleii* (*c*. AD 600):

> If any propose a journey, then let him take to him in hand this wort Artemisia,
> and let him have it with him, then he will not feel much toil in his journey.
> And it also puts to flight devil sickness; and in the house in which he, the man
> of the house, hath it within, it forbiddeth evil leechcrafts, and also turneth
> away the evil eyes of evil men.

And the belief continued. In the early years of the twentieth century in Somerset, it was said that if you put mugwort in your shoes you could run all day without getting tired. The same author records that in 1906 a Somerset man told her, 'If yew do pick'n right there idn't nothing yew can't wish vor.'

Mugwort was infinitely useful in the house (maybe a sprig or two was kept aside for sustaining long journeys). Its dried leaves have been served as a substitute for tea; it has flavoured beer, and protected clothes from moths. The herb was strewn on floors to repel fleas and smoked in lieu of tobacco – with the added benefit of helping to restore a lost appetite.

The past importance of mugwort has not been entirely forgotten. The plant is still celebrated in the Isle of Man: it is the symbol worn by everyone on Tynwald Day (the day of the opening of the Manx parliament); on a recent visit, the Queen conformed to tradition and wore a sprig of mugwort. It is also enjoying a revival in its use by acupuncturists, following in the Chinese tradition.

In the past, though, mugwort was above all a woman's herb, highly valued in an entirely practical way, as the following eighteenth-century remedy, from the Gunton Household Book testifies:

For a poor Country woman in Labour to hasten their birth

Take 3 handfuls of Mugwort, 12 cloves whole boyle them in a pint of white wine half an hour, then Strein it and let the party drink it blood warm at a draught, you may gather mugwort and dry it in a chamber and soe keep it all the year which is as useful as the green is

Mullein
(*Verbascum thapsus*)

Husbandmen of Kent do give it their cattle against the cough of the lungs, and I, therefore, mention it because cattle are also in some sort to be provided for in their diseases.

William Coles, *Adam in Eden* (1657)

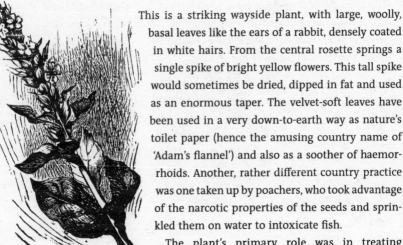

This is a striking wayside plant, with large, woolly, basal leaves like the ears of a rabbit, densely coated in white hairs. From the central rosette springs a single spike of bright yellow flowers. This tall spike would sometimes be dried, dipped in fat and used as an enormous taper. The velvet-soft leaves have been used in a very down-to-earth way as nature's toilet paper (hence the amusing country name of 'Adam's flannel') and also as a soother of haemorrhoids. Another, rather different country practice was one taken up by poachers, who took advantage of the narcotic properties of the seeds and sprinkled them on water to intoxicate fish.

The plant's primary role was in treating pulmonary complaints. In folk medicine, both leaves and flowers have been made into an infusion valued for coughs and colds, whether in humans or cattle (the plant was once called 'bullock's lungwort'). It was important to strain the flowers and leaves through muslin to avoid any hairs, which could cause itching and irritation to the mouth. The leaves, which have a pleasant, light scent when crushed, were boiled in milk to produce a remedy for pulmonary tuberculosis; this tonic was especially common in Ireland where the plant was also used to treat diarrhoea, kidney complaints, stings and sores. An infusion of the flowers was said to promote sleep.

Pechey in 1694 reports that mullein was 'used for Diseases of the Breast, for a Cough, and Spitting of Blood, and for the Gripes' in official medicine. John Moncrief's slightly tricky, eighteenth-century remedy for diarrhoea recommends 'the Smoke of Mullein taken thro' a hollow Chair'. Kemsey in 1838 advised the plant for fluxes and for swellings.

Nineteenth-century medical herbalists used mullein for bronchitis and catarrh and also, externally, for treating inflammation, as do medical herbalists in this country today.

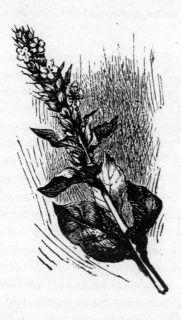

Navelwort
(*Umbilicus rupestris*)

It groweth upon Westminster Abbey, over the doore that leadeth from Chaucer's tombe to the old palace.

John Gerard, *The Herball; or, Generall Historie of Plantes* (1597)

Navelwort grows primarily in the west of Britain where it can be found tucked into the cracks and crevices of walls and stone banks. It was once much more widespread. The plant is called navelwort because of the dimple in the bright green leaf at the point where it joins the leaf stalk. 'Dimplewort' is a Devonian variation of the name, and of course the generic name *Umbilicus* refers to the same feature. The shiny, round leaves have also earned the plant the country name of 'wall pennywort'. When young and fresh, the leaves may be included in a salad.

It is not surprising that navelwort leaves have formed the basis of various children's games. In one game, two leaves were spat on and stuck together. The leaves were then thrown into the air and observed closely when they fell to the ground: if they stayed stuck together, then wet weather was coming; if they fell apart, dry weather could be expected.

Especially in the west of Britain where it is common, navelwort has been harnessed by folk medicine for the treatment of wounds and chilblains. For the latter, the 'skin' was peeled from the underside of the leaf and the exposed leaf tissue was rubbed on the chilblain. Sore breasts were similarly treated. Even the leaf 'skin' had a value; in Cornwall, it was applied like a plaster to an embedded thorn and, in a day or two, would draw it out. Warts and corns were also rubbed with navelwort leaves; in Worcestershire the plant is called 'corn-leaves'. In Wales, burns were soothed with a mixture of navelwort and unsalted butter and, in the nineteenth century, navelwort was used 'by the peasantry' for treating sore eyes. The herb was apparently a remedy for epilepsy in the west of England. In the Isle of Man, it seems to have been particularly highly valued: there it was used to treat bruises, scalds, whitlows and erysipelas (a particularly nasty skin infection).

Pechey in 1694 tells us that in official medicine navelwort is good for 'Inflammations, and St Anthony's fire [erysipelas]' and recommends an ointment prepared from the herb for treating chilblains, 'kibes [sore, cracked skin]' and scrofula. Kemsey was still advocating it in the nineteenth century for the same ailments, but thereafter it was dropped from official practice. Modern medical herbalism in this country makes little or no use of the plant.

We can still find vestiges of the use of navelwort in folk medicine. This Wiltshire family's recipe for a healing ointment has been handed down through many generations, and was used within living memory.

Grandmother's ointment

2lb mutton- or deer-fat

3oz beeswax

$^1/_2$ pint salad oil

2 handfuls elderflowers, gathered fresh

2 handfuls of the inner bark of the elder

2 handfuls of the inner bark of the elm

2 dozen young, green ivy leaves

2 handfuls of laurel leaves

2 handfuls of the hart's tongue fern

2 handfuls of houseleek

2 handfuls of navelwort

2 handfuls of wild geranium [HERB ROBERT]

2 handfuls of scrophularia [FIGWORT]

Boil this very slowly together in just enough water to cover it for a long time, then strain it through muslin. It must be well mixed and melted together in the oven before it is potted and tied down. It will keep for years and is excellent for burns, broken chilblains or any kind of sores.

Mrs M. M—, Wiltshire (1998)

Nettle
(*Urtica dioica, Urtica urens*)

I hate thee nettle.
What's thy place
In earth's economy?
I care not I ne'er see thy face
Nor folks that act like thee.

James Rigg, *The Poet to the Nettle* (1897)

The nettle is a very vigorous and variable plant, which makes it a great survivor. For thousands of years, it has flourished as a weed of cultivated ground, and it is probably one of the few wild plants that everyone in Britain is aware of. As Culpeper said in 1653, it can easily be found on the darkest night. Although its sting has given it a bad press, it deserves better because it is an invaluable plant; many of its past applications are extremely surprising.

The nettle plant contains strong fibres, some of them as much as three inches long individually, and they have been used at least since the Bronze Age for making cloth and cord. The poet Thomas Campbell (1777–1844) commented in his letters on the relative lack of English interest in nettle cloth:

> In Scotland, I have eaten nettles, I have slept in nettle sheets, and I have dined off a nettle tablecloth. The stalks of the old nettle are as good as flax for making cloth. I have heard my mother say that she thought nettle cloth more durable than any other species of linen.

The use of nettle fibre for clothing was not just a Scottish curiosity. A famous Hans Christian Andersen fairy tale tells the story of a girl who had to weave eleven nettle shirts in order to break a spell that had been cast over her brothers, turning them into swans. It has been estimated that eighty-eight pounds of nettles are needed to make one shirt.

During the First World War when cotton was scarce, nettle fibre was collected on a huge scale in Germany and Austria, for the manufacture of cloth for military uniforms. Captured German overalls were analysed and found to be composed of 85 per cent nettle fibre as well as 15 per cent ramie fibre (from a tropical member of the nettle family). In 1916 in Germany, 2,700 tonnes of nettle fibre were collected, and the natural supply could no longer keep up with demand. Attempts were made to cultivate nettles for this purpose, but with mixed success. During the Second World War, green dye prepared from nettles was used in Britain for camouflage uniforms. There were even plans for the construction of aircraft wings from nettle fibre.

There were serious food shortages in 1940s Britain, and many people resorted to using nettles in cooking. For many this was simply a continuation of an old tradition. The young growing tips may be steamed and eaten like spinach, but care must be taken to gather only young nettles because older plants are toxic. In the past, this was common knowledge and enshrined in many popular sayings, for example that the devil used nettles in May to make his shirts. Many traditional recipes emphasize that young nettles only should be used, such as this one from the Scottish Highlands for nettle broth:

> Gather young nettles from the higher part of the wall where they are clean. Wash the tops in salted water and chop very finely. Have some good stock boiling – chicken stock is best – in which you have cooked a sufficient quantity of barley. Add the nettles, simmer till tender, and season to taste.

The nettle is a prime example of how in the recent past food and medicine overlapped. It was commonly known that nettles were good for the health. Within living memory, a nettle pudding was made in East Anglia from young nettle tops in aspic or egg white. This was a spring pudding, used as a pick-me-up after the winter. Samuel Pepys records in his diary in 1661 eating nettle pudding and finding it very good. Other springtime tonics included nettle beer prepared from the roots and nettle tea:

> Great emphasis was placed on keeping the bowels open and the pores closed and of cleansing the blood after the rigours of winter, and so in the spring we were sent to gather young nettles. Nettle tea we had to drink to purify our

blood, Grandpa (unwillingly) for his sciatica and Aunt Rose for her pleurisy. I wondered how it knew which it was supposed to do.

Mrs E. M—, Essex Age Concern essay (1991)

Nettles are excellent in the treatment of anaemia because of their high iron content, and were often used to counter the effects of heavy periods. For this they are particularly effective, since they have blood-staunching properties as well as being iron-rich. In the manuscript notes kept by an eighteenth-century surgeon–apothecary in Dalkeith, there is an entry concerning a patient whose heavy periods had returned six times in three months. She was 'prescrib'd nettles, knowing how she dislik'd all shop medicines'.

Country people with arthritis and rheumatism eased the pain with nettles, an application that is now being vindicated by the discovery of anti-inflammatory polysaccharides in the plant. In a small recent trial (C. Randall et al. and J. Roy) of people who had osteo-arthritis at the base of the thumb, rubbing daily with a stinging nettle was shown to produce better pain relief than in the control group. Although it sounds heroic to beat the aching parts with stinging nettles, it does apparently bring great relief. There are still elderly people in East Anglia who practise this. It is thought that the Roman nettle (*Urtica pilulifera*) was introduced to this country for similar use by Roman troops.

The following story illustrates the importance of accurately preserving the details of how plants were used in the past. In an eighteenth-century book on farriery, there is a strange piece of advice to ensure a horse becomes pregnant. It claims that the mare should be beaten with nettles before the stallion arrives. I mentioned this to a Norfolk horseman who had spent sixty years with shire horses, leading a stallion around from farm to farm, often sleeping with it at night. He looked at me with disbelief, and then his face cracked into a smile and he laughed with sheer delight at the stupidity of such learned authors.

'They books, they get it ALL wrong. You beat the mare AFTER the stallion has been!'

Of course this makes much more sense, since the stinging nettle would make the mare's hindquarters contract.

There are numerous other folk medical applications for nettles. They have been used for nosebleeds, and the juice to treat burns and rashes and as a gargle. The juice has even been dripped into the ear for earache and, in the eighteenth century, a concoction of chopped nettles and egg white was applied to the temples to cure insomnia. Nettles have even had a role in slimming. An anonymous twentieth-century pamphlet tells us that 'twenty to thirty crushed nettle seeds taken night and morning, is the best remedy for stout people, which will prevent burdensome fat surrounding the kidneys.'

Nettles were used for a wide variety of ailments in official medicine. Salmon in 1693 states that 'used as a pot herb they loosen the belly, cleanse the Reins [kidneys] and expel the Stone [large urinary stones]'. He recommends them too for diseases of the lungs. Nettle leaves, he adds, are 'antidotes against Hemlock and Henbane', but he makes no mention of their role in treating bleeding. Pechey in 1694 similarly emphasizes nettle's efficacy for kidney and lung complaints, but adds that the juice or crushed herb put up the nostrils is good for stopping a nosebleed. By the nineteenth century, the nettle is still in official use 'to open the pipes and passages of the lungs'.

In the nineteenth and early twentieth centuries, medical herbalists in this country have prescribed nettles for coughs and shortness of breath. Currently the number of ailments treated with nettles is impressive: allergies, anaemia, arthritic problems, heavy menstrual bleeding, low milk production and skin conditions. The list now includes benign prostate enlargement – a use now vindicated by recent research. The future for the humble nettle certainly looks promising.

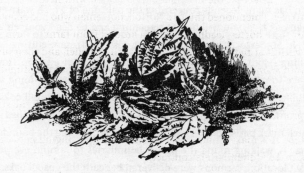

Oak
(*Quercus robur*)

Wae's me! Wae's me!
The acorn is not yet
Fallen from the tree,
That's to grow the wood,
That's to make the cradle,
That's to rock the bairn,
That's to grow to a man,
That's to lay me.

'The Cauld Lad of Hilton', from *Popular Songs and Nursery Rhymes*,
ed. James Orchard Halliwell (1849)

This species of oak is the quintessentially English tree and our culture has held it in high esteem for many centuries. Deciduous woodland is the natural climax vegetation for much of Britain and before the advent of man the oak would have formed extensive areas of forest. Natural oak woodland is now scarce; there are fragments remaining in Scotland and Ireland, and a few of our ancient woodlands, such as Hatfield Forest, survive in England. We have an impressive legacy of ancient specimen oaks, many of them planted in parkland.

Britain has many legends concerning the oak, one of which warns that if you fell an oak tree, you will hear it screaming and be dead yourself within the year. In Somerset, it was believed that oak trees resent cutting – never mind felling – so it is bad luck even to travel near coppiced oaks. However, if you have to cut one down, it is wise to sing psalms while doing so and carry a Bible in your pocket. As a result of this reluctance to fell oaks, they became prominent boundary markers; this is the origin of the so-called gospel oaks, which mark parish borders. When the annual 'beating the bounds' took place, that is, walking round the parish boundaries to remind everyone of their exact location, sermons were delivered beneath the gospel oaks.

Several individual oak trees have become famous for their historical associations. The Boscobel Oak in Shropshire, in which Charles II hid after the Battle of Worcester, gave rise to the tradition of Royal Oak Day on 29 May. It is also known as Oak Apple Day, when sprigs of oak are worn in memory of Charles' escape. The oak tree in which Robert Kett hid before he led a famous rebellion against the enclosure of common land in 1549 still stands, and is known as Kett's Oak. In Sherwood Forest, the Major Oak, said to be Robin Hood's hiding place, is so important to the area as a tourist attraction that it has recently been cloned to preserve it for the future. Near Dunkeld in Scotland is the Birnam Oak, thought to be the last remaining tree of Birnam Wood, made famous in *Macbeth*. The spirit of the oak itself became identified with the Green Man, a symbol of man and nature. In carvings, the Green Man is usually depicted surrounded by oak leaves.

Ancient trees were seen as having great powers. It is considered auspicious to dream of oak; this can foretell long life and wealth. In Devon, acorns were used to foretell the outcome of a love affair. Two acorns were floated on water; if they drew together, then the pair would marry.

In folk medicine, oak played a role in symbolic healing, of fevers in particular. This was achieved by taking the sick person to a crossroads where an oak was planted; the illness was then 'transferred' to the tree. Oak trees growing at Berkhampstead, Hertfordshire, in the nineteenth century were famed for this healing power. The patient was taken to one of the trees, a lock of their hair was nailed to the trunk and wrenched out with a jerk so that the hair, and hopefully the fever too, were transferred to the tree.

In more practical folk medicine, ground acorns in milk sometimes served in the treatment of diarrhoea but it was the bark of the oak that was particularly effective in many illnesses. An infusion of bark was prescribed for rheumatism and a gargle was prepared from the bark in the Scottish Highlands. It was also widely used for these ailments in Ireland, as well as for hardening the feet in the summertime and for toothache and ulcers.

In official medicine, Gerard in 1597 recommended oak apples (galls formed on oak by wasps) ground in white wine vinegar to remove skin blemishes and to dye hair black. An ink could also be obtained from the galls. Culpeper in 1653 advocated the distilled water of oak buds for treating inflammations. In the seventeenth century, a bath in which oak bark had been soaked was advised for healing the wounds of those who had been 'cut for the Stone [large urinary stones]'. Grated acorn in white wine was said to be good for a stitch, as were roasted acorns ground with cinammon for a rupture. Kemsey in 1838 states that a decoction of oak bark was used for treating diarrhoea, as a gargle and as a wash for piles.

Nineteenth- and early twentieth-century herbalists utilized oak bark's 'astringent' qualities to check diarrhoea and as a gargle for sore throat. Today medical herbalists in this country use it similarly; as well as for tonsillitis and haemorrhoids.

The economic uses of oak have been diverse and numerous. Its timber is durable and strong, making it extremely valuable. Apart from its obvious role in the building of houses and boats, oak has been exploited as a source of fuel, of charcoal, for smoking fish, for tanning leather and for dyeing. It has been estimated that the roof of the great Hall of Stirling Castle required two hundred oak trees. A stick of oak was often used to preserve yeast for brewing; it was dipped in the culture and thoroughly coated with it, then dried for future use. A very humble application of the mighty oak occurred in Scotland, where oak twigs served as toothbrushes.

Onion
(*Allium cepa*)

To dream of eating onions means
Much strife in thy domestic scenes,
Secrets found out or else betrayed,
And many falsehoods made and said.

T. F. Thiselton Dyer, *The Folk-lore of Plants* (1889)

Like GARLIC, the onion's exact origin is obscure. We know that onions were eaten in Egypt about 3000 BC. The Norse Sagas tell how they were used to assess the gravity of wounds, in a kind of triage: they were fed to the injured man, and if his wounds subsequently smelt of onions, he was given up for dead and attention turned to others in a less serious state. In Britain, they have formed part of our diet for as long as there are written records. Onion had a reputation as an aphrodisiac, and to dream of onions, as in the rhyme above, could foretell discord in one's love life. Alternatively, an onion dream could also predict illness.

Onion is a notable exception to the generalization that only native plants were used in folk medicine. It was however widely available and this is quite likely the reason why it features in such a large number of folk remedies. In a recent collection of remedies used within living memory, it is one of the most commonly mentioned plants.

The widely held belief that onions could fend off infection has been passed down from generation to generation, from the days when bunches of onions were hung up in an attempt to stop the spread of plague. Mr M—, of Wymondham in Norfolk and in his seventies, who was brought up in Ayrshire by his grandmother, recalled in 1987 being told as a small boy about a village that was almost wiped out by a fever when his grandmother was a child. His forebear's household was one of the few to survive because, according to his grandmother, 'it was all hung about with onions'. Even today, many people believe that a cut onion on a saucer will remove infection from the air.

A great number of common ailments such as coughs and colds were treated with onions prepared in various ways. Onions cooked in milk provided a cure for colds and fevers and the juice of the onion was widely used as a cough medicine, but specially prepared, as in this recipe:

1lb nice onions, chopped
1lb demerara sugar
1 lemon

Chop onions, mix sugar and juice of one lemon. Leave in cool place for a day or two and strain off syrup into a container. Excellent for bronchitis or chest coughs. I have used this since I was young and I am now 92 years old.

Mrs W. B—, Essex Age Concern essay (1991)

An alternative preparation, this time for bronchitis, was to make a thick onion gruel:

'Onions chopped and cooked slowly in milk. Well drained and the stock used for making a thick white sauce. All returned to the pan where salt and a very generous amount of pepper added. Made very hot and then served in a basin with a large knob of butter (which was homemade). Father would tuck a handkerchief under his chin and really enjoy his supper.'

Mrs D. H—, Essex (1991)

A very simple remedy for earache was to place a small, roasted onion in the ear. The warmth was soothing and apparently the treatment was often effective. Onions were also rubbed on chilblains, insect stings and minor burns. Even the transparent 'skins' from the fleshy scale leaves (layers) of an onion were employed in folk medicine, as a kind of natural elastoplast. It is clear now why these remedies worked. Studies have shown that onion contains a whole host of formerly unknown chemicals, including allicin, which has antibiotic properties, and allylpropyldisulphide, which is found to be effective in the treatment of asthma.

In official medicine, Gerard in 1597 recommended onion for treating the bites of mad dogs, for baldness, scalds and fevers. Pechey in 1694 tells us that 'Old Women cut a raw Onion, and infuse it in Water all Night; and the next Morning give the Water to Children, to kill the Worms, with good

Success.' By the nineteenth century, the only use of onion suggested by Kemsey in the *British Herbal* is as a cough medicine.

Coughs and colds are still treated with onion by our modern medical herbalists. They also use it to poultice sores and as an aid to oral health. New applications have been found for the humble onion; studies have shown that, like GARLIC, it can be helpful in fending off angina and heart attacks. When all the family's coughs and colds have been cured, here is an unusual way of using up the spare onions:

Where gilt frames become dull, freshen them up this way!

To half a pint of water add sufficient flowers of sulphur to give a golden tinge and in this boil 4 or 5 bruised onions. Strain off liquid and when cold apply to frames with a soft brush. When dry they will look as good as new.

J. D—, Great Waltham (1991)

Orpine
(*Sedum telephium*)

We have heard of its being used in some country districts as a decoration for a fireplace-screen or chimney-board, a framework of wood being covered with the plant. We are told that if this be sprinkled with water about once a week, it will continue fresh and green-looking for some months.

F. Edward Hulme, *Familiar Wild Flowers* (c.1910)

This is a scarce plant of woodland edges, which may or may not be truly native to Britain. It has succulent, rounded leaves and pretty, starry, rose-coloured flowers and was once widely grown in gardens. Among its many country names are 'live long' and 'midsummer men'. This last name refers to its use in love divination, in which orpine has a long history. At least since the seventeenth century, sprigs of orpine would be brought into the house in the evening on Midsummer's Day. One sprig represented the man, one the woman. They were placed in cracks in the joists of houses, or, more recently, jammed in empty cotton reels. If in the morning the two sprigs leaned towards each other, all would be well, and the lovers faithful; if they leaned away from each other, then one or other lover would be unfaithful.

The main medicinal use of orpine was as a wound-healer: the generic name *Sedum* means 'to assuage'. In official medicine, Culpeper in 1653 recommended the plant for burns, ruptures and wounds and Pechey in 1694 tells us that "Tis excellent for Easing Pain, both in fresh Wounds, and old Ulcers.' By the nineteenth century, it was still advised for fluxes, inflammation and wounds. Today's medical herbalists rarely use the plant.

Orpine was sometimes used in folk medicine, although it was probably never common enough in the wild to have been used widely. It was grown in gardens in the eighteenth century as a wound-healing plant and, in the nineteenth century, it was described as 'a popular vulnerary'. It may well have been the 'heal-all' included in a Cambridgeshire garden in the early years of the twentieth century as first aid for the family. The 'wrong' (lower) side of the leaf was used to draw out pus, the 'right' (upper) side to heal it:

> '... regarding the Heal-all leaf ... it was green all year round as far as I can remember ... it was used for all sorts of cuts and infections. A lot cheaper then than what we have to pay today for little ailments.'

Mrs E. R—, Quy, Cambridgeshire (1990)

Johnson in 1862 describes orpine providing a treatment for piles and diarrhoea in domestic medicine. The young leaves may be eaten as salad, and the roots can be pickled.

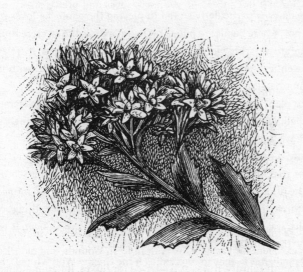

Ox-eye Daisy
(*Leucanthemum vulgare*)

This large, bright daisy of grassland and road verges is easily spotted growing en masse when driving down the motorway. In Classical times it was dedicated to the moon goddess Diana, hence its vernacular name 'moon daisy'. Diana was seen as a protectress of women and children, so the belief arose that it was a herb for women. The moon daisy was still employed in twentieth-century Somerset, in a spell to bring back an unfaithful lover. In Christian times the name was changed, and the flower dedicated to Mary Magdalen. Gerard in 1597 refers to it as 'maudlinwort' and it is still called maudlin in some parts of the country.

This large daisy is particularly suited to playing the game 'he loves me, he loves me not', where petals are pulled off one at a time; the last remaining petal gives the answer. This widespread game was still remembered in Ireland in the late twentieth century; in England it is more often played with the smaller common DAISY.

The entire plant has an acrid taste and in earlier times was extremely useful in repelling fleas. Despite this, the leaves can be used, sparingly, in salad. They have 'a slightly aromatic flavour, when fresh'.

Medicinally, the plant's uses have varied but it seems to have been particularly good for treating coughs and asthma. In folk medicine in the Scottish Highlands, the juice was mixed with honey for a cough cure and an infusion drunk for asthma; in Ireland, for coughs in general and also for bathing sore eyes. The juice was also utilized as a wound-healer. Infused in beer, it was employed by 'the country people' for treating jaundice.

In official medicine, Pechey in 1694 called it the Greater Wild White Daisy. 'The Flowers cast forth Beams of Brightness', he says, and he recommends an infusion of the whole plant for asthma, consumption and difficulty of breathing, as well as an external or internal application for wounds and ulcers. The herb has another attribute, too, which is slightly puzzling: 'A Decoction of the Herb cures all Diseases that are occasion'd by drinking cold Beer when the Body is hot.' The famous eighteenth-century physician from

Edinburgh, William Buchan, wrote a book called *Domestic Medicine* (1769), which ran to innumerable editions. This extract from the third edition of 1774 shows that Pechey's belief was still held in Buchan's time:

> Nothing is more common than for people when hot, to drink freely of cold small liquors. This conduct is extremely dangerous ... It would be tedious to enumerate all the bad effects which flow from drinking cold thin liquors when the body is hot. Sometimes this has occasioned immediate death. Hoarseness, quinseys, and fevers of various kinds are its common consequences.'

A hundred and fifty years later, Kemsey recommends ox-eye daisy simply as a wound-healer. Nineteenth- and early-twentieth-century herbalists applied it internally for asthma and coughs and externally as a wash for ulcers and wounds. It seems now to have fallen from use among medical herbalists in this country.

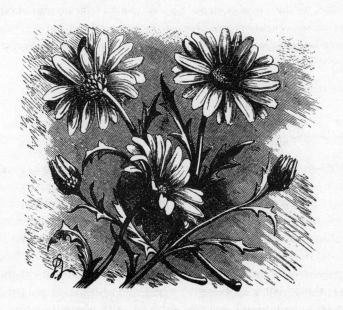

Pellitory-of-the-wall
(*Parietaria judaica*)

> ... a good old woman—
> ... did cure me,
> With sodden ale and pellitorie o' the wall;
>
> Ben Jonson, *The Alchemist*, III, iv, 144–146

As its name suggests, this member of the nettle family typically grows in the niches of stone walls and high hedges. It occurs throughout Britain, but is uncommon in Scotland. In official medicine, it was famous for treating gravel and stone (urinary stones) and dropsy. Culpeper in 1653 heartily recommends it for these conditions and goes on to list a large number of other uses: bruises, coughs, earache, skin conditions, sore throat and suppressed menstruation. Salmon in 1693 was a staunch advocate of it, because it brought him back from the brink of serious illness:

> A Syrup of the juice and honey cures the Dropsy to admiration. Therewith, my Father cured me of the Dropsie Anasarca, when I was a Youth, and the hope of life but small; I took 2 or 3 spoonfulls of this Syrup every Morning and Evening for a Month together, and became well, without so much as once purging.

The herb's uses in folk medicine have been varied, including by gypsies to treat ulcers, sores and piles. Its application for urinary complaints seems to have been borrowed from official medicine: there are few convincing records of its folk usage in this way. Mary Thorne Quelch, writing in 1941, describes it as 'one of the old remedies which have not been surpassed, and sufferers from stone, gravel and dropsy, or from any disorder which causes suppression of the urine, will find help from this homely herb'. It was drunk as an infusion, either on its own or mixed with WILD CARROT and parsley piert (*Aphanes arvensis*), and was also said to be 'the certain cure for whooping cough'.

The plant continued to be used primarily for gravel and stone and present-day medical herbalists still use the plant for kidney conditions of many kinds, thus continuing the herbal tradition.

There were some less prosaic uses for pellitory too. Apparently when burnt the plant gives off the smell of hellfire, and so in mediaeval times was burnt to drive off the devil. Could this be related to the use of the plant in Ireland, where it is called peniterry? There it was invoked by scared school-boys to save them from punishment:

> Peniterry, peniterry, that grows by the wall
> Save me from a whipping, or I pull you roots and all

Britten and Holland (1886)

The last word has not yet been written on this plant. It is known to contain sulphur and to be rich in potassium nitrate (hence the smell of hellfire?) and these made the plant useful in cleaning the glass lamp-covers of the past. Yet another practical use of this inconspicuous plant was reported by Anne Pratt in the nineteenth century. The leaves scattered in granaries were said to destroy corn weevils.

Pennyroyal
(*Mentha pulegium*)

This member of the mint family is now very scarce, having once been abundant. In 1946, Mary Thorne Quelch described it as 'common on the sides of ditches and in marshlands in many parts of Britain. Here in the south it flourishes amazingly.' Sadly, no longer.

Like other mints, pennyroyal has been used as a culinary herb and brought into cultivation. Gerard in 1597 states that pennyroyal is used by sailors to sweeten their drinking water when at sea, a use which can be traced back to the natural historian Pliny the Elder (AD 23–79). The plant had a reputation as an insect repellent, and was picked and brought into houses for this purpose; the specific name *pulegium* comes from the Latin *pulex*, meaning 'a flea'. Pechey in 1694 mentions that 'The fresh Herb wrap'd in a Cloth, and laid in a Bed, drives away Fleas; but it must be renewed once a Week.' To keep mosquitos at bay, fresh pennyroyal was rubbed onto the skin.

In folk medicine, the herb was employed as an abortifacient, although, unsurprisingly for such a sensitive subject, records of this are few and hard to find. There is evidence of its use in this way from several areas of the east of England, and in other areas it was known as an emmenagogue (provoking menstruation), a term often used as a euphemism for abortion. Pennyroyal also, like other mints, alleviated coughs and colds; in the west of the country, the plant was called 'organ' and tea prepared from it was given for chills. An infusion was considered a pleasant and refreshing drink and was traditionally carried out to the fields for Devonian harvesters, while sailors there used it to 'sweeten' their drinking water at sea. In the Isle of Man, the herb was pounded with meal to provide a dressing for burns.

Dioscorides in the first century AD noted that pennyroyal provokes menstruation and labour. Official medicine in this country used it for these purposes. Gerard in 1597 tells us that it 'provoketh the monthly termes, bringeth forth ... the dead childe'. Pechey in 1694 adds other roles for the plant, in treating coughs, dropsy, gripes, jaundice and stone (large urinary stones). But by the nineteenth century, it was little used in official medicine.

Kemsey writing in 1838 says that it is 'now justly considered of little or no value: this is the College account'.

Nineteenth-century medical herbalists meanwhile still prescribed pennyroyal for 'obstructed menstruation' and as an infusion for flatulence and sickness 'as it is very warming and grateful to the stomach'. Today, medical herbalists in this country recommend pennyroyal for indigestion and minor respiratory complaints. Two millennia after Dioscorides, we now know that pennyroyal contains the compound pulegone, which powerfully stimulates uterine contractions, provoking menstruation and causing abortion. It should be avoided during pregnancy.

In Yorkshire it used to be called 'pudding-yerb', because it was used to flavour black puddings there [Britten and Holland]. Combined with honey and pepper it once formed a well-known stuffing [Grieve]. This plant is another example of the overlap in the past between food and medicine. It has been suggested that in India many women knew of the contraceptive benefits of certain plants and would add them to the daily diet [Riddle]. It is not inconceivable that pudding-yerb was used in the same way in this country. As one early twentieth-century writer rather delicately puts it, 'Pennyroyal Tea is an old-fashioned remedy for colds and menstrual derangements.' A district nurse in Yorkshire in the 1950s records that pennyroyal was used 'to get a woman to abort if she had too many children' [Nurse S.]. Significantly it was taken with Holland's Gin (see JUNIPER) and was used at the time a period was expected, so that the woman would not know whether she had become pregnant or not. This would make the method more acceptable to many.

Periwinkle
(*Vinca* species)

The periwinkle grows in woods and shady places throughout Britain. It spreads by means of runners, which readily root to form a continuous carpet of shiny, evergreen leaves and beautiful, purple-blue flowers. The generic name comes from the middle Latin *pervincula*, meaning 'to bind about', and the plant lends itself to the making of garlands and cords. Following the overthrow of William Wallace, who fought the English king for Scottish rule, his fellow rebel Simon Fraser wore a garland of periwinkle on the way to Wallace's execution in 1306.

Periwinkle has for most of recorded time had magical associations, remembered still in its country name 'sorcerer's violet'. In Apuleius Platonicus's *Herbarium*, written in the second century AD, the herb is recommended for devil sickness, envy and terror. When gathering the plant, the harvester should say:

> I pray thee, *vinca pervinca*, thee that art to be had for thy many useful qualities,
> that thou come to me glad, blossoming with thy mainfulness; that thou outfit
> me so that I be shielded, and ever prosperous, and undamaged by poisons.

In folklore, there is a tradition that periwinkle reinforces the bond between husband and wife if they eat the leaves together and Culpeper refers to this idea in 1653. In the more recent past, periwinkle planted in a couple's first garden was said to ensure a happy marriage.

Chewing the leaves was recommended in folk medicine to staunch bleeding, especially from the nose. Boils, bruises, cuts, skin irritations and sores were all treated with periwinkle, or 'cutfinger' as it is also known. Chewing the leaves was also said to prevent nightmares.

''Tis a famous Vulnerary', proclaimed Pechey in 1694, and he advocates its use in official medicine for bleeding at the nose, dysentery, heavy periods and piles, as well as for poulticing 'a Scrophulous Tumour'. By the nineteenth century, periwinkle was still officially recommended: 'the leaves chewed stays bleeding. The decoction is used for staying fluxes', wrote Kemsey in 1838.

Periwinkle had a reputation for curing cramp. William Coles in the seventeenth century recorded the story of a friend 'vehemently tormented with the cramp for a long while which could be by no means eased till he had wrapped some of the branches hereof about his limbs'. Periwinkle also had a reputation for curing cramp in folk medicine. In Somerset, an infusion of the leaves was drunk, but in other areas a piece of the plant was placed in the bed, or wrapped around the body, as described above.

Medical herbalists in the nineteenth and twentieth centuries have treated bleeding, and especially heavy periods, with periwinkle, as well as mouth ulcers and sore throats. Today medical herbalists in this country still recommend it for staunching bleeding and for gingivitis (gum disease), mouth ulcers and sore throats.

Periwinkle has recently been shown to contain a substance, vincamine, which increases the blood supply to the brain (could this explain its use in preventing nightmares?). Following this discovery, periwinkle is now used in the treatment of some forms of dementia. A cousin of our British periwinkle, the Madagascar periwinkle (*Vinca rosea*), has recently become famous for its beneficial effects on some types of cancer. The vinca-alkaloids isolated from it have been used in the battle against childhood leukaemia and Hodgkin's disease.

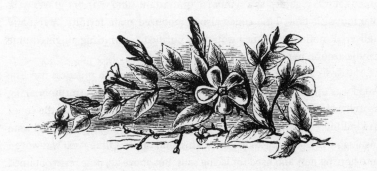

Pine

(*Pinus sylvestris* and other species)

The Scots pine is the only pine tree native to Britain and five thousand years ago was widespread throughout the country, in particular covering large areas of northern Scotland. Today the only remnants of natural pine forest are in the Scottish Highlands, in the remains of what was once the great Caledonian forest. The characteristic, asymmetrical crown of the Scots pine (*Pinus sylvestris*) and its reddish bark mark it out from other species. But in pine forests of all kinds, the lovely smell of the needles underfoot and the sound of the wind in the trees are both evocative of wild, open spaces. A walk in a pine forest is undoubtedly good for the soul.

In much of East Anglia as well as Dorset, pine was extensively planted as windbreaks in the eighteenth and nineteenth centuries. The tree is said to have been planted in the Cotswolds in areas sympathetic to the Jacobite cause. Old drovers' routes were often marked out with pine trees, making them important landmarks.

As one would expect, it is Scotland that has used the plant the most. There the tree has been used symbolically in many ceremonies. Like other evergreens, it was regarded as a symbol of immortality and warriors' graves were planted with pine. Pine cones also symbolized male fertility. A recently delivered mother in Orkney would be 'purified' by whirling a lighted pine candle around her bed.

The Scots had numerous ways of putting the pine to practical use. The wood was often employed in boat-building, building and furniture-making as well as being an important source of fuel. Children still gather the cones as kindling; cones were sometimes known as pine 'apples'. Pine roots were invaluable in thatching and rope-making, and the root fibre itself was woven into herring nets and used for lacing sails. But above all, pine resin obtained from making cuts in the bark seems to have been highly prized. Uncovering the resin-rich roots of ancient pines trapped in bogs was a long job, but worth it. They were used as torchlights, burning fiercely but quickly. The job of replenishing the torch was usually given to the youngest member of the household. Night-fishing was sometimes carried out by the light of these pine torches. Paints, tars and varnishes were all obtained from pine resin.

In folk medicine, the resin also provided an antiseptic dressing; the following incident took place in the 1930s in England.

> I grew up in a small village at the edge of a forest ... During summer, children walked without shoes and one day I had a rusty nail sticking in my foot. I pulled it out myself and went on playing. After some days my foot became painful and I noticed pus coming from the wound. Granny went to the nearby woods and collected resin from the pine trees. This was put on a little linen pad, softened on the warm kitchen range and put onto my sore. I could soon feel a drawing sensation. When checked after some days, the wound was beautifully clean and it had healed nicely.

Mrs B—, Essex Age Concern essay (1991)

The same lady remembers a cough medicine prepared from the very young shoots of pine, matured with sugar on a sunny windowsill. A very similar remedy was employed in Scotland. Also in Scotland, pine bark was used to treat fevers and its buds for scurvy. A pure and simple aid to speedy recovery for convalescents was to walk in pine woods and breathe in the fragrant air.

Various species of pine have been used in official medicine since Classical times. Pine was recommended by Pechey in 1694 for the treatment of fluxes as well as kidney stones, lung diseases and scurvy. In addition, he tells us that 'The Nuts have a delicate taste, and are good for Coughs and Consumptions, and for Heat of Urine. They increase Milk, and provoke Venery.' Resin was collected to treat wounds, ulcers and diseases of the lungs at that time, and resin from various species of pine was still listed in the *British Pharmacopoiea* of 1932.

Today's medical herbalists use Scots pine needles, as well as an essential oil obtained from them, as a respiratory antiseptic; the seeds are used for bronchitis, tuberculosis and urinogenital problems. Oil distilled from the needles is also used as a rub for muscle stiffness and arthritic problems. Care should be taken since pine can produce an allergic reaction in some people.

Poplar
(*Populus* species)

Skirting the stream, that softly choirs,
The Beech has lit her farewell fires
Beneath the Poplar's amber spires.

Whose leaves, when fitful breezes wake,
All pattering, dancing, shimmering shake,
Like big rain o'er a sleeping lake.

James Rigg, *In October* (1897)

Of this large family, only two types of poplar are native to Britain, the black poplar (*Populus nigra*) and the aspen (*P. tremula*), but numerous other species have been introduced for screening, timber and wind protection, because they are fast-growing. Lombardy poplars (*P. nigra* 'Italica') in particular were planted in great numbers in cities, often to hide unsightly buildings. The white poplar (*P. alba*), which used to be called the 'abel', has grown in England since the thirteenth century, but is not thought to be a true native.

All poplars share the same characteristic, delicate tremble of their leaves in the wind. The aspen's leaf stalk is flattened at right angles to the leaf blade, so that the leaf shivers in the smallest air current. It is believed that the trembling of poplar leaves on a still day in summer indicates the approach of rain, so that the poplar has sometimes been called 'the weather tree'. There is a legend that Christ's cross was made from poplar or aspen wood and since then the leaves have shivered with shame. Perhaps because of this, in some parts of Britain there is a prohibition against making farm implements or boats from aspen wood. Similarly, on St Michael's Day in Scotland, poplar wood would be excluded from the firewood pile used for cooking. Paradoxically, this legend has also made the wood blessed in the eyes of some, so that teething rings in the Scottish Highlands were sometimes made from aspen wood.

Medicinally, the poplar had a variety of uses, especially as a painkiller. In official medicine, a famous ointment called populeon was prepared from poplar buds to treat inflammation and pain and to dry up milk at weaning. Gerard in 1597 warns that white poplar bark 'is reported to make a woman barren', but he recommends it particularly for sciatica and gives this translation of an old Latin verse by Sammonicus:

An hidden disease doth oft rage and raine
The hip overcome and vex with paine
It makes with vile aching one tread slow and shrinke
The bark of White Poplar is helpe had in drinke.

Culpeper in 1653 suggests poplar juice to ease earache, and the leaves bruised in vinegar for gout. Pechey in 1694 similarly tells us that the buds of black poplar are good for easing pain, and are also used by women 'to thicken and beautifie their Hair'. John Moncrief in his book *The Poor Man's Physician* (1741) states that 'Green leaves of Poplar-tree, bruised and applied, cureth swollen knees'.

Poplar does not seem to have been used much in folk medicine. Within living memory in Somerset, an infusion prepared by boiling white poplar bark was administered as a cure for fevers, indigestion and night sweats. This might however be a remedy 'borrowed' from the learned tradition.

Poplar is now known to contain salicylates (populin and salicin), which have anti-fever and analgesic properties like those of aspirin. Today's medical herbalists use aspen to alleviate the pain of arthritis as well as diarrhoea and urinary tract infections.

The wood of black poplar has been used for centuries. It is resistant to splitting and this makes it eminently suitable for making into barrel staves and packing cases. The bark was often used to make fishermen's floats. An inscription found on an old plank of poplar states its case:

Though heart of oak be ne'er so stout,
Keep me dry and I'll see him out.

Poppy
(*Papaver rhoeas*)

Through the corn my charmed eye
Doth catch the Poppy's scarlet dye

James Rigg, *The Poppies in the Corn* (1897)

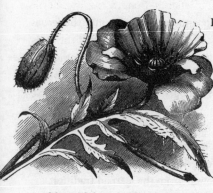

Despite all the odds, the field poppy has survived the onslaught of pesticides and is still a common sight at least at the edges of our arable fields. In earlier times, before the immense changes in British agriculture, the poppy grew among wheat and corn in great numbers. Working in the fields, the Land Girls of the Second World War had a handy solution to the problem of their restless babies. Unlike its eastern relative the opium poppy (*Papaver somniferum*), our own poppy is only mildly sedative and an infusion of the flower petals in milk would be given to the infant to help it sleep while the mother continued with her work. An alternative method of quieting a young child was to dip a dummy in the seeds, and give it to the baby to suck, also very useful when teething.

The poet Abraham Cowley wrote that the poppy 'is scattered over the fields of corn, that all the needs of man may be easily satisfied, and that bread and sleep may be found together'.

Since the two world wars, the poppy has become a powerful symbol of remembrance. They were cultivated between the wars as a crop in Flanders for their seeds and oil, and used in cooking. Poppies growing en masse can seem almost blinding in their intensity; soldiers reported seeing red for days after marching through the poppy-filled countryside.

Folklore seems to have been ambivalent about the plant long before it became tinged with sadness. There was a superstition that it was unlucky to pick the flowers, and that to do so could cause a thunderstorm, or the picker could be struck by lightning, be blinded, get a headache or develop warts. Why all these superstitions arose is unclear. It has been suggested that they may have been devised in order to stop children trampling the corn while they picked poppies. The soft petals were irresistible to children who would make 'dollies' from poppies by folding down the petals to reveal the head and would then tie a grass sash round the middle. Pieces of stem were used as arms.

The flowers are pollinated by bees. They cannot 'see' red, but their eyes are sensitive to the ultraviolet light that is reflected from the surfaces of the petals, and this is what attracts them. The flowers produce no nectar, but the jet-black stamens produce abundant pollen. The whole plant, but especially the seed capsule when it forms, exudes a white, milky sap. The ripe seed capsule resembles a pepper pot, with tiny holes under the rim through which the seeds are shed. This capsule has been likened in the past to the shape of a button, or 'cop', which has given rise to such country names as 'coprose' and 'cup rose'.

In folk medicine, the plant has had many positive applications in addition to being a great boon to the Land Girls. Earache, insomnia, neuralgia and toothache have all been treated with wild poppies. Chewing the seeds in Norfolk was a way not to provoke, but to cure headaches, especially hangover headaches; the poppy was even called the 'headache flower'. The more well-to-do adapted this folk remedy and in the seventeenth- and eighteenth-century Gunton Household Book, there is a remedy for a 'surfeit': 'Take a great many of ye field Red Poppies and steep them in Sack and Brandy.' There's more than a hint of the 'hair-of-the-dog' about this solution.

The cultivated opium poppy was much more widely used in official medicine than our native field poppy. Salmon in 1693 tells us that 'the *Garden* and *Wild* or *Corn Poppy*, have much the same Virtues, but the Wild is accounted *the weaker*.' Both Gerard in 1597 and Culpeper in 1653 recommend the wild poppy for treating the pain of pleurisy. Syrup of field poppies, used to treat pain and as a cough mixture, remained in the British Pharmaceutical Codex until as recently as 1949.

Modern medical herbalists still prescribe syrup prepared from the flowers to treat coughs and insomnia. While much safer than the notorious opium poppy, our wild poppy plant is still toxic and should not be eaten; it contains some of the same alkaloids as the opium poppy, but not the morphine. The seeds alone are non-toxic.

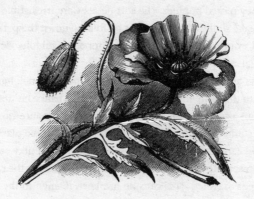

Primrose
(*Primula vulgaris*)

One of our early spring flowers, the primrose was once abundant in our hedgerows and wood margins, but is now far more localized. This decline may be partly down to picking of the flowers and transplanting to gardens, but it is more likely to be the result of change in woodland management and the relative scarcity of coppicing, which produces a variably shaded habitat that suits the plant. The delicate primrose blossoms were made into wine by our forefathers; they certainly couldn't be gathered in sufficient quantity today.

Primroses have an ambivalent folklore reputation; in the Isle of Man, for example, they are called 'sumark' and are lucky flowers. The famous glens of the Isle are still carpeted in primroses in the spring. The flowers are picked on May Day eve and scattered in front of houses, because they are loved by the 'little people'. They were also scattered in Ireland – by the byre to prevent fairies stealing the cow's milk. Yet in many counties, Norfolk included, it is regarded as unlucky to bring the flowers into the house. A primrose flowering in the winter was taken as an omen of death and it was unlucky to bring into the house a single bloom.

Yet conversely, bringing them into the house could have its advantages. The primrose has been associated with the hatching of eggs, both goose and hen, and it was said that if a bunch of primroses was gathered and brought into the house, the equivalent number of eggs would hatch. Traditionally a broody hen's clutch would number thirteen, so a minimum of thirteen primroses had to be gathered. A 'pottage' included primrose as its basic ingredient and a delicious-sounding dessert with saffron, honey and almonds would also be concocted – which definitely made it worth bringing a plant into the house.

In the nineteenth century there was an attempt to institute a national 'Primrose Day' in memory of Disraeli, as it was his favourite flower. His supporters marked the anniversary of his death, 19 April, for some years by wearing primroses, but sadly the custom soon died out.

Somehow it seems apt that in folk medicine the primrose is such a great soother. Healing salves for skin conditions and burns were prepared from the flowers, and the leaves infused formed a soothing eyewash. Within living memory, sore throats were treated in Lewis with an infusion of primrose flowers. The juice from primroses, and from COWSLIPS too, was used in Ireland to remove wrinkles; the crinkly leaves of both species served as a handy reminder of this role.

In official medicine, the primrose was used differently. Pechey in 1694 recommended it for 'Melancholy Disease, and for Fluxes of the Belly', while Salmon in 1693 suggested it for a huge variety of conditions, including gout, migraine, palsy, toothache, and 'all diseases of the Brest and Lungs'. Official use of primrose had almost died out by the nineteenth century, although Kemsey in 1838 states that 'a fine salve for green [fresh] wounds may be made from the leaves of primrose.' The plant is little used in modern-day official herbalism.

Recipe for a primrose ointment

Pick primroses from a sunny bank, when in full bloom. Pull them out of their stems and chop finely. Take an equal quantity of unsalted butter once-washed from the churn. Melt the butter in a small saucepan. Add the chopped primroses, and simmer slowly till reduced to half the quantity. Strain through muslin, pot and tie down. The residue in the muslin is useful to cure bad cuts.

Lotions and Potions: Recipes of Women's Institute Members and their Ancestors (1955)

Puffball Family
(*Lycoperdaceae*)

There are a number of different puffball species of varying sizes that are native to Britain. They all have in common a more or less spherical shape and the characteristic ability when ripe to 'puff' large clouds of brownish-yellow spores into the air. This fungus has attracted a large number of country names: in Suffolk they are 'devil's soot bags', in Norfolk they are 'bulfers' or 'bulfices'. Before they ripen, young puffballs are delicious sliced and fried in butter.

Some puffballs grow to the size of a football and early man cannot have failed to notice them. In excavations in Orkney of a two-thousand-year-old site, a collection of puffballs was found in a midden. The quantity suggested that they had been deliberately gathered but, since they were mature puffballs and not good to eat, they were probably used medicinally.

In folk medicine, puffballs were an important source of first aid for man and beast until well into the twentieth century. Every farm In Norfolk had a dried puffball hanging in the kitchen or outhouse for emergency use. Similarly in Suffolk: 'I knew an old horsekeeper who always kept a puffball in his stable, in case of cuts to horses or men.' Barbers' shops too kept a supply near at hand in case a customer was accidentally nicked by the razor. The spores dusted onto cuts stopped bleeding, and a poultice made from the chopped-up puffball helped wounds to heal quickly and cleanly. In some areas, they were believed to prevent tetanus.

A lady now in her seventies told me a remarkable story. When she was a child, her dog cut a large blood vessel in its leg on broken glass. She rushed to her uncle's house, and he fetched a puffball, dusted on the spores, bound the chopped 'bulfice' on the leg and told his niece that all would be well. Despite losing a lot of blood, the dog gradually made a complete recovery. Folk medicine used puffballs too for treating burns, piles and warts. Nellie, a 'wise woman' from Gloucestershire, also clearly knew about the puffball's special qualities:

'Whenever we went out in the meadows in summer, Nellie would exhort us to look for a bulfice [puffball] for her, so that she could dry it, and then have plenty of the powder which she had taken from the inside to put on cuts, grazes, etc.'

Mrs C. H—, London (2001)

Puffballs were used in official medicine not only to stop bleeding but also to ease chafed skin. Parkinson in the seventeenth century reports that country surgeons would string up lines of puffballs for use when required. Their medicinal function continued into the nineteenth century; Johnson in 1862 describes them as haemostatic (retards bleeding) and adds that they may be eaten fried in slices with egg and breadcrumbs. The use of puffballs in official herbalism had largely died out by the early twentieth century. Nowadays medical herbalists in this country rarely use the plant.

How fortunate it was for beekeepers when it was discovered that the spores have an anaesthetic property if inhaled in quantity. In a similar practice to the one used by modern apiarists, the spores would be puffed into hives and wild nests to stupefy the bees, allowing the honey to be collected.

Purple Loosestrife
(*Lythrum salicaria*)

There is a willow grows aslant a brook,
That shows his hoar leaves in the glassy stream;
Therewith fantastic garlands did she make
Of crowflowers, nettles, daisies, and long purples ...

Shakespeare, *Hamlet*, IV, vii, 165–170

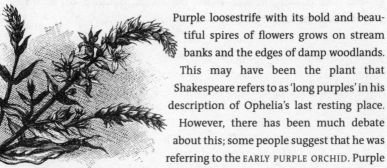

Purple loosestrife with its bold and beautiful spires of flowers grows on stream banks and the edges of damp woodlands. This may have been the plant that Shakespeare refers to as 'long purples' in his description of Ophelia's last resting place. However, there has been much debate about this; some people suggest that he was referring to the EARLY PURPLE ORCHID. Purple loosestrife is perhaps a likelier candidate since the riverside is its usual habitat.

A woman brought up in the Cambridgeshire fens in the last decades of the nineteenth century recalled her childhood days of playing down by the dykes and gathering flowers. Purple loosestrife was among them: 'Only the old iron-'ards defeated us, for try as you may you can't pick these flowers with your bare hands, though their great long purply-red flowers were very tempting. I've heard my husband say as their proper name were "iron-hards" because the roots were so hard that when the men were doing the dykes out, if they hit one o' the roots o' this plant, it were so tough and hard it 'ould bend their shovels.'

The plant has not been prominent in folk medicine in Britain, but in Ireland its Gaelic name translates as 'wound plant'. Although there is little direct evidence of it as a remedy for wounds, we do know that the plant was used there for treating diarrhoea and dysentery.

In official medicine the record is more straightforward. Culpeper in 1653 recommended 'Loosestrife, with spiked heads' for eye conditions and wounds. Later herbalists continued to use the plant as a wound-healer and also for 'fluxes of the belly'. In the nineteenth century it was 'much gathered for medicinal purposes' in Lancashire, where it was called 'red Sally'.

Today's medical herbalists in this country prescribe purple loosestrife for the same ailments as past generations – diarrhoea and dysentery, ulcers and wounds. It is also used to alleviate heavy periods. Recent research has shown the plant to have antibiotic action, especially against the micro-organism (*Rickettsia*) that causes typhus.

If purple loosestrife with its tough roots was ever wrested from the ground, it would sometimes be used to tan leather, in place of oak bark. The root is rich in tannin, which preserves leather.

Ragwort
(*Senecio jacobaea*)

The leaves of this plant are much divided, giving it a tattered appearance – hence its common names of ragwort or ragweed. Its bright yellow, daisy flowers are a common midsummer sight in pastures, especially relatively poor ones, so it has been described as 'a good crop with bad farmers'. The plant is toxic to animals, and to horses in particular. They do not touch it when grazing, but it is more difficult to avoid if caught up in their hay, and farmers and horse owners put a great deal of effort into eradicating it from the land. It is said that ragwort reached Scotland in the fodder of the horses brought into that country by the hated English Duke of Cumberland in the eighteenth century; it has been christened 'stinking Willie' there in his memory. The entire plant has a very strong, bitter smell when crushed and, in the Hebrides, corn stacks were sometimes layered with ragwort to deter mice and rats.

It is not all bad news for ragwort; there is one creature for which ragwort is the plant of choice. The striking black and yellow caterpillar of the cinnabar moth feeds almost exclusively on its leaves, and its body is well camouflaged among the flowering stems.

Ragwort has, in fact, proved useful to mankind. Rope was sometimes made from its stems and used in thatching in the Scottish Highlands. Its tough stems were also used in basketmaking, and dyes of bronze, green and orange have all been obtained from the plant.

In folk medicine, the plant was used to treat horses and humans alike when they suffered from quinsy – an old-fashioned term for a sore and swollen throat. A poultice was made from the plant for this condition. Ragwort was also applied to boils to bring them to a head and, in the eighteenth century, for swellings of the breast. In some parts of Britain, a sprig of ragwort was carried as a protection against infection; for example when visiting anyone with an infectious illness. It was highly valued in Ireland and was employed in treating numerous ailments, including burns and scalds, colds, coughs and cuts, as well as rheumatism and sore throats.

In official medicine, the plant was considered a good remedy for healing wounds and for aches and pains, as well as swellings of the throat. Gerard in 1597 tells us that it also 'taketh away the old ache in the huckle bones called Sciatica'. A century later, Pechey says that 'It cures Ulcers, Inflammations, and a Fistula. Being applied hot to the Belly, in the form of a Cataplasm, it cures the Gripes.' Kemsey in 1838 reports that ragwort is good to heal sores.

Nineteenth-century medical herbalists used ragwort for treating rheumatic pains, sciatica, sores, ulcers; an ointment 'prepared from the fresh plant is excellent for inflammation of the eyes'. Ragwort is now known to contain poisonous alkaloids, and for this reason is today used by medical herbalists only as an external application to ease pain and inflammation.

For some reason, ragwort was thought to be favoured by the fairies. They used it to shelter from the rain and rode on branches of it from one island to another. Witches too rode on plants of ragweed, as Robert Burns, in his poem *Address to the Deil* tells us:

> ... on ragweed nags,
> They skim the muirs an' dizzy crags,
> Wi' wicked speed ...

Ramson or Wild Garlic
(*Allium ursinum*)

Eat leeks in Lide [March] and ramsins in May
And all the year after physicians may play.

C. N. French, *A Countryman's Day Book* (1929)

This plant of damp woodland is especially abundant in the west of Britain, where it can form large colonies. It was once considered to be of great importance in folk medicine as illustrated by the seventeenth-century saying quoted above. It was believed that ramsons could ward off infection, in much the same way as the ONION.

In the Scottish Highlands, ramson poultices were applied to infected wounds and an infusion was used to strengthen the blood. The strong-smelling leaves were also utilized in Scotland to repel midges. The bulbs would be pickled on the Isle of Man in the spring, in dark brown sugar and rum, and brought out in the winter as a remedy against coughs and colds. In Ireland, the plant was considered a panacea, to treat a wide range of ailments: 'Nine diseases shiver before the garlic' is a Sligo saying. There it combatted coughs and colds, indigestion and toothache, as well as boils and infected sores. Many people in Ireland during the influenza pandemic of 1918 carried ramsons in their pocket to ward off infection.

In official medicine, cultivated GARLIC seems to have been used rather than the wild ramson, and the same is true in modern medical herbalist practice in Britain.

Although ramsons are strong smelling, they are mild to eat. The leaves make a delicious addition to cream cheese, and when finely chopped provide a lovely onion flavour for an omelette. In recent times in the Scottish Highlands, they were boiled as a vegetable, as they were in England in Gerard's time: 'The leaves of Ramsons are stamped and eaten with fish, even as we do eate greene sauce, made with Sorrell.' It seems a shame that people do not make more of them.

Raspberry
(*Rubus idaeus*)

The raspberry is native throughout Britain, growing especially in damp woodland. One of its older names is 'hindberry', meaning 'the berry eaten by deer in the woods'. In some places it has escaped from cultivation. Its attractive, white flowers resemble those of the BRAMBLE, but its prickles are not as tough or as large as those of the blackberry. Raspberry leaves have a characteristic coating of dense, white hairs.

The best-known attribute of the raspberry is its delicious fruit, which were undoubtedly an important food source in times past. The Romans certainly enjoyed them – the remains of raspberries have been found in their latrines alongside Hadrian's Wall. The fruit also flavoured punches, and is still made into refreshing country wines and cordials. Mixed with barley, strawberries and sugar, they produce a delicious, rose-coloured wine. The raspberry is cultivated on a wide scale in Scotland where the damp climate seems to suit it.

Raspberry was and still is a medicinal plant. Until very recent times, raspberry vinegar soothed sore throats and a cooling raspberry drink was said to calm a fever, but its most important role in folk medicine was to ease delivery. An infusion of the leaves taken throughout the latter stages of pregnancy is thought to strengthen the uterine muscles. However, if taken in the early months of pregnancy it can cause an abortion, and was used at least unofficially for this purpose. Raspberry-leaf tea was also taken for period pain, and was thought to increase maternal milk. It was also recommended for bouts of diarrhoea and, in the Scottish Highlands, as a wash for wounds and ulcers.

In official medicine, the herbals seem to indicate that the raspberry was not widely exploited. Gerard describes the plant in 1597, but gives no uses for it. Pechey in 1694 states that raspberry syrup is good for fevers, and gives the recipe for a drink prepared from raspberries mixed with other ingredients, which 'is a Cordial for Women before Delivery'. Salmon in the seventeenth century mentions raspberry's usefulness against fevers and describes the ripe fruit 'which mightily please the Stomach'.

Modern medical herbalists still recommend taking raspberry-leaf tea in the last ten weeks of pregnancy to encourage easy labour. The same infusion is also prescribed for diarrhoea, as an eyewash for conjunctivitis and as a cleanser for ulcers. There is little folklore attached to this plant, although dreaming of raspberries is said to be a good omen for a love affair.

Raspberry wine

To every quart of well-picked raspberries, add a quart of water. Bruise the fruit thoroughly and let it stand for two days. Strain off the liquor, and to every gallon put three pounds of lump sugar. When dissolved, put the liquor in a barrel, and when fine (cleared) which will be in about two months, bottle it and to each bottle add a tablespoonful of brandy.

The Woman's Treasury for Home and Garden, ed. A. J. Macself (c.1920)

Red Campion
(*Silene dioica*)

This striking plant of shaded hedgerows has been given an enormous number of country names. Geoffrey Grigson in his book *The Englishman's Flora* records more than sixty of these. Many include the words 'Robin', 'Rob' or 'Jack' and evidently associate the plant with goblins such as Robin Goodfellow and Jack o' Lantern. In some parts of Britain, there were prohibitions about picking this plant: if one did, misfortune or even death could follow. In Wales however, where the plant is known as 'snake's flowers', picking it could lead to snakebite. Another of its country names, 'bachelor's buttons', has been given various interpretations. Gerard in 1597 suggested the flowers resemble buttons that were fashionable in his day, but another sixteenth-century writer, Robert Greene, implies that it was used by women to attract men: 'I saw Batchelers buttons, whose vertue is to make wanton maidens weepe when they have worne it fortye weekes under their Aprons for a favour.'

Red campion hybridizes readily with the white campion (*Silene alba*), a common naturalized weed of arable land. The hybrids produce flowers in varying shades of pink.

Red campion seems to have been relatively little used in medicine. Culpeper in 1653 lumps all the campions together, and says that a decoction of the herb in wine is good for inward bleeding, for kidney troubles, and 'helps those that are stung by scorpions, or other venomous beasts'. He recommends it too for ulcers and sores.

The juice of the plant is corrosive in the fresh state and has been used in folk medicine to treat warts and corns and continued to be (under the name of 'Robin Hood') in the 1950s in Somerset. Rather surprisingly, in Sussex it was also used as a tonic. In the twentieth century, red campion wine, made by boiling oranges, lemons, red campion flowers and leaves with barley and sugar, was still considered 'a healthful drink'.

Charles Bryant in his *Flora Dietetica* (1783) was very much in favour of a related species, the bladder campion (*Silene vulgaris*), suggesting that it should be exploited as a vegetable. When cooked the plant is quite delicious, but the book's recommendation seems to have fallen on deaf ears, and the plant was not regularly included in the household diet.

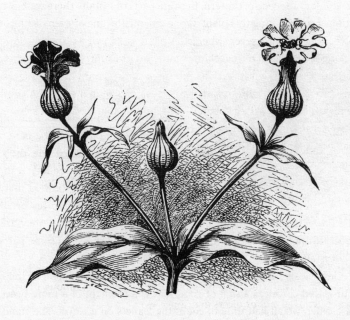

Red Clover
(*Trifolium pratense*)

Over then, come over, for the bee has quit the clover
And your English summer's done.

Rudyard Kipling (1865–1936), *L'Envoi*

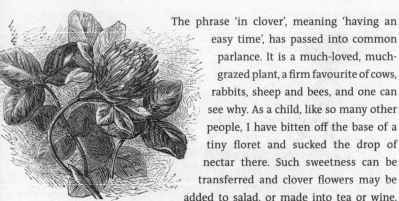

The phrase 'in clover', meaning 'having an easy time', has passed into common parlance. It is a much-loved, much-grazed plant, a firm favourite of cows, rabbits, sheep and bees, and one can see why. As a child, like so many other people, I have bitten off the base of a tiny floret and sucked the drop of nectar there. Such sweetness can be transferred and clover flowers may be added to salad, or made into tea or wine. The flower stems are tough but, particularly in white clover, they are as sweet-tasting as the leaves. Indeed, white clover is known in some parts as 'honeystalks'.

Clover leaves have held a fascination for us all; the emblem of the rare four-leaved clover as a sign of good luck is a remnant of a more peaceful past, when we all had time to count the leaflets on a clover. The standard three-leaved clover was regarded as a symbol of the Trinity, and believed to have the power to ward off evil. Dreaming of clover is seen as a good omen and it was used in love divination in Cambridgeshire, but there a leaf with two leaflets was favoured:

A clover, a clover of two,
Put it in your right shoe;
The first young man you meet,

In field, street or lane,
You'll get him, or one of his name.

The plant can also be a serviceable weather forecaster. If its leaves 'rise up', it is a sign of bad weather on the way – an idea that dates back to the writings of Pliny the Elder (AD 23–79).

Apart from its value as a food plant for our livestock, and as an important source of nectar and honey, man has found a variety of roles for the red clover. In folk medicine, an infusion of the blossoms with honey was used to treat coughs and purify the blood; a similar infusion served in Yorkshire and Ireland to treat bowel cancer. An anonymous pamphlet from Yorkshire contains the recommendation: dipping a 'wet a rag in the tea, this apply to the cancerous sore'. Both flower and leaves could be infused to make a liniment for soothing skin rashes or the leaves could be chewed for toothache in the Isle of Man.

Gerard in 1597 refers to clover as 'three-leafed grass or medow trefoile'; Culpeper adds in 1653 the (confusing) name of honeysuckle, and records the plant's application for treating inflammation and wounds. Salmon in 1693 describes similar uses of clover as 'astringent, strengthening and vulnerary'. He tells us that 'A Clyster made of the Decoction and Honey eases fretting pains of the Guts.'

Present-day medical herbalists use clover to treat coughs and skin conditions. It has oestrogenic properties and may in the future prove useful for menopausal problems. It has a known contraceptive effect on sheep. Perhaps a clover-rich field is not such a good idea after all.

A delightful clover story – a little fanciful perhaps – has been recorded from Papa Stour in the Shetland Islands. If the breeze was coming off the land at twilight, fishermen at sea were guided back to shore by the strong, sweet smell of red clover coming off the fields.

Restharrow
(*Ononis* species)

Four pounds of the rootes first sliced small and afterwards steeped in a gallon of Canary Wine ... and so set to boyle in a Balneo Marie for 24 hours is as daintie a medicine for tender stomachs as any the daintiest Lady in the land can desire to take.

John Parkinson, *Theatrum Botanicum* (1640)

Restharrow used to be a common weed of pasture, but is now rather more difficult to find. It is a great shame because its flowers are like miniature sweet peas and of a beautiful crimson colour. The leaves have a resiny scent when crushed. Unlike most of our native members of the pea family, this is a woody perennial with tough stems and – at least in one species – prickly spines. The plant acquired the name of restharrow because its tough, long roots were capable of stopping a horse-drawn plough (the harrow) in its tracks. These same spreading roots make the plant a valuable stablilizer of sand dunes.

Official medicine found considerable use for the root, and boiled it in vinegar for toothache and also for kidney stones. Salmon in 1693 recommends it for jaundice, piles, toothache and the falling sickness (epilepsy).

The plant does not seem to have played a significant role in folk medicine, but the Irish managed to find a role for it: the juice of the leaves was rubbed onto chapped and rough hands.

By the nineteenth century, restharrow had gained a reputation for being an effective diuretic, and medical herbalists still prescribe the plant for urinary problems. The root has a dual role: when fresh, it acts as a diuretic, but when dried this effect is reversed and it helps to cut down urine flow.

Restharrow has also been valuable as a food source. The root tastes sweet with a liquorice-like flavour and would be chewed with relish, satisfying the thirst on a hot day. One of its alternative names is 'wild liquorice'. It could also be boiled and eaten as a vegetable, the young, tender shoots sweetening the breath. The flowers are still occasionally picked to decorate salads.

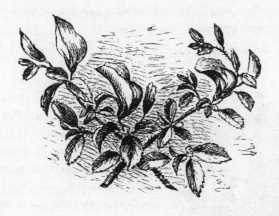

Ribwort Plantain
(*Plantago lanceolata*)

We used to call the spikes 'Jack-straws' and many a good game I have had with them fighting my fifty against my neighbour's fifty.

Margaret Plues, *Rambles in Search of Wild Flowers* (1892)

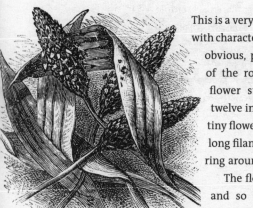

This is a very familiar weed of waste ground, with characteristic, long, pointed leaves with obvious, parallel veins. From the centre of the rosette of leaves springs a tall flower stalk, sometimes as much as twelve inches long, with a black head of tiny flowers at the end. The stamens have long filaments and stick out in a delicate ring around the flowerhead.

The flower stalks are tough and wiry and so have lent themselves readily to children's games. There are many variations, but everyone will recognize the general principle. In one game, one plantain is knocked against another; whichever is 'beheaded' first is the loser. In another version, the base of the stalk is wrapped once round the stem and folded back on itself; it can then be slid up the stem rapidly, knocking off the flowerhead, which can be 'shot' at a target. Many children call this game 'soldiers', and the plant is in fact called 'soldiers' in some parts of the country. There is an interesting connection between this game and the very distant past: one of the old names for ribwort plantain is 'kemps', derived from the Anglo-Saxon *cempa*, meaning soldier.

The ribwort plantain has been used in folk medicine, although not as widely as its cousin the GREATER PLANTAIN. Both were used above all as wound-healers. In the Scottish Highlands, the leaves of ribwort plantain were applied to cuts to stop bleeding and, for a graze, the leaf would be moistened with spit. As so often in folk medicine, it would be the upper surface of the leaf that was used for healing. Generally the underside of a leaf was used to 'draw' an injury (to bring out any pus), and then the smooth upper surface would be applied to complete the healing (see also ORPINE). In Ireland, ribwort plantain was also taken internally in an infusion for coughs and liver complaints, and as a drink for delicate children.

Plantains were utilized also in official medicine for healing. Salmon in 1693 tells us that the juice 'stops the Courses and heals all inward griefs of the body'.

In modern herbalism, ribwort plantain is employed in similar ways to its relative, the GREATER PLANTAIN: to treat bruises, catarrh, fractures, haemorrhoids and ulcers.

There is some folklore associated with this plant. In Shetland, it was used in love divination: the curious lover would remove the florets and put them under a stone; if new florets opened before the old ones had withered, the outcome of a current relationship would be marriage.

Grazing animals find ribwort appetizing and it is a regular constituent of hay. Farmers believed that ribwort plantain could cause fermentation and even cause hayricks to catch fire if it formed too high a proportion of the hay. It was therefore sometimes known as 'fireleaves'.

Rosebay Willowherb
(*Chamerion angustifolium*)

Rosebay willowherb was first described in Britain by Gerard in 1597; its spires of reddish-purple flowers are, in his words, 'brave floures of great beauty'. The plant now has an extraordinarily wide distribution; it is one of the few wild flowers that have increased in commonness and range over the course of the last century. This is partly as a result of its ready colonization of newly opened areas, such as cleared woodlands and bomb-sites. It also thrives in areas that have been burnt, hence its once popular name of 'fireweed'. 'London, paradoxically, is the gayest where she has been the most blitzed,' reported the *New York Tribune* in 1944. 'There is the brilliant rose-purple plant that Londoners call rose-bay willow herb ... It sweeps across this pockmarked city and turns what might have been scars into flaming beauty.' The fluffy seeds, which each plant produces in abundance, once airborne can form veritable blizzards on windy days. The flowers wilt very quickly when they are picked.

The soft, downy seeds were used in Scotland in much the same way as thistledown, for stuffing mattresses. The fluff was at one time exploited commercially, according to Thomas Green's *The Universal Herbal*: 'The down of the seeds, mixed with cotton or fur, has been manufactured into stockings, etc.' The young, tender stems were eaten as a vegetable and the leaves, if carefully dried, make a tea substitute that apparently is hard to distinguish from the real thing.

The plant seems to have been little used in medicine. Parkinson in 1629 calls it the 'Willowe flower' and says: 'There is no use hereof in Physicke that ever I could learne, but is onely cherished among other sorts of flowers, that serve to decke and set forth a Garden of varieties.'

Although Britain seems to have made little medicinal use of rosebay willowherb, it has been used in other European countries and in North

America too, for asthma, childhood skin problems, gut irritations and whooping cough. Some of these applications have been imported into present-day medical herbalism in Britain.

Rosebay willowherb is well known to beekeepers as a good source of nectar. In North America, apiarists sometimes follow behind the loggers, knowing that as the fireweed colonizes the newly open land, it will boost honey production.

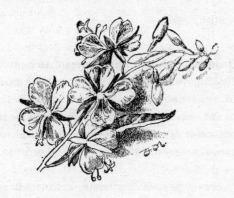

Rowan or Mountain Ash
(*Sorbus aucuparia*)

Rowan, ash and red thread
Keep the devils frae their speed

Traditional Scottish rhyme

The rowan, or mountain ash, is a small, elegant tree producing vivid, orange-red berries. It grows in all parts of Britain, but especially favours the uplands and mountainous areas. The name rowan is thought to be derived from the Old Norse *rune*, meaning 'charm', and the tree was held in great regard because of its protective powers. Countrywide, people would utilize the tree in all manner of inventive ways in order to bring these powers to bear.

Rowan was frequently planted near houses and byres to safeguard the occupants from both witches and fairies (although a rowan would never be planted near an apple tree because it was believed that one would kill the other). The wood of a baby's cradle might have some rowan worked into it; protective necklaces for children were made from rowan berries; and fishermen would sometimes wear rowan amulets to protect them from harm when at sea. In Scotland, the crossbeam in the chimney is known as a 'rantree', because it was usually made from rowan.

Keeping crops and animals safe was next on the list. In Hereford, oxen yokes were made from rowan wood to ensure that the animals would not be bewitched. Farmers in Strathspey drove their sheep and lambs through rowan hoops on May Day, with the farmer following immediately behind. A sprig of rowan might be tied to an animal's tail; the farmer's herding stick itself might be made from the wood; and in nineteenth-century Devon it was customary to hang rowan wreaths around the necks of sick animals to prevent them from getting worse.

Such customs have now largely died out and the sight of a rowan tree growing by the door of an old house is a reminder of a once more superstitious and ritualized past, when life was so precarious that people would do everything they possibly could to protect themselves.

Medicinally, rowan was used in a variety of ways all over the country, but especially in folk medicine. In seventeenth-century Wales the berries were eaten as a cure for scurvy and in eighteenth-century Moray the bark was used as a purge. An infusion of the leaves was considered in Ireland a good remedy for rheumatism; alternatively, the leaves could be burnt and the smoke inhaled for asthma. Various preparations of apple and rowan berries were good for whooping cough, and the berries pulped and sieved provided a gargle. The inner bark of the rowan also served in Wales to expel a retained afterbirth.

Relatively little use seems to have been made of rowan in official medicine. Pechey in 1694 says of 'The Sorbe, or Quickentree' that 'The berries yield an acid Juice, which purges Water excellently well; and is very good for the scurvy. The Liquor which drops from the wounded Tree in the Spring, cures the Scurvy, and Diseases of the Spleen.'

Twentieth-century herbalists made a gargle from the berries, and treated diarrhoea with the bark. Present-day medical herbalists treat diarrhoea, haemorrhoids and sore throats with rowan. Interestingly, we now know that the rowan has antibiotic properties.

The berries are extremely versatile in the kitchen and were, and still are, made into jellies and drinks. The jelly is particularly good with venison. The seeds are toxic, and these should always be removed if the berries are used in cooking or medicine.

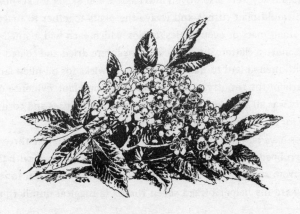

Rush
(*Juncus* species)

I'll sing you one, oh;
Green grow the rushes, oh!
What is your one, oh?
One is one and all alone and ever more shall be so.
Green grow the rushes, oh!

Traditional English counting rhyme

There are several species of rush growing in this country, the most wide-spread being the common rush of pond edges and marshy areas, *Juncus effusus*. It is a unique and easily recognized plant, with spiky, cylindrical 'leaves' (strictly speaking, the stems) and bunches of insignificant, brownish flowers that are easily detached by running a finger up the stem. Colonies of rushes often survive as a marker long after a pond has drained away.

Because of their strength and flexibility, rushes are ideal for weaving and plaiting, and are still used to make chair-backs and seats. In the Scottish Highlands, fines imposed by the Church were sometimes paid in rushes, which were then used to thatch the roofs, to make chair-backs and to strew on the floor. They were also woven into baskets and 'skeps' for keeping bees. Children would plait rushes and weave the plaits together to make dolls' cradles, small mats or even babies' rattles, which each had a small pebble inside to make a clatter. Summer-cut rushes were dried and coated several times with melted lard to make rushlights, or wicks for oil-filled lamps. In some parts of the country where rushes were abundant, evidence of their versatility was all around – rush candles, thatch for houses and corn stacks, matting for human dwellings, baskets, hats, ropes and toys.

Rushes have played a small part in folk medicine. In Devon, three rushes could be rubbed on warts, then thrown away, taking the warts with them. A sufferer from shingles in nineteenth-century Devon was taken to running water, where his helper picked seven rushes (a magical number), rubbed them over the afflicted area, and threw them into the water, which carried away rushes and shingles together. In Ireland, the ashes of rush were used to treat shingles, ringworm and chickenpox.

Official medicine seems to have had no time for the rush – 'as good let them alone as taken' was Culpeper's verdict in 1653 – nor does it figure in modern-day herbalism.

Vestiges of the part that rush played in people's lives are still in evidence. Rush-bearing ceremonies, especially in the north of England, continue to this day. In times past, rushes would be strewn across church floors to provide some softness underfoot, as well as warmth and a fresh scent. This strewing ceremony is relived, usually on a local saint's day, even in the twenty-first century; a procession of villagers bearing rushes woven into shapes such as crosses and hearts complement the proceedings.

When in Cornwall, listen for the word 'rish', meaning 'tally'. It is thought that beads strung on a rush may have been employed in an old method of counting, and the saying 'I'll begin a new rish' is sometimes used, in the sense of 'turning over a new leaf'.

St John's Wort
(*Hypericum* species)

So then about her brow
They bound Hypericum, whose potent leaves
Have sovereign power o'er all the sullen fits
And cheerless fancies that besiege the mind;
Banishing ever, to their native night,
Dark thoughts, and causing to spring up within
The heart distress'd a glow of gladdening hope,
And rainbow visions of kind destiny.

Alfred Lear Huxford, quoted Anne Pratt, *Wild Flowers* (1898)

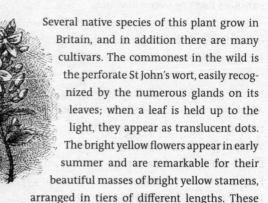

Several native species of this plant grow in Britain, and in addition there are many cultivars. The commonest in the wild is the perforate St John's wort, easily recognized by the numerous glands on its leaves; when a leaf is held up to the light, they appear as translucent dots. The bright yellow flowers appear in early summer and are remarkable for their beautiful masses of bright yellow stamens, arranged in tiers of different lengths. These provide pollen for a large number of different insects, which fertilize the flowers while feasting. The strange smell of the crushed plant has been likened to wet fur.

This beautiful plant has always been associated with the power of good. Richard Banckes in his sixteenth-century *Herball* tells us, 'If it be putte in a Mannes house there shall come no wycked sprite therein.' In the distant past, it may have been used to celebrate the midsummer solstice, and with the advent of Christianity it was dedicated to St John the Baptist, whose feast day was Midsummer Day (24 June). It was said in Aberdeenshire that placing a sprig of St John's wort under the pillow on St John's Eve would ensure life for another year.

However, it is as a remedy for depression that St John's wort is justly famous. There is an old story told in Scotland of a young shepherd boy who after nights alone on the mountainside was clearly losing his mind. St Columba suggested putting packages of St John's wort in the lad's armpits and groin, and his sanity was restored. Does this tale represent a forerunner of the main role the plant has today?

Writing in the early twentieth century, Michael Moloney tells us that 'the herb is recommended by the chief herbalist in County Waterford as an excellent remedy for "an airy fit", i.e. to dispel the clouds of melancholia and other forms of insanity'. In the Isle of Man, we know it was regarded as a tonic for low spirits. The plant's application as a remedy for depression has continued in the European continent through to the present time, but this use has only recently been rediscovered in Britain. The plant is now referred to as 'the sunshine herb', in recognition of the good it has done for so many people.

St John's wort has been used in folk medicine to treat a wide variety of other ailments, from burns and warts to fractures. In Scotland, it was utilized for urinary infections and to rid children of worms.

In official medicine, the plant was used primarily as a wound-healer. A beautiful, deep red liquid can be prepared by steeping the flowers in olive oil, and this was used on all kinds of injuries. Gerard in 1597 recommended this especially for deep wounds. Salmon in 1693 advocated the plant as a vulnerary and also for easing delivery. Of the seed, he says, 'being drunk in Broth or Wine for 40 daies together, it is said to help the sciatica, Palsie, and Falling-sickness'. The flowers of St John's wort were an ingredient of General Wade's Balsam in the eighteenth century, of which one manuscript writer claimed, 'There is not cut of iron Nails which is not Mortall but it Heals in Eight Days time by applying it with a Feather cotton or Injectione provided you use nothing else to it first.'

Kemsey in 1838 was still recommending the plant for wound-healing, and for spitting of blood and for fevers. Nineteenth- and early-twentieth-century medical herbalists in this country prescribed St John's wort as a wound-healer and for coughs and urinary conditions. In modern medical herbalism, the plant is still favoured as a healing agent for burns and wounds, as well as a pain-reliever for cramp and nerve pain. It is used to treat menopausal symptoms and to relieve mild to moderate depression.

The herb's value in treating anxiety and depression only relatively recently again came to the attention of the orthodox medical profession in this country. Now, as a result of numerous clinical trials, it is accepted as effective in mild and moderate depression. As usual with a plant remedy, actual analysis of how and whether it works is a very costly and complex process. As recently as 2000, a leading authority wrote that 'The most important actives of even such a significant herb as St John's wort are still under discussion.' Current research into the plant's strong anti-viral properties suggests that there may in future be a role for this plant in the treatment of HIV and AIDS. Perhaps St John's wort has still more favours in store for mankind.

Scarlet Pimpernel
(*Anagallis arvensis*)

No heart can think, no tongue can tell,
The virtues of the pimpernel.

Country saying, quoted Sybil Marshall, *Under the Hawthorn* (1981)

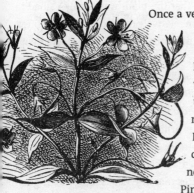

Once a very familiar weed of our cornfields, the scarlet pimpernel is now more often found as a garden and wayside weed. Its small, bright scarlet flowers open wide in the sunshine and close when the weather is grey, giving it the country name of 'poor man's weatherglass'. Regardless of the weather, the flowers close by about three o'clock in the afternoon, which is handy for telling the time. Pimpernel is a member of the primrose family, and closely related to YELLOW LOOSESTRIFE.

In sixteenth-century Scotland, the pimpernel had a strange role in diagnosis. Detailed in a manuscript of Gaelic medicine is a test to determine whether a wounded man will survive. He is given a drink of pimpernel leaves: if he vomits, then the outlook is hopeless. If he does not vomit, and the solution of pimpernel and water seeps through the wound, then the outlook is favourable.

The application of pimpernel was a little more straightforward in other areas of official medicine. It was considered a most effective blood-stauncher, wound-healer and tonic for consumption. In 1731, John Moncrief in *The Poor Man's Physician* recommends a simple measure for staunching bleeding: 'Take Pimpernel and hold it betwixt your Teeth, and you shall not bleed so long as you hold that.' The seventeenth- and eighteenth-century kitchen book, the Gunton Household Book, included the following suggestion:

To staunch bleeding at ye nose Take ye herb calld Pimpernell, bruise it and put
it into ye nose and often renew it till it staunch, ye herb Periwinck [PERIWINKLE]
will do ye same.

In the nineteenth century, the herb was described by one surgeon as
valuable for drawing out such objects as thorns from the flesh, relieving
intestinal blockages and cleansing ulcers, but by the twentieth century it
was realized that the plant had toxic properties, which halted more widespread use. Today scarlet pimpernel is little used in this country by medical
herbalists and because of its toxicity it is not recommended that it be taken
internally for long periods.

The proverb quoted above suggests that the plant was highly valued in
folk medicine, but records of its usage are relatively few. Dog- and snakebites,
kidney trouble, rheumatism, sore eyes and stings could all be treated with
pimpernel and, like many plants, it was also employed as a cure for warts.
In Wales, the plant was used against melancholy, which is interesting in view
of the plant's generic name: *Anagallis* is thought to be derived from
Dioscorides' name for the plant, *Anagelao*, meaning 'to laugh aloud'. A
Somerset name for the plant is 'laughter-bringer'.

Perhaps the value of the plant for country folk lay not only in its medicinal use but also in its aura of magic. A manuscript on magic, preserved in
the Chetham Library at Manchester, states that 'the herb Pimpernel is good
to prevent witchcraft, as Mother Bumby doth affirme' and that the following
lines must be said, 'this fifteen dayes together, twice a day, morning earlye
fasting, and in the evening full' as the plant is gathered:

Herbe pimpernell, I have thee found
Growing upon Christ Jesus' ground:
The same guift [sic] the Lord Jesus gave unto thee,
When he shed his blood on the tree,
Arise up, pimpernel, and goe with me,
And God blesse me,
And all that shall were thee.
Amen.

Tantalizingly, we know no more about Mother Bumby.

Scots Lovage
(*Ligusticum scoticum*)

The Scots lovage, as its name implies, is native to the northern half of Britain only. Its leaves are similar to the garden lovage (*Levisticum officinale*), but its flowers are white rather than yellow. All around the Scottish coast, the plant was gathered and eaten raw or cooked as a vegetable. It was considered a valuable tonic and a protection against scurvy. In the eighteenth century, it would be added to lamb broth, mixed with ALEXANDERS and given to patients suffering from consumption. It was also said to be good for expelling wind.

In official medicine, it is the garden lovage that is normally used, rather than the wild species. However, it is known that Dr Sutherland gathered Scots lovage for his Edinburgh Physic Garden in the eighteenth century, which suggests that at least in Scotland the native lovage may have been utilized. Sutherland had studied at Leiden University under the famous professor of medicine, Dr Hermann Boerhaave. Back home in his native Orkney, he gathered some of his *materia medica* in the wild, from a glen called the Guills of Scalpa. Scots lovage was still growing there when the traveller Patrick Neill visited at the beginning of the nineteenth century.

Otherwise, it seems to have mainly been the yellow-flowered garden lovage that was used in official medicine. Culpeper recommends it for fevers, indigestion and a number of other complaints. It was also used for asthma, the 'gripes', as an emmenagogue and as a diuretic. Modern medical herbalists still use garden lovage for period pain, as well as for indigestion and urinary tract complaints.

It would seem that Scots lovage was used to calm the nerves: 'They called [it] the Cajoler's Plant, since its soothing property gave quiet to the mind.' Recently the garden lovage has been found to contain compounds that are sedative and anti-convulsant, so perhaps its wild cousin really can induce peace of mind too.

Scurvygrass

(*Cochlearia officinalis, Cochlearia anglica*)

As its name implies, this coastal plant was widely used to prevent and treat scurvy. Its juicy, bright green leaves were eagerly picked in springtime after a long winter, when fresh fruit and vegetables would have been scarce. It is now known to be very rich in vitamin C. The high intake of salt and alcohol in the diet of the average seventeenth- and eighteenth-century Englishman made him particularly susceptible to scurvy because these interfere with the absorption of vitamin C.

Captain Cook is known to have taken quantities of scurvygrass on his famous voyages, but it is likely that it would not have kept for much longer than a few weeks. Official medicine wholeheartedly recommended it, but advised that if cooked into a 'decoction' it would lose its efficacy, therefore it was best to take it raw. Ironically, it was therefore more than likely that poorer people, who could not afford doctors' prescriptions and ate freshly picked scurvygrass instead, would have benefited the most from the plant.

Scurvygrass was utilized in folk medicine not only to treat scurvy but other skin conditions in general, as well as boils and cuts, colic, constipation and cramps. The plant was also very nutritious. An early eighteenth-century story relates how two men were trapped on a rock off the Hebridean Isle of Fladder: 'This rock affords a great quantity of scurvy-grass, of an extraordinary size, and very thick; the natives eat it frequently, as well boiled as raw.' The two men 'fell to eating this scurvy-grass, and finding it of a sweet taste. They ate a big basketful of it, which did abundantly satisfy their appetites until their return home.'

Folk medicine certainly knew what it was doing when it came to scurvy-grass. In the Scottish Highlands, it was eaten for breakfast as recently as the nineteenth century. The herb was gathered from the wild in some quantity, although those rich enough to afford a garden for herbs had a scurvygrass bed. The plant was of obvious importance to sailors and fishermen, and one of its Gaelic names translates as 'the sailor'. It was often for sale on the dockside, where this seventeenth-century street-cry would be heard:

> Hay'ny wood to cleave,
> Will you buy any scurvy grass?

Among the rich, the plant was superseded eventually by imported lemons and limes. A truly luxurious, seventeenth-century drink against scurvy included 'sea scurvygrass', garden scurvygrass, watercresses, brooklime, wormwood, horseradish, lemons, oranges and beer.

Scurvygrass was recommended in official medicine not only for scurvy. A saline tincture of scurvygrass, says Salmon in 1693, 'is a famous remedy against the scurvy, dropsie, jaundice, gout and stone'. In the nineteenth century, it was still being officially advocated by Kemsey for foul ulcers and diseases of the skin, as well as scurvy.

Present-day herbalists still recommend scurvygrass as a spring tonic and for treating spots, pimples and mouth ulcers.

Sea Holly
(*Eryngium maritimum*)

I came on that blue-headed plant
That lovers ate to waken love,
Eryngo; but I felt no want,
A lovesick swain, to eat thereof.

Andrew John Young (1885–1971), *Eryngo*

This distinctive, silvery, prickled plant with beautiful, bright blue flowers grows in sand dunes and shingle around our coast, but is rare in Scotland. The roasted roots have a chestnut flavour and were once eaten with some gusto, because of their reputation as an aphrodisiac. Shakespeare alludes to this property:

... let it thunder to the tune of Green
Sleeves, hail kissing-comfits and snow eringoes;

The Merry Wives of Windsor, V, v, 18–19

A seventeenth-century Colchester apothecary, Richard Burton, developed an industry from making candied sea-holly roots called 'eryngoes', a corruption of its botanical name. The roots were dug from a depth of six feet, peeled, cut into slivers, twisted like barley sugar and preserved in thick syrup. These candies became very popular as a tonic and the production of eryngoes continued until the 1860s.

Another sea holly species (*Eryngium campestre*) that is native to continental Europe was often used in official medicine instead of the native British one. Both species were grown by Gerard in the sixteenth century in his herb garden, no doubt for making his own eryngoes: 'The roots condited or preserved with sugar ... are exceeding good to be given to old and aged people that are consumed and withered with age, and which want natural moisture: they are also good for other sorts of people that have no delight, nourishing and restoring the aged, and amending the defects of nature in the yonger.' He also advocated sea holly for liver conditions, cramps, convulsions and the 'falling sickness'. Here is Gerard's recipe:

The manner to condite Eryngos

Refine sugar fit for the purpose, and take a pound of it, the white of one egge, and a pint of cleere water, boile them together and scum it, then let it boile until it be come to a good strong syrrupe, & when it is boiled, as it cooleth add thereto a sawcer full of Rosewater, a spoonful of Cinnamon water, and a graine of Musk, which have been infused together the night before, and now strained: into which syrrupe being more than half colde, put in your rootes to soke and infused until the next day: your rootes being ordered in the maner hereafter following

These your rootes being washed and picked, must be boiled in fair water . . . then must they be pilled Cleane as ye pil parsnips, & the pith must be drawn out at the end of the root . . . let them remain in the syrup till the next day, and then set them on a fire in a faire broad pan until they be very hot, but let them not boile at all: let them remain over the fire an hour or more . . . This done, have in readiness great cap or royall papers, whereupon strow some sugar, upon which lay your roote . . . these papers you must put into a stouve or hothouse to harden . . . in this manner if you condite your rootes, there is not any that can prescribe you a better way.

Over the centuries, other ailments were treated with this plant. Culpeper in 1653 added to the list of sea holly's virtues its efficacy against jaundice, kidney disorders, King's evil (glandular tuberculosis), 'melancholy of the heart', wounds and 'for them that have their necks drawn awry, and cannot turn them without turning their whole body'. Pechey in 1694 details similar uses, adding that the roots are good for 'Consumptive People' and that 'used in the form of a Cataplasm, and applied to the Belly, it prevents Abortion'. By the nineteenth century, the list of applications is much shorter. Kemsey in 1838 states that 'the root removes obstructions in the viscera, and is diuretic and good for the jaundice. The roots bruised and applied outwardly is good for the king's evil.'

Modern medical herbalists prescribe sea holly mainly as a diuretic. Apart from its popular use as an aphrodisiac, sea holly was little used in folk medicine. In the Isle of Man, its juice was used for ear infections and, in the Irish Aran Islands, it was used against worms in children.

Plutarch tells the story that if a goat bites off a piece of sea holly it will cause her, and the rest of the herd, to stand stock-still, until the sea holly is removed. It's an ancient belief but one that could still be tested.

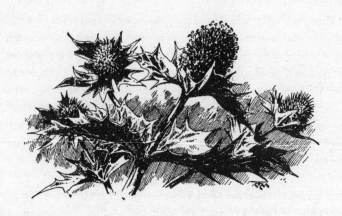

SEAWEEDS

'O God of the Sea,
Put weed in the drawing wave
To enrich the ground,
To shower us with food.'

Chant recorded in Scotland

Seaweed was an important part of the economy in many coastal areas of Britain. So important was it in parts of Scotland that libations of ale or of porridge were ceremonially poured into the sea, to the accompaniment of chants like the one quoted above, to ensure a good harvest of seaweed. And a good harvest was certainly needed. Seaweed was eaten, either raw or cooked, by man and beast. It was harvested as manure for the fields, it was dried and burned and the ashes, known as kelp, were used for soap-making and glass-making. Agar was extracted from the plant, and iodine too, for medicinal use. In the nineteenth century, 'it is said that the beds of sea-weed on the island of North Uist, one of the Hebrides, let for £7,000 a year, while the quantity of kelp made in Scotland alone amounted annually to twenty thousand tons.'

Although the commercial importance of seaweed as a source of soda for glass-making has declined, it now has great value as a source of agar, which is a component of many processed and thickened foods, as well as bases for pills and ointments, cosmetics, pastes and glues of all kinds and dissolvable thread used in surgery. It is vital too as a culture medium for laboratory growth of pathogens. Tess Darwin in her fascinating book *The Scots Herbal* (1996) quotes the surprising statistic that over a thousand tons of seaweed a year was harvested in Orkney alone during the 1970s.

Coastal communities had, and still have, many general and medicinal applications for seaweed; variations depend on the type of seaweed. Many seaweeds were used when wet as soothing plasters on burns and wounds, and in recent years seaweed dressings have been applied to leg ulcers. This account from Ruby E— of Essex in 1991 is impressive:

'A small white pad was placed on the ulcer and I thought to myself what good will that do. I had to return to the treatment room after three days and when they took the pad off I was stunned; the ulcer was covered in seaweed and no pain. Then I had a second one on and the ulcer was then filling up with tiny granules and after three times the hole in the ulcer filled to the top and within a week all cleared and I have never had another one since; so seaweed is a good cure for quite a number of things.'

Various seaweeds were used in folk medicine. As a food and as a tonic, seaweed was a great help to poorer coastal communities. Carrageen (*Chondrus crispus*), dulse (*Palmaria palmata*), green laver (*Ulva lactuca*) and tangle (*Laminaria* species), which grows in broad ribbons attached to rocks, have all formed staple foods for many an impoverished family.

Carrageen was made into a healthy, blancmange-like food, which could be eaten by anyone but also given to consumptives. In recent times, it was soaked in honey and warm milk to provide a remedy for a child's chesty cough. This seaweed is still used commercially as a thickening agent in some foods, such as ice cream, and medical herbalists still prescribe it for bronchitis, acid indigestion, cystitis or as an emollient to soothe a sore throat.

Dulse was widely regarded as a tonic in Scotland, so much so that in Orkney it was said that eating the seaweed protected a person from 'all maladies except Black Death'. Both in Scotland and Ireland, it became a treatment for a wide range of ailments, including constipation, headaches, scurvy, worms and skin diseases as well as fevers. In the Hebrides in the seventeenth century, a dulse poultice was used to expel the afterbirth. C. Pierpoint Johnson, writing in 1862, states that: 'It has long had a reputation among the lower classes in Scotland and Ireland as an antiscorbutic and "sweetener of the blood".'

Green laver is one of the more palatable of the common seaweeds and has been eaten by coastal communities for centuries. It has gently laxative properties. It was applied in the Hebrides as a cooling poultice to ease headache, and was said to induce sleep. In Caithness, green laver was made into a jelly that sailors took to sea to eat with their oatcakes. In coastal parts of Britain, 'laver bread', as this seaweed is sometimes called, is still eaten today.

The tough, broad ribbons of tangle grow attached to rocks beyond the tidal zone and are often washed up after storms. Its surprisingly tough 'stems' used to be dried and made into knife-handles. Like dulse (see above), it was a staple food among the poorer people in seventeenth-century Scotland:

> Scrapt haddocks, wilks, dulse, and tangle,
>
> And a mill o' guid sneeshin' to prie;
>
> When weary wi' eatin' and drinkin'
>
> We'll rise up and dance till we dee ...

'The Blythesome Bridal', seventeenth-century song

Tangle, like wrack, was also a source of kelp. In the west of Scotland, tangle was eaten as a tonic or for constipation or loss of appetite. The stalks were roasted and chewed as a tobacco substitute and were also sometimes chewed raw by children.

Wrack (*Fucus* species) is familiar to all – it is the brown, branched seaweed that is often washed up on beaches. Writing in the eighteenth century, Charles Bryant tells us that *Fucus* is 'collected by the sailors, and people along the sea-coasts, as salad herbs, and are esteemed excellent antiscorbuticks [anti-scurvy agents]'. Bladderwrack (*Fucus vesiculosus*) provided an effective arthritis treatment in Scotland. The seaweed would be held under the hot tap when running a bath, and the contents of the vesicles (bladders) would dissolve into the bathwater and help to soothe the pain. A lady now in her sixties remembers being sent as a child to the coast, to collect a jar of seaweed and another of seawater for her grandmother. The seaweed was heated in the seawater and applied while hot to bunions, corns and other painful areas, as well as being used as a footbath to ease arthritic toes.

A rub prepared from bladderwrack and rum was used in Yorkshire for bowed legs. It can be effective too for strains and sprains. Mary Thorne Quelch in 1941 relates the story of a man who was injured on a beach; he used bladderwrack juice to ease the pain in his damaged leg sufficiently to enable him to hobble out of the way of the rising tide. Within living memory in Cornwall, a jelly was made by boiling wrack, other seaweeds and RAMSONS, to serve as a rub for aching limbs and inflammations. In Ireland, the muci-laginous content of the bladders was swallowed for a sore throat.

Seaweeds were not widely used in official medicine. In the seventeenth century, Pechey described wrack as good for inflammation when used fresh and, in subsequent centuries, it was used for scrofula and to aid weight-loss.

Wrack is sometimes employed today by medical herbalists in the treatment of rheumatic conditions and of goitre; its iodine content is significant in this last respect.

Like many other plants mentioned in this book, seaweeds were regarded as both food and medicine. Various seaweeds are still eaten, especially in the West of Scotland. Although it is unlikely that they will ever again occupy the central role in food that they once did, some of the old recipes are surely worth preserving. In her fascinating book *The Scots Kitchen*, Marian McNeill gives no fewer that six recipes. Here is her recipe for a Dulse Dish, from the Isle of Barra:

> Wash the dulse carefully and let it simmer in water till very tender. Strain, cut small, and put into a pan with a little butter, and make thoroughly hot. Add salt and pepper to taste . . . A jelly may be made by letting the dulse simmer in milk until dissolved and set aside to cool.

According to Martin Martin, visiting the western Isles in the early eighteenth century, dulse was regarded as 'loosening' and good for the sight, as well as for the stomach.

For weather forecasting, any seaweed will do. Hang a strip of it up in the porch; if it remains dry and brittle, this indicates good weather but, when it becomes moist, rain is expected.

Selfheal
(*Prunella vulgaris*)

The wayside blue and innocent heal-all ...

Robert Frost (1874–1963), *Design*

With its square stem and opposite leaves, this is a typical member of the mint family. It grows in grassland throughout Britain, where its character-istic, stubby flowerheads can be difficult to spot. They are only an inch or so long and need close inspection to appreciate them. The sepals are tipped with bronze, forming a striking contrast to the royal-purple flowers. Country names such as 'pickpocket' and 'poverty pink' reflect the belief that the plant was an indicator of poor soil; it was even said that the plant was responsible for impoverishing the soil on which it grew, hence the name 'heart-o'-the-earth', which is known throughout Britain.

In folk medicine, the fresh leaves were used to heal boils, cuts and infected fingers; the latter ailment gave the plant the vernacular name of 'carpenter's herb'. As recently as the Second World War, the herb was used by charcoal-burners in Kent for treating cuts and bruises. Country writer Doris E. Coates in 1976 recalls gathering selfheal in her childhood and calls it 'a very aptly named plant in that cuts, bruises and grazes of all kinds seemed to respond to bathing in an infusion of the leaves and flowers'.

Selfheal tea has also been used to treat coughs. The Irish valued the plant highly and there it was also utilized as a heart tonic. As comparatively recently as the nineteenth century in Hampshire, children were warned not to pick the flower, otherwise the devil would carry them away. It seems that the plant had an even more important role in folk medicine than written records suggest; it was too precious to be picked just for pleasure.

There is no doubt about the role of selfheal in official medicine. The early herbal writers recommended it enthusiastically for treating wounds. Gerard in 1597 tells us that it is as good as bugle, 'and in the world there are not two better wound herbs as hath been often proved'. Culpeper agrees: 'It is an especial remedy for all green wounds to close the lips of them and to keep the place from further inconvenience.' The plant also provided a gargle for sore throats. In his *English Physitian* is the following passage, which would seem to demonstrate that ritual healing was not just confined to folk medicine:

> The Root, Crollius says, that being dryed, and rubbed upon an aking Tooth till it fetch blood, and then put into a pierced Willow, and the hole stop with a peg of the same Willow, it will ease the pain of the Teeth by a magnetick power.

In the nineteenth century, selfheal was still being recommended by Kemsey for wounds, sores and ulcers. Modern medical herbalism utilizes selfheal in a rather more straightforward manner, mainly as a gargle and wound herb. Recent research in China has shown that the plant has a quite strong antibiotic action against a wide range of pathogens.

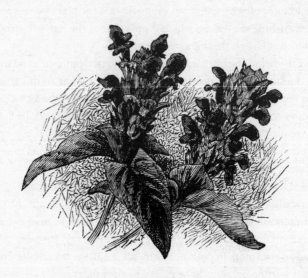

Shepherd's Purse
(*Capsella bursa-pastoris*)

I would stare 'till my eyes started out of their sockets,
Were I sure I should know how you fashion your pockets,
Or how you can pack 'neath each green tiny fold
Your round living treasures – more precious than gold!

James Rigg, *To the Shepherd's Purse* (1897)

Although you wouldn't think so to look at it, shepherd's purse is a member of the cabbage family. This very common and tenacious weed has tough, wiry stems that enable it to survive a certain amount of trampling at the edges of paths and tracks. Its characteristically heart-shaped seed capsules were thought to resemble mediaeval peasants' purses, hence its commonest name. In Scotland, it is 'an sporran'.

Another peculiarity about the seed capsules is that, once ripe, they break easily in half. Several children's games exploit this: in one, a child challenges another to pick a seed case; if it breaks, the child is told that it has broken its mother's heart. Another game is to watch as a child breaks the seed capsule and the 'coins' (seeds) fall out, then to accuse them of theft:

Pick pocket, penny nail,
Put the rogue in jail.

In folk and official medicine, shepherd's purse played an important role as a blood-stauncher, especially during heavy menstruation. Several of its country names have emerged from this property, including the straight-to-the-point 'staunch'. Pechey in 1694 summarizes the plant's application in folk medicine: "Tis outwardly used by the Common People, to heal Wounds, with good Success.' In a hand-written collection of notes from the nineteenth century is the following entry:

> A Drink made from the Shepheard's Purse is Good for my Complaint. Ointment of the same is Good for Wounds.

It would seem that even in her own notes, the lady concerned was too delicate to spell out her (presumably menstrual) problem. Shepherd's purse was also used to treat diarrhoea, among other complaints. Its importance in folk medicine is indicated by one of its country names, 'permacety'; this is derived from spermaceti, the whale-oil base of many valuable official ointments in the past. Few could afford such an expensive and exotic ingredient, but the humble shepherd's purse was freely available to all as a substitute.

Official medicine recommended the plant as a wound-healer but, as time went by, also employed it for a host of other ailments. Gerard in 1597 simply says of the plant that 'it staieth bleeding in any part of the body'. Culpeper in 1653 adds to the list diarrhoea, earache, inflammations and jaundice. Salmon in 1693 includes catarrh and fevers. The herb's popularity declined and by the nineteenth century is not even mentioned by Kemsey.

In medical herbalism in this country in the nineteenth century, the plant was used to treat kidney complaints and diarrhoea, but its use for staunching bleeding was not forgotten. During the First World War, when the plant drugs of choice for stemming bleeding could no longer be imported, herbalists used shepherd's purse instead. Modern herbalists still use it for heavy periods and other forms of bleeding and also for cystitis.

As a food source, the plant had its uses. The leaves may be eaten as a vegetable, and are said to improve the flavour of other greens if cooked with them. The seeds would be ground into flour or given to cage birds. They were certainly eaten as long as 2,000 years ago. A body of a man found in Danish peat bogs in 1950 proved to be about 2,400 years old. He was called, after the village from which his discoverers came, 'Tollund Man' and his remarkably well-preserved stomach contents showed that shepherd's purse formed part of his last meal.

Silverweed
(*Potentilla anserina*)

Honey under ground,
Silverweed of spring.
Honey and condiment
Whisked whey of summer.
Honey and fruitage
Carrot of autumn.
Honey and crunching
Nuts of winter.

Alexander Carmichael, *Carmina Gadelica* (1900–1971)

This creeping plant has possibly the most beautiful leaves of any of our native flora. They resemble silver feathers, smooth-silky and incredibly soft to the touch. On long marches, Roman soldiers in Britain would wear the leaves in their boots to prevent the excessive sweating that could give them sore feet. The custom has survived right through into the present century, at least in East Anglia, and is reflected in the alternative names of 'chafe grass' and 'traveller's joy'. 'Midsummer silver' is another of its country names, and in eighteenth-century Surrey the leaves were woven into garlands to decorate churches.

Gerard in 1597 was clear that the name silverweed came from 'the silver drops that are to be seene in the distilled water thereof when it is put into a glasse, which you shall easily see rowling and tumbling up and down in the bottom'. Place a leaf in a tumbler of water and the underside appears like the silvered surface of a mirror. Leave it a few hours, and the bubbles trapped by the long hairs are released into the water; the leaf no longer appears silver, but the glass is coated with tiny, silvery air-bubbles, which can indeed be made to 'roll and tumble'. Maybe this was the basis of Gerard's statement.

In folk medicine, the leaves were crushed in vinegar and applied to the soles of the feet to reduce fevers and fluxes of all kinds. An infusion of the leaves was used as a cosmetic to improve the complexion; one method was to steep the leaves in buttermilk for nine days. Pechey wrote in 1694, 'The Women in England use the distill'd Water of it to take off freckles, Spots and Botches from the Face, and when they are Sun-burnt'. A similar wash was used in the days when smallpox was widespread, to heal the pitted scars left by that disfiguring disease. In Irish folk medicine, silverweed has also been utilized for bleeding piles, diarrhoea and heart trouble.

Silverweed was once employed in official medicine for a wide variety of ailments. According to Salmon in 1693, 'It stops all sorts of Fluxes of the Belly, spitting of Bloud, Catarrhs, Fluxes of the Womb, pissing Bloud, heals Ulcers of the Reins and Bladder, breaks the Stone, cures Wounds, eases the Toothach, and abates the heat of Fevers.' Gradually its use declined and, by the nineteenth century, it was used simply as a cosmetic and gargle.

Modern medical herbalists in this country prescribe an infusion of silverweed as a mouthwash and for diarrhoea and bleeding haemorrhoids.

Silverweed was an important food-source in the past. Before the introduction of the potato, the plant was cultivated for its roots in the Scottish Highlands and Islands. It was claimed in North Uist that a man could nourish himself by growing the plant on a plot of land that was only as long as the man was tall. The roots were roasted and eaten like turnips or grated and made into a flour-substitute. In the seventeenth century, the roots were evidently eaten in England too:

> The Root of it, which they call Moors, in Yorkshire, about Settle, are eaten by the Boys in Winter; for they taste sweet, and are as pleasant as Parsnips. Hogs dig them up and eat them greedily.

Sorrel

(*Rumex acetosa*)

This member of the dock family has characteristic, spear-shaped leaves, which taste refreshingly bitter. The plant is common on acid heathland and as a weed of pasture, where sheep and cattle eat it readily. Sorrel has a fine reputation as a food for humans, and it is increasing. Reminiscing on a fenland childhood, one lady recalls: 'One pocket was allus full of carrots, and the other of cock-sorrel leaves for chewing.' My own children call the plant 'vinegar leaves' and, when they were small, enjoyed chewing them on a hot, thirsty walk.

The leaves lend a delicious piquancy to soups and salads or a green sauce may be prepared from the herb, to accompany meat and poultry. The leaves have also been used as a natural meat tenderizer and wrapped around tough meat while it is cooking. The diarist John Evelyn, writing in 1720, says that 'Together with salt, it gives both the name and the relish to sallets from the sapidity, which renders not plants and herbs only, but men themselves pleasant and agreeable.' What more could one ask of a plant?

In folk medicine, the plant was used as a tonic and, particularly in the north and west of Britain, as a remedy for scurvy. Fevers and, in parts of Scotland, consumption too were treated with it. Like its cousin the DOCK, sorrel is recommended for minor wounds and bruises. Irish applications of it were numerous and included burns, cancer, heart trouble and jaundice. Even animals benefited:

'I have an excitable King Charles spaniel who has a heart condition and she gets chopped sorrel leaves in her meals to calm her.'

Mrs P. M—, Selkirk (2002)

Sorrel had a reputation in official medicine as a cooling tonic and appetite stimulant that was also useful 'against the Plague', according to Salmon in 1693. One anonymous eighteenth-century physician states that sorrel 'is useful in spitting of blood, and in a stinking breath'. It seems to have had other, impressive powers. An eighteenth-century Norwich doctor, Edward Rigby, observed that wild rabbits, which breed phenomenally, fed largely on sorrel. He therefore planted a patch in his garden and ate it in salad. He fathered twelve children – the last when he was seventy years old – so maybe he proved himself correct. Modern medical herbalists occasionally employ the plant as a mild laxative and diuretic.

A variety of practical uses were found for sorrel. The juice has served in lieu of animal rennet to curdle milk and could also remove rust stains from linen. The plant also had a small role as a dyestuff. Surprisingly, the root when boiled gives a beautiful, red colour and the leaves were sometimes used in Scotland as a mordant (dye-fixer).

Sorrel soup

1 stock cube

1 tablespoon rice

1 bunch of herbs as available from following: mint, comfrey, sorrel, borage, yarrow, dandelion, basil, rosemary, parsley, marigold leaves or flowers, nasturtium leaves or flowers, nettle.

Dissolve stock cube in one pint boiling water. Add rice, boil five minutes. Add finely chopped herbs, boil five minutes more.

Mrs P. R—, Selkirk (2002)

Sow Thistle
(*Sonchus oleraceus*)

When sowes have pigs, they do most greedily desire it, because they know by
a certain natural instinct, wherewith most brutes are indued, that it doth very
much increase their milk.

William Coles, *Adam in Eden* (1657)

Sow thistle is thought to have been
introduced by the Romans for cooking,
since the earliest records we have of its
seeds all come from Roman settle-
ments. The common name of sow
thistle does, however, imply that it was
also fed to pigs: in fact, many animals
relish it. Edward Topsell, in his *Historie of
Four-footed Beasts* (1607) tells us how the
plant acquired one of its country names, 'hare's
lettuce': 'When hares are overcome with heat, they
eat of an herb called ... hare's-lettuce, hare's-house, hare's-palace: and there
is no disease in this beast the cure whereof she does not seek for in this
herb.' In Wales, the association with pigs was stronger, and sow thistle was
considered uniquely effective in healing a wound made by a hog.

Although it looks prickly, the plant is in fact quite soft and juicy, with
small, relatively harmless prickles fringing the leaves. The stems are smooth,
broad and hollow and, when broken, ooze white 'milk', like dandelion juice.
This sap has been used to treat warts, again like DANDELION. An East Anglian
country name for this plant is ''Tis an' t'Ain't' [a thistle].

In official medicine, the plant was advised for treating gravel and stone
(small and large urinary stones) and to increase the milk of nursing mothers.
Culpeper in 1653 has other recommendations too: 'Three spoonfuls of the
juice taken ... causes women in travail to have so speedy a delivery, that

they may be able to walk presently after.' Also, perhaps more believably, he adds that it is a good face cleanser, bringing lustre to a woman's skin. By the nineteenth century, Kemsey regarded sow thistles as 'cooling and somewhat binding, and are very fit to cool a hot stomach and to ease gnawing pains. A decoction of the leaves and stalks causes abundance of milk in nurses, and their children to be well coloured, and prevents milk curdling in the breast. The bruised herb or the juice, may be profitably applied to all hot inflammations, as also for the heat and itching of the piles or other parts'.

The plant is rarely used today in medical herbalism, but it remains a valuable tonic for domestic and farm animals. People still eat sow thistle however, as they have done for generations. The leaves may be added to a salad, or prepared as a vegetable. Like spinach, it is best cooked with minimal water, butter and lemon juice.

Speedwell, Bird's-eye or Germander
(*Veronica chamaedrys*)

Heath Speedwell
(*Veronica officinalis*)

... Dear tender, fragile flow'r
That from the azure vault once drew thy dow'r!
... Emblem of Friendship – rarest gem of blue –
From me thou ever hast affection true.

James Rigg, *To the Common Speedwell* (1897)

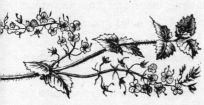

The tiny, bright blue flowers of this common weed of lawns and pastures are one of the cheering sights of spring and early summer. The blossoms are very fragile and drop their petals almost at once if picked. This property may have led to the names 'remember me', which was used in Yorkshire, as well as 'speedwell' which means 'farewell'. Irish folklore offers an alternative explanation: a sprig of the plant should be worn on a journey to keep the wearer safe, and 'speed him well' on his way.

Why the plant should be called bird's-eye speedwell is less clear; only a few birds have blue eyes. Maybe the simplest explanation is that the prominent, white centre of the otherwise blue flower may have suggested an 'eye'. 'Cat's eye' and 'angel's eye' are alternative country names. In Somerset, there was a warning that the flowers should not be picked; if you did, a bird would peck your eyes out. It was also believed that if you picked the flowers, you could bring about a storm.

The name 'sore eyes' is more easily explained, because an infusion of the flowers was widely employed in folk medicine to ease tired and inflamed eyes. It shares a country name with EYEBRIGHT, the white-flowered *Euphrasia*, which is also used for eye conditions. Bird's-eye speedwell also served for treating epilepsy, jaundice and worms, as well as easing the sore breasts of nursing mothers. In Cumbria, it was sometimes used as a tea substitute and was known as 'poor man's tea'.

In official medicine, the less common heath speedwell (*Veronica officinalis*) was the species mainly used. Salmon in 1693 extolled the virtues of this plant as a wound-healer, a reputation that lasted at least into the nineteenth century, when Kemsey recommended it for green wounds, sore eyes and ulcers.

Although in the early twentieth century the heath speedwell was still prescribed by medical herbalists for coughs and skin complaints, today they make little use of either species in this country. This decline may be due to lack of efficacy or it may be a result of the words of one French phytotherapist, who declared in 1935 that 'the infusion [of speedwell] has no more virtue than the hot water used to prepare it'. However, time might prove him wrong, since it is now known that bird's-eye speedwell contains a number of medicinally active compounds.

A Gaelic name for one species, thyme-leaved speedwell, translates as 'herb of the whooping cough'. Interestingly, speedwell contains the glycoside scutellarin, named after the skullcap (*Scutellaria*), which is much used for its calming effects. Only time and further research will tell whether it was right to drop this herb from our *materia medica*.

Spurge
(*Euphorbia* species)

For love of God do take some laxative;
Upon my soul that's the advice to give . . .
Centaury, fumitory, caper-spurge
And hellebore will make a splendid purge.

Chaucer, *The Nun's Priest's Tale*, 178–198

Several species of spurge are native to this country and many more still are grown in our gardens. Spurge is thought to be the same word as 'purge', and not surprisingly therefore the plants have had a reputation as excellent purgatives. Chaucer's character (see above) was recommended to take 'Catapuce' (caper spurge) as a purge after his bad dream. A relatively mild purge in that instance, but some of the spurges had an action so powerful that they were dangerous.

In Ireland, this has led to some rather dubious practical jokes. A man in Galway was dosed by his friends with Irish spurge (*Euphorbia hyberna*) and 'ran up and down the street like a madman, and swelled so big that his friends had to bind him with hay-ropes lest he shall burst'.

Spurges were employed in country medicine mainly in the treatment of skin conditions, and warts in particular. The different kinds of spurge have usually not been distinguished in records of folk medicine. The latex that exudes from all parts of the plant when it is bruised is thick and white – this was painted on the offending wart; it is still found useful today. A more unusual application of the sun spurge is implied by its Wiltshire name of 'Saturday night pepper'. In the Isle of Man – and perhaps in Wiltshire and elsewhere – it was found that juice of sun spurge had the effect of making the tip of the penis swell. Writing about caper spurge (*E. lathyris*) in 1892, North-American botanist Charles F. Millspaugh claimed that 'the laity in England are said to use one capsule to cause catharsis, and the women, several to produce abortion'. Clearly these plants are of great value in small doses, albeit perilous otherwise.

In official medicine, Gerard tells us in 1597 that spurge juice served to cure 'all roughness of the skinne', as well as callouses, carbuncles, scabs and warts. Parkinson in 1640 warns of the corrosive nature of spurges: 'Three or four droppes of the milke taken fresh is often put into a dry figge, which is taken by strong country people; but it requireth some caution in gathering of the milke that they stand with their backes and not their faces to the winde, and especially that they touch not their face or eyes with their hands.' This was good advice because the sap can cause severe irritation of the skin and even blindness if it gets into the eyes. Beggars made good use of this sap to raise blisters on their bodies and elicit pity.

In 1693, Salmon warns against Greater Spurge, as a powerful purge 'but is seldom used'. The seeds, however, he recommends for dropsy, jaundice and a number of other conditions, 'but by reason of the heating and burning quality thereof, are always used with caution'. Nowadays because of their toxicity our native spurges are not used in medical herbalism in this country.

However, they can still be friends to gardeners and fishermen. It is said that if you bury seeds of caper spurge in mole runs, the mole will be repelled and find someone else's lawn to dig up. Every gardener should encourage spurges because they apparently raise the temperature of the soil and so assist the growth of more tender plants. As for the fishermen – the Irish spurge used to be thrown into the river by the fishermen of Kerry in order to stupefy fish. Its effects would be noticeable for several miles downstream.

Stonecrop
(*Sedum acre*)

There from his rocky pulpit, I heard cry
The Stonecrop: See how loose to earth I grow,
And draw my juicy nurture from the sky:
So draw not thou, fond man, thy root too low.

Reverend R. W. Evans, quoted by Anne Pratt, *Wild Flowers* (1898)

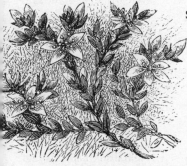

Stonecrop grows on harsh ground – on gravel paths, roadsides and shingle and in low walls. Its small and neat, succulent leaves and upright, stout stems with tiny, yellow star-flowers brighten up many a lay-by. It is very shallow-rooted and needs only a tiny amount of soil in which to grow, so that it does appear to 'sit' on the stones. Its generic name may be derived from the Latin verb 'to sit'. Like its cousin the HOUSELEEK, it was sometimes deliberately planted on thatched roofs to protect the house from lightning.

The plant's peppery taste explains perfectly its country names of 'wall pepper' and 'biting stonecrop'. Despite, or because of, its taste, it was often added to salads. John Evelyn, the seventeenth-century diarist, confirms this: 'When young and tender, [it] is a frequent ingredient in our cold sallet.'

In the recent past, stonecrop was an important plant for first-aid treatment of cuts and wounds. Its succulent growth made it highly suitable for poultices and for 'juicing'. The juice has indeed been used in folk medicine to treat a wide variety of skin conditions including dermatitis, erysipelas and shingles. In Ireland, it served to treat worms. The seeds of the related English stonecrop (*Sedum anglicum*) were sometimes applied with a linen cloth on cases of 'the itch'.

Official medicine too has exploited the plant, for scurvy and the King's evil (scrofula) and, in the sixteenth and seventeenth centuries, it was a vital ingredient in a 'treacle' for killing worms. In the nineteenth century, the plant was still in use for treating ulcers and 'scorbutic disorders' (scurvy symptoms), but soon after the plant seems to have fallen from use in official circles (although it is still favoured in continental Europe). Present-day medical herbalists in this country seldom prescribe it.

Perhaps this game also disappeared at the same time: children would take stonecrop stems and strip them of their leaves. The stems were then scraped over one another to produce a fiddle-like sound – the plant had the local name of 'crowdy-kit', crowdy being an alternative name for fiddle.

Strawberry, Wild
(*Fragaria vesca*)

Doubtless God could have made a better berry
But doubtless God never did.

Dr William Butler (1535–1618)

The majority of us are familiar only with the large cultivated strawberry and find it difficult to fathom that the tiny wild strawberry, greatly superior in flavour, was many years ago the only edible strawberry there was. For ancient man, it must have been a welcome addition to the summertime diet.

The strawberry had probably been brought into cultivation by the time the Romans arrived in Britain and, together with raspberries and hazelnuts, the remains of strawberries have been found in the Roman latrines at Hadrian's Wall. One of the earliest written references to the strawberry is in a manuscript of 1265, which describes a 'Straberie' fruit; this older form of the name suggests that it comes from the old verb 'straw', meaning 'strew'. This may be an allusion to the way in which the runners and fruit are strewn across the ground.

By the sixteenth century, the strawberry was deemed – quite rightly so – to be a fruit of exceptional deliciousness with unsurprisingly erotic associations. It became traditional for lovers to exchange bracelets made of wild strawberries threaded on grasses. They appear as a food for pleasure in Hieronymous Bosch's painting *The Garden of Earthly Delights* (c.1504) and, in the sixteenth century, farmer and poet Thomas Tusser clearly rates the strawberry very highly:

Wife, into the garden, and set me a plot
With strawberry roots of the best to be got,
Such growing abroad among thorns in the wood,
Well chosen and picked prove excellent good.

Many people preferred the native strawberry for its delicate flavour and it was frequently brought from the wild into the garden. The wild variety was sufficiently common, in the region around Bath in the seventeenth century, for local children to collect and sell them, in boxes made from the bark of ash trees.

The strawberry plant had several different uses in folk medicine. In the Scottish Highlands, it helped to prevent tartar building up on the teeth. The leaves could be warmed up and applied to inflammations or an infusion of the leaves used for diarrhoea. In Cornwall, a folk song recorded in 1698 shows that girls rubbed strawberry leaves on their skin to improve the complexion.

In official medicine, Gerard in 1597 recommends a poultice of strawberry leaves for inflamed wounds, and states that 'a decoction thereof strengtheneth the gummes, and fastneth the teeth'. Parkinson in 1629 advocates distilled strawberry water for 'passions of the heart, caused by perturbations of the spirits'. The same water also helps spots, and he suggests that the leaves are good for gargles and for diarrhoea. The famous Swedish naturalist Carl Linnaeus enjoyed wild strawberries and thought that they cured his gout. In Culpeper's opinion, 'It is so harmless an herb, you can scarce use it amiss.' The seventeenth- and eighteenth-century Gunton Household Book suggests this recipe for treating jaundice:

Take Strawberry roots leaves and Red Strings altogether as they grow, wash them and boyle them in reasonable strong beer very well, and give ye patient to drink morning and evening a good draught.

In the nineteenth century, Kemsey also recommends taking strawberries for the liver: the leaves and roots were boiled in water and wine to make the medicine. He describes strawberries as 'cooling and refreshing. [They] cool the liver and blood, assuage inflammation, and help the urine.'

Today's medical herbalists, at least in Britain, use the plant rarely, but it can be employed to treat diarrhoea and dysentery. At home, the cut surface of a strawberry may be used to remove slight sunburn and to clean away discoloration from the teeth.

Sundew
(*Drosera rotundifolia*)

Syne we keek thro' the lens at the spangled sun-dew
Wi' her witchin' tiara o' di'monds sae clear –
Invitin' the doom'd thochtless midge tae its bier.

James Rigg, *The Hunt for the Staghorn Club-Moss* (1897)

This small, rare plant of boggy areas is one of our few native insect-eating plants. It has a unique appearance: its round, flat, pad-like leaves are covered with stiff, glandular hairs, each of which holds a droplet of a sticky secretion that is ideal for trapping a small insect. The sight of these many droplets caught in the sunlight doubtless is what has given the plant its name of sundew, as well as endowing it with an aura of magic. The 'dew' remains on the plant even in the hottest sunshine. In the Isle of Man, sundews were used as love-charms, and a piece of the plant was secretly slipped inside the clothing of the desired person. That this is an old use of the plant is indicated by two of sundew's mediaeval names, 'lustwort' and 'youthwort'.

The entire plant is very bitter and its juice was sometimes used as a rennet-substitute to curdle milk. In Scotland, where the plant is abundant in bogs and wet moorland, sundew was used in a number of ways in folk medicine. The juice was mixed with milk to remove freckles and unbecoming signs of suntan, as well as corns and warts. In the Scottish Highlands, the plant provided a remedy for headlice. Sundew served in the Glencoe area of Scotland as a treatment for asthma and whooping cough.

Official medicine made use of sundew too. According to William Turner in his *A New Herball* of 1568, 'Our Englishmen nowadays set very much by it, and holde that it is good for consumptions and swooning, and faintness of the harte.' The drink prepared from it became in time a celebrated liqueur that was taken just for pleasure. In Gerard's time, it was called Rosa Solis, meaning dew of the sun. Its use as a liqueur persisted in France as 'Rossoli'. The seventeenth- and eighteenth-century Gunton Household Book gives this recipe for a 'Restorative' made from Rosa Solis, as this plant was sometimes called:

> Take ye herb yt growth in ye meadows and low marsh grounds and mossy and
> in noe other Place. It must be gathered betwixt ten of ye clock in ye morning
> and three in ye afternoon in wch time it beareth most dew wch ye herb it self
> is full of strength nature and vertue, wherefore in any case you must not wash
> it neither touch it wth ye hand at gathering but Pull it up Stalk roots and all,
> for if you either wash or touch it wth your hand its vertue will goe away.

In the fifteenth- or sixteenth-century *Regimen Sanitas*, a Gaelic text used by some families of the Highland medical practitioners, sundew leaves boiled in asses' milk were recommended for whooping cough. Culpeper likewise in 1653 advised it for diseases of the lungs and states that: 'There is a usual drink made thereof with aqua vitae and spices frequently, and without any offence or danger, but to good purpose used in qualms and passions of the heart.' Pechey in 1694 tells us that: 'Botanists differ about the Virtue of this Plant: Some commend it for a Consumption, the Plague-wounds, and the Falling-sickness: But others, with good Reason, forbid the inward use of it … many Superstitious Things are reported of this Plant, which I designedly omit.'

However, time has proved that the sundew has indeed some very valuable medicinal properties and that Pechey's sceptics were wrong. The plant contains anthraquinones, which are 'anti-microbial, anti-spasmodic and also cough-suppressing'; they are used by present-day medical herbalists to treat whooping cough, asthma and coughs in general.

One final thing: the ancient Celts employed sundew to dye their hair. The entire plant will yield a bright yellow dye if mixed with ammonia, but the root alone produces a purple dye. We do not know the Celts' preferred colour – perhaps it was a mixture of both?

Sweet Violet
(*Viola odorata*)

Beauty clear and fair
    Where the air
Rather like a perfume dwells;
  ... Where the violet and the rose
  ... Their blue veins and blush disclose,
And come to honour nothing else:

John Fletcher (1579–1625), *Beauty Clear and Fair*

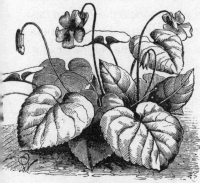

This is the sweet-smelling violet, so beloved of poets and mythmakers. It can, if conditions are favourable, form small colonies, which are a wonderful sight and scent en masse. Partly because it flowers early in the year and partly on account of its lovely scent, the violet has inspired more poetry than most of our wild flowers. It is also the subject of extensive lore and legends.

Dreaming of violets is said to foretell prosperity, and yet these flowers are sometimes associated with death, especially the death of the young. When speaking of Ophelia, Shakespeare said:

    Lay her in the earth;
And from her fair and unpolluted flesh
May violets spring!

Shakespeare, *Hamlet*, V, i, 232–234

The Romans and Greeks designated violets as the flowers of love and used them in many ways, both symbolic and practical. Wearing a crown of violets was believed to fend off intoxication. They also used an infusion as a sleeping draught or a comforting drink to soothe anger.

Violets have been used since earliest recorded times in official medicine. They are mentioned in a tenth-century herbal, and were used here in Britain as the Romans did, to procure sleep. Six centuries later, Gerard recommends violets for inflammations, especially of the chest. He says that violets make a 'Plate, which is most pleasant and wholesome, especially it comforteth the heart and other inward parts'. Apothecaries during Charles II's reign sold a conserve called 'Violet Plate' as a pleasant laxative. Culpeper in 1653 advocates violets for inflammations too, but also for piles in an unusual remedy – of violets fried with egg yolks and applied to the offending haemorrhoids. At the end of the seventeenth century, violets were prescibed by both Salmon and Pechey for catarrh, fever, headaches and pleurisy, but there is only a two-line entry in Kemsey's *British Herbal* (1838): 'The leaves of the violet are gently laxative. The syrup is used as a purgative to infants.'

Modern medical herbalists in Britain prescribe violets for catarrh and coughs, and also as a supportive treatment for breast and stomach cancer. The role of sweet violet in treating cancer is somewhat controversial. Evidence for its effectiveness is largely anecdotal, but it became fashionable in British herbalism during the early twentieth century. There is now some supporting evidence of anti-cancer effects of violet in experiments using mice. At the very least, applications of violet leaves might provide a soothing remedy, but they should not be acclaimed as a cancer cure.

The *Woman's Treasury for Home and Garden* (c.1930) gives the following recipe for violet cough syrup:

> Pick the petals from their calyces and use one ounce. Boil for five minutes in a pint of water with eight ounces of sugar. Strain through muslin, bottle and use in one-teaspoonful doses as occasion demands.

Violet syrup could be purchased in chemist shops in the 1940s, but many people made their own.

In folk medicine, violets were used for treating skin conditions or simply as a cosmetic. This piece of good advice was recorded by the Reverend John Lightfoot in Scotland in the eighteenth century: 'Anoint thy face with goat's milk in which violets have been infused and there is not a young prince on earth who would not be charmed with thy beauty.'

The scent of the flowers has been used to revive people who have fainted; the blooms were made into balls for this purpose. Headaches were treated with an infusion of violets. Perhaps they were mood-changers too: in *The Diary of a Farmer's Wife 1796–7*, thought to have been written in the eighteenth century, we read how the best solution for a grumpy husband is to make him a violet pudding.

The most common folk-medical application however has been in the treatment of cancers and ulcers, although what were termed cancerous growths in the past were not necessarily the malignant tumours that we would today describe as cancer. The flower buds were eaten to ease the pain of a cancer or an infusion was drunk. Poultices of violet leaves were also applied. In parts of the Scottish Highlands, flowers of the related dog violet (*Viola canina*) were boiled in whey to treat fevers.

Endlessly valuable, violet flowers have been stuffed into small pillows for a scented slumber, made into wine or crystallized and eaten, along with those delicious, traditional chocolates, violet creams. The flowers are still used in cosmetics, perfumes and soaps, although a synthetic version of the chemical responsible for violet scent often takes the place of the actual flower.

Tansy
(*Tanacetum vulgare*)

I believe that Asia does not produce a plant of greater fragrance than tansy ...

Dr Hermann Boerhaave (1668–1738)

Tansy is not native to Britain and it is thought that it was brought over from Europe to cultivate for medicinal use. It is commonly found near old buildings where it would have been deliberately planted. In midsummer, tansy produces a flat bunch of yellow, button-like flowerheads, which consist entirely of disc florets so that they appear like the inner ring of a daisy without its 'petals'. The flowers are known as 'buttons' in Yorkshire. If gathered in full bloom, they keep their colour for months; it has been suggested that this gave rise to the name tansy, from the Greek *athanatos*, meaning 'immortality'. The entire plant is pungently aromatic when crushed; it was brought into the house to keep away mice as well as insects, and layered with clothes to repel moths. It was also used in farriery as an insect repellent, and gave a fine shine when rubbed into a horse's coat. The leaves could also be rubbed over the surface of meat to deter flies and over corpses to deter worms.

The intestinal worm was not safe from tansy either. In folk medicine, an infusion of the plant would be taken to rid both humans and animals of the dreaded creatures. It was wise to be careful of the strength of the infusion though, since the plant is toxic in high concentrations. An early-twentieth-century manuscript by Mark R. Taylor records this remedy:

Cure for threadworm – boil the flowers or foliage of tansy weed and drink the infusion. Dose – a wineglassful each morning.

Headlice could also be treated with a tansy infusion. The plant was an important 'woman's herb' in folk medicine, utilized to treat period pain and procure abortions; in apparent contradiction to this last use, couples who wished to have children also ate the herb.

Tansy was also highly favoured for warding off fevers: simply placing a leaf in the shoe was thought to achieve this. Alternatively, in Orkney, people would stick a sprig of tansy between their upper lip and nose, so that as they inhaled its aroma the fever would be kept at bay. Gout was eased with tansy poultices or infusions of the flowers and seeds. In the Outer Hebrides, a tansy infusion was drunk for insomnia. Tansy flowerheads and marigold petals together were infused and drunk for bronchitis in Buckinghamshire in the twentieth century. Mrs M. H— recalled in 1985 that in Yorkshire, tansy was used as a heart tonic.

In official medicine, tansy was sometimes used in similar ways. Culpeper in 1653 advises it for preventing miscarriages and adds, 'Let those women who desire children love this herb, it is their best companion, their husbands excepted.' On the other hand, he says that it promotes the courses (periods). He recommends it too as a digestive and for gout and kidney stones, and the seeds for killing worms in children. Two hundred years later, Kemsey states that tansy 'is now used chiefly for expelling worms'.

We now know that the whole plant, and especially its essential oil, is toxic; for this reason its internal use is not advised. Modern medical herbalists use tansy with caution for treating worms. It must be avoided during pregnancy.

The flavour of tansy is unusual, which is not surprising since its leaves are so pungent. Eggy cakes called 'tansies' were cooked with this herb and were traditionally eaten on Easter Day. Gerard in 1597 says of these that they 'be pleasant in taste and good for the stomache'. An eighteenth-century recipe for a 'tansy' includes eggs, salt, spinach juice, tansy juice, sugar, cream, bread and butter. Perhaps the recipes have changed with the passing of the years, or people's tastes have changed, but by the nineteenth century tansies and tansy puddings are described by botanist Anne Pratt as 'sufficiently nauseous and bitter to be eaten by way of penance. Many country people, however, eat the puddings with much relish.' Here is a modern-day recipe given by Jennifer Westwood for a tansy, based on a seventeenth-century one, that readers, at their own risk, can judge for themselves:

1 teaspoon tansy juice
300 ml double cream
4 eggs (use only 3 whites)

240 g spinach boiled in 2 tablespoons water without salt

30 g caster sugar

30 g butter

juice of 2 oranges

nutmeg

pinch of salt

Drain the spinach, pressing it well (discard the leaves). Stir the tansy juice and the sugar into the spinach juice. Beat the eggs, cream, salt and nutmeg together, then beat the tansy/spinach juice into the mixture. Heat the orange juice and keep it warm. Fry the tansy on both sides as for an omelette, but turning so that both sides are lightly browned. Serve at once, pouring the warm orange juice over.

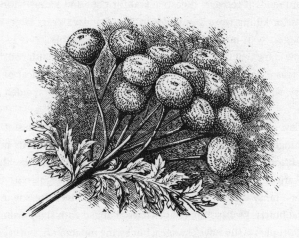

Teasel
(*Dipsacus fullonum*)

The Water that is receiv'd in the hollowness of the Leaves, is good for Inflammations of the Eyes …

John Pechey, *The Compleat Herbal of Physical Plants* (1694)

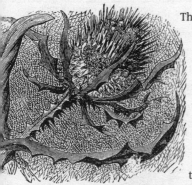

The teasel is a striking plant with tall, very upright stems and bright green leaves that clasp the stem in pairs, each pair forming a cup-like cavity between them. The water that lodges in this cup was considered to be magically powerful, a belief which goes back at least to the time of Pliny the Elder (AD 23–79). Its generic name *Dipsacus* is derived from the Greek *dipsao*, meaning 'to thirst'; this characteristic of the plant has also given rise to the names 'Venus's bath' and 'our lady's basin'.

Teasels were vital tools in nineteenth-century textile mills. The thistle-like flowerheads were used to comb (tease) wool before spinning. The arms of the Clothworkers' Company were three teasel heads, reflecting the plant's huge importance in the industry. Eventually carding machines took over the teasel's role although the plant was still being cultivated in the early decades of the twentieth century in southwest England. Here, they were used for raising the nap on cloth: the dried teasel heads were attached to the surface of a cylinder, which revolved against the surface of the material. Teasel heads are still employed to comb the green baize of billiard tables, a process where their flexibility gives them superiority over any machine. This is not the whole story of teasel's value to man though.

In folk medicine, the water from the teasel 'cup' was collected to treat sore eyes, improve the complexion and remove warts. As Gerard noted in

1597, 'certain little magots' are often to be found in the seedheads and these too were credited with magical powers to cure ague. The grubs had to be wrapped in a bag and worn by the sufferer. Gerard tried this himself when he had a fever and declared that he found it no good at all. A more mundane application of teasel was to boil the roots in order to make a poultice for abscesses and to treat warts.

In official medicine, Culpeper mentions in 1653 the use of teasel-cup water as a good cosmetic and eye lotion; the roots he adds are good for cankers, fistulas and warts. Pechey in 1694 records the use of boiled teasel root in addition for treating 'Ulcers of the Fundament [the buttocks]'. Medicinal exploitation of the plant seems to have declined after this, and modern medical herbalists in this country prescribe it rarely.

The value of teasel in fulling (the process of cleaning cloth and drawing out the fibres to thicken it) has persisted, however, albeit on a much reduced scale, and it is still cultivated in Somerset for this purpose. Flower arrangers value teasel since the dried heads keep their colour indefinitely.

Thistle
(various species)

The thistle now is older,
His stalk begins to moulder,
  His head is white as snow;

Richard Watson Dixon (1833–1900), *Willow*

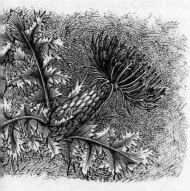

There are numerous species of thistle in this country, perhaps none more striking than the Scotch thistle (*Onopordum acanthium*). This is a magnificent, architectural plant with characteristic, spiny wings along its stems and large, solitary flowerheads that are familiar from Scottish heraldry. It is naturalized throughout Britain, and thought possibly to be native to East Anglia.

Numerous other thistles have been claimed to be *the* Scotch thistle, and the debate continues. Tradition tells us that the thistle became the symbol of Scotland after an invading barefoot Danish army trod on them; their subsequent shrieks alerted the nearby Scots, who raced to defend their land and eventually defeated the Danes.

The windborne seeds of all thistles can travel great distances, sometimes helped by man. Once established, they are hard to eradicate from agricultural land and, according to local proverbs, the timing of cutting them down is critical.

Cut them in June,
They'll come again soon.
Cut them in July,
They're sure to die.

Gerard tells us in 1597 that thistledown was gathered by the poor to stuff their beds and is 'also bought of the rich upholsterers to mix with feathers and down they do sell, which deceit would be looked unto'. An eighteenth-century botanist, John Bartram, reported that a Scots minister brought with him to North America his thistledown-filled bed. When he arrived in the New World, he found that feathers were plentiful and preferable, and so thistledown was replaced by feathers. The discarded thistle seeds grew and flourished, and that was how the Scotch thistle reached North America. In more recent times, the nature writer Richard Jefferies said that: 'thistle down is sometimes gathered to fill pillow-cases, and a pillow so filled is exquisitely soft'.

There are a small number of records of the Scotch thistle being used to treat cancer. One isolated report from England from a gypsy related that the treatment had a successful outcome.

In the nineteenth century, Kemsey writes, 'All thistles provoke the urine, and are said to help a stinking breath, and to strengthen the stomach.' Although many records of the use of thistle do not distinguish between the numerous species, one thistle does stand out as distinctive – the 'blessed thistle' (*Cnicus benedictus*). This yellow-flowered species is not native to Britain, but has been cultivated for centuries and has become naturalized occasionally as a weed of wasteland. It was used in official medicine to treat a great range of illnesses, including mad dog bites and other wounds, pleurisy, indigestion, and fever including the plague; it 'powerfully resists the Plague,' according to Salmon in 1693. Beatrice in *Much Ado about Nothing* (III, iv, 66–67) is advised for her sickness: 'Get you some of this distill'd Carduus Benedictus, and lay it to your heart'. The plant was given to nursing mothers to increase their milk, and was so even in the 1930s. Present-day herbalists prescribe the blessed thistle as a tonic, for fevers, and for wounds and sores.

The milk thistle (*Silybum marianum*) was utilized very similarly in official medicine and occurs occasionally as a naturalized weed. It has characteristic, white veins in its leaves, which have given rise to the legend that the Virgin's milk leaked onto the leaves when she was feeding the Infant Jesus. Another of its names is Marian thistle. Like the blessed thistle, this species has been recommended to increase milk in nursing mothers. Modern herbalists employ it to treat liver complaints and help repair the damage done to the liver by chemotherapy.

Most thistles have been used as food at some time. The flowering heads of both the Scotch and the milk thistle were boiled and eaten like miniature globe artichokes. A thistle tea was made in the Scottish Highlands that had the added bonus of helping sufferers of depression.

Thyme
(*Thymus* species)

Mark where the dry champaign
Swells into cheerful hills; where Marjoram
And Thyme the love of bees, perfume the air,
There bid thy roofs, high on the basking steep,
Ascend; there light thy hospitable fires.

John Armstrong, *The Art of Preserving Health: A Poem* (1744)

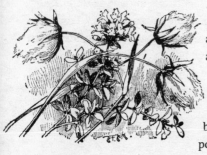

Although mostly familiar to us today as a garden herb, anyone who has walked among banks of thyme in the wild will never forget the scent and the sound of the bees humming above it. Thyme is common throughout upland Britain, but less so in the lowlands; it thrives in poor pastures because it survives grazing by sheep. The sheep of the South Downs are said to taste better for grazing on thyme.

The romantic landscapes in which the herb grows may have contributed to its symbolism, which is romantic and evocative. Fairy haunts are said to be where thyme grows, and it is also said to have been among the plants laid in the manger for the Christ-child. Thyme has also been associated with death and is often planted on graves, especially in Wales. The Oddfellows (one of Britain's oldest Friendly Societies) carry a sprig of the plant at funerals.

It is likely that because of its strong scent thyme would have been one of the earliest plants used to flavour food, and its medicinal properties would have been discovered much later. There is a widespread tradition that wild thyme should not be brought into the house – again a dark association with illness or death – and for this reason, infusions of the herb were prepared outside.

In folk medicine, thyme was used as a gargle for sore throats and an infusion for coughs and colds. Thyme tea was considered good for depression, for headaches and in preventing bad dreams. In the Hebrides in the nineteenth century, indigestion was treated with thyme.

Official medicine also recommended thyme for headache and lethargy, as well as coughs. The herb was also considered to 'force the Courses [periods], and Urine'. Oil of thyme was found to be effective in relieving the pain of toothache.

Modern-day medical herbalists prescribe thyme for asthma, coughs, hay fever, skin infections and sore throat. The herb has been shown to have strong antiseptic and antifungal properties. One of the constituents, thymol, is familiar to many as an ingredient of 'glycerine of thymol', which was until recently widely used as a gargle. Other ingredients of thyme have been shown to have antispasmodic properties, justifying its role in treating coughs.

Thyme's scent and flavour have made it indispensable in the domestic sphere. It is often added to country liqueurs, and with dates and barley makes a good wine. Honey from thyme-fed bees is exceptionally delicious. Dried thyme has been used to perfume household linen and it was an important constituent of herbal tobaccos. Should that not be enough, the stem tops of thyme produce a purple dye.

Tormentil
(*Potentilla erecta*)

Every Man tans & dresses his own Leather and makes his own Shoes. He tans
it with the Roots of Tormentil for there is scarcely a tree to be seen in the Island
to afford Bark.

Letter from John Lightfoot (1772) to his patron, regarding the Isle
of Skye

Tormentil grows on sandy heaths, and its small, four-petalled, bright yellow
flowers appear in late spring and early summer. Its stems are almost as fine
as hairs yet wiry too, so that the plant forms a springy cushion. In country
areas in the past, the plant was a common substitute for tea, and regarded
as a healthy tonic.

Its generic name is derived from the Latin for 'little torture', suggesting
its value in relieving the complaint it cures best – the griping pains of the
intestines. 'Tormenter', short and to the point, is one of its best-known
country names.

In herbalist's terms, the plant is astringent and has therefore proved a
useful country remedy for diarrhoea in man and animals. Dr Moffat, of
Midlothian, told in 1995 how the chopped remains of tormentil recovered
from medical waste at the site of the Soutra mediaeval hospital in Scotland
were always found in association with the eggs of whipworm, a human-gut
parasite, suggesting that the herb may have been used to treat worms as
well as diarrhoea. A drug company in North America recently investigated
this plant as a diarrhoea remedy for children. They searched for an 'active
principle' and thought they had found it; however, in trials it made the
diarrhoea worse. This is an example of a herb working in a more complex
way than at first supposed: the effect of using only one of its many
compounds proves to be completely different from using an extract of the
whole plant.

Another widespread folk remedy based on tormentil was for controlling bleeding. In Cornwall, tormentil roots were chopped and applied to cuts to staunch and heal them. Other remedies included ones for sunburn and fevers; in Gloucestershire, tormentil provided a soothing bath for sore feet and in Scotland the plant helped sufferers of 'sea-scurvy' by fastening the teeth.

As in folk medicine, official medicine used the plant mostly against diarrhoea. In the late-seventeenth century, both Salmon and Pechey are full of praise for tormentil: 'There is no Remedy more proper for Fluxes of the belly and Womb, than the Roots of Tormentil.' Gerard in 1597 also recommended a decoction of the root, held in the mouth, for toothache. A man in eighteenth-century England gained a great reputation for his tormentil cures and became such a local celebrity that the Bedfordshire landowner Lord William Russell gave him a piece of land on which to grow the plant.

Today's medical herbalists use tormentil for diarrhoea, staunching bleeding and as a mouthwash for infected gums and mouth ulcers.

The closely related species creeping cinquefoil (*Potentilla reptans*) was used in much the same way as tormentil medicinally, mainly to treat diarrhoea and fevers. It was regarded as having magical power and reputedly kept witches at bay. Creeping cinquefoil was a component of many spells in the Middle Ages, including ones for love divination. Tormentil too had a connection with the supernatural: in Orkney, its roots were used in the ritual of exorcism.

Both plants were of great use to fishermen. Tormentil root was used for tanning leather, which was especially useful in areas where trees – the more common source of tannin – were relatively scarce. In the Western Isles, fishermen tanned their nets using tormentil roots, or 'red roots', so called because they were a source of a bright red dye. Creeping cinquefoil was mixed with various other herbs such as marjoram and thyme, then boiled with corn and used on the nets as fish bait, which was believed to ensure a good catch – a little bit of magic again.

Traveller's Joy
(*Clematis vitalba*)

The cuckoo shouts all day at nothing
   In leafy dells alone;
And traveler's joy beguiles in autumn
Hearts that have lost their own.

A. E. Housman, *Tell me not here, it needs not saying* (1922)

John Gerard was the inventor of the name 'traveller's joy'. This woody climber was once very common, extravagantly garlanding hedgerows and banks with masses of flowers and fluffy seedheads. It is not quite as abundant these days because so many hedges have been grubbed up over the years; it can still be found in woodland and wasteland throughout Britain, although it is less common in Scotland. Its clusters of greenish-white flowers are not spectacular, but they are sweetly scented, smelling of vanilla. Another of the plant's names is 'old man's beard', from its white fluffy seedheads. The generic name *Clematis* is derived from the Greek *klema*, meaning 'vine branch'.

Sections of the stems used to be smoked in lieu of tobacco by schoolboys, who gave it names such as 'whiffy cane'. Its characteristic, stringy bark has been used in rope-making and, in Devon where the plant is common, the wood served to make the bottoms of crab pots. It was also used in basket-making. Farmers had an ingenious use for the tough stems; they were twined round farm gates to fasten them, a use which may have given rise to the name 'with-bind'.

The plant has played only a minor role in folk medicine. In Warwickshire, a loop of twined traveller's joy would be placed around the neck of a child suffering from convulsions and, in Gloucestershire, an infusion of the leaves eased rheumatism.

The story is no different in official medicine. Gerard in 1597 says of it, 'These plants have no use in physicke as yet found out, but are esteemed only for pleasure, by reason of the goodly shadow which they make with their thicke bushing and clyming, as also for the beauty of the floures, and the pleasant sent or savour of the same.' Yet it is reported in the nineteenth century that the leaves were 'formerly used by herbalists in rheumatism'. A decoction of the roots and stems was used in the early twentieth century as a treatment for itch. Today's medical herbalists do not advise the plant to be taken internally, but a preparation of the leaves is sometimes used externally to treat arthritis.

Beggars in the Middle Ages sought out the plant for its caustic juice. As in many other members of the buttercup family, the juice is an irritant; beggars knew this only too well and would deliberately raise blisters on their skin to elicit sympathy. On a very different note: the plant was known as 'virgin's bower' in some areas, also sometimes just called 'love', and was included in bridal bouquets as a symbol of binding the couple together.

Valerian

(*Valeriana* species)

It is of a great esteem in the Northern parts, where they never make any pottage or broath for any one that is sick, but they put some of this herb therein, be the disease what it will, and is called of them, The Poor Man's Remedy'.

William Coles, *Adam in Eden* (1657)

There are two native species of valerian, both of which are distributed throughout Britain. The common valerian (*Valeriana officinalis*) grows in grassland and is a tall, graceful, hairless herb, with divided basal leaves. Marsh valerian (*Valeriana dioica*), confined as its name suggests to damp areas, is a smaller plant, with undivided basal leaves. Both have pale pink or white flowers.

Valerian is fascinating to cats: when they smell the crushed leaves or root, they become excited and will roll on it and eat it with a great passion. It has a similar attraction for rats and has been used as bait by rat-catchers. It was said that the Pied Piper of Hamelin hid pieces of valerian root on himself to persuade the rats to follow him. The smell of the dried root is a strange one but nevertheless, in the sixteenth century, it was placed among clothing to sweeten them and, much later, was used as a basis for perfumes. It is mainly this strong-smelling root that has been used medicinally.

The plant has been used as a wound-healer for cuts and festered fingers in folk medicine. Its main use has been as a tonic. Gerard in 1597 tells us that country people so valued the plant in his day that 'some woman Poët or other hath made these verses.

They that will have their heale
Must put Setwall in their keale.'

'Setwall' is an old name for valerian; Chaucer uses it, describing one character as 'sweete as any Setwall'.

In official medicine, Culpeper in 1653 recommends valerian for a wide variety of conditions including croup, headache, the plague, wind and wounds. Pechey in 1694 describes similar uses for the plant and adds that 'it purges upwards and downwards'! An eighteenth-century manuscript in private hands in Norfolk recommends for kidney and bladder stones the roots of 'setwell', sliced and steeped with lemon juice and flavoured with marshmallow syrup. In the Gunton Household Book, there is a recipe for 'a good healing salve' composed of valerian and WOUNDWORT.

The Italian nobleman Fabio Colonna (1567–1650) claimed to have cured his epilepsy using valerian and published his findings in 1592; after that, the plant gradually became famous, particularly on the Continent, as a treatment for nervous diseases. By the nineteenth century in Britain, Kemsey says that it was 'employed in chronic headaches, epilepsy, hysterics, and in general nervous complaints'.

It is now known that valerian has a sedative effect on the central nervous system and is a good herb for treating insomnia. It was of particular value during the air raids of the First World War to soothe the 'overwrought nerves of civilian men and women'. The herb was cultivated for medicinal use in parts of Britain, but demand exceeded supply. A Board of Agriculture leaflet (no. 288) issued in 1915 states that: 'The foreign root was selling in January, 1914, at 30s. per cwt., English being worth about four times that price, 1s to 1s 3d per lb., and prices are about the same at the present time. Very little valerian is now cultivated in this country.'

Recent pharmacological studies are beginning to explain the action of the plant. Some of its constituents are now known to act directly on the part of the brain concerned with emotional response, while others have a direct sedative action. Present-day medical herbalists use valerian root for treating stress, muscle tension and insomnia, and many preparations including valerian root are now widely available to soothe anxiety and insomnia.

Even animals can be affected by valerian, as a recent story about some well-rested goats can confirm. The goats had escaped into a water meadow and were grazing on the plant growing there, much to the concern of the owner. The plant turned out to be valerian and the goats slept for twenty-four hours, but showed no ill effects. In the nineteenth century, there was still sufficient demand for the plant for it to be cultivated. The leaves were fed to cattle after the roots had been harvested for medicinal use. Hopefully no roots were included.

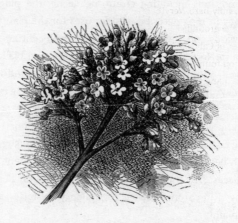

Vervain

(*Verbena officinalis*)

Al-hale, thou holy herb, Vervin
Growing on the ground;
On the Mount of Calvary
There was thou found;
Thou helpest many a grief,
And stanchest many a wound.
In the name of sweet Jesus
I take thee from the ground.

Elizabethan MS, Chetham Library, Manchester

This delicate and inconspicuous plant bears slender spikes of pale lilac flowers. It is hard to understand why our ancestors regarded such a modest and unassuming plant as immensely powerful. Since pre-Christian times, it has been credited with magical and religious powers and was used in love philtres and in foretelling the future. In Elizabethan times, it was recommended to recite the prayer above while gathering the plant. Witches included it in their spells; equally, it could be employed against witchcraft:

Vervain and dill
Hinder witches from their will ...

Vervain was known as a holy herb and was sacred to the Druids. Its reputation persisted through the centuries. Carrying vervain was said to protect the bearer from the barking of dogs and the bites of snakes; bound on the head it would cure headaches. The use of vervain as an amulet continued in rural England into the nineteenth century; it was tied around the neck of sickly children to help make them strong. In Devon, it was claimed that a mixture of the juices of vervain, dill and ST JOHN'S WORT anointed on the eyes on three successive days would enable a person to see the spirits of the air. The plant is so highly valued in the Isle of Man that it is often referred to simply as 'the herb'. In that same island, it also goes by the name of 'Nan Wade', after a famous Manx witch.

It is unclear to what extent the plant was utilized in practical medicine. In recent folk medicine, a preparation of the roots was used to treat wounds, fevers and eye conditions. An infusion of the whole plant has been used to soothe sunburn. Whether these are the vestiges of earlier, wider use is hard to ascertain.

In official medicine, the picture is confusing. One old English manuscript gives a recipe for a wound ointment in which vervain is combined with BETONY, a similarly revered plant; the author says of vervain, 'How good he is to mannys helpe'. Gerard in 1597 mentions vervain's use against fevers and the plague, but is disparaging of it as a remedy, 'for it is reported, that the Divell did reveal it as a secret and divine medicine'. On the other hand, Culpeper in 1653 recommends it for a wide variety of ailments including fevers, headaches, jaundice, ulcers and wounds. Pechey in 1694 suggests it for a similar list of illnesses and it was also said that: 'A Garland of Vervain put upon the Head, extirpates all Pain.' In the Gunton Household Book, a recipe is given for a salve called 'Gratia Dei' for treating all sores, new and old. It is composed of vervain, betony and SCARLET PIMPERNEL.

By the nineteenth century, Kemsey was still officially recommending vervain for 'jaundice, dropsy, and the gout, coughs, shortness of breath, and wheezings. Made into an ointment with hog's lard and a little honey, it is good for old ulcers, and the piles.' Our present-day medical herbalists mainly prescribe vervain for headaches, nervous exhaustion and for premenstrual tension. Although the plant is known to contain an array of interesting compounds, much research remains to be done. A leading authority on plant medicine, Professor Edzard Ernst, recently stated that vervain is likely to repay further investigation because of its anxiety-reducing and sedative effects. Perhaps one day we will come to understand better why vervain was regarded in the past as an all-powerful panacea.

On a lighter note, vervain was once used to repel rats. Is this how the Pied Piper finally got rid of his rodent followers after he had attracted them with VALERIAN?

Watercress
(*Rorippa nasturtium-aquaticum*)

I ha'e an itching to express
My thanks to thee – wee Watercress …
Thou'rt no a plant to tak' the e'e
Or wauken up a poet's glee:
Sae, plain this truth to you I'll blab –
Your strong appeal is to the gab!

James Rigg, *To the Water-cress* (1897)

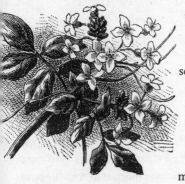

Watercress is still a common plant of streams and ditches throughout Britain. At one time, it was a very important source of green salad, valued for its flavour as well as its medicinal properties. It was also a source of supplementary income for many country people over the centuries, who gathered it and sold bunches of it beside their own produce at the local market. There was a tradition that watercress should be eaten only when there was an 'R' in the month; as a result it was not gathered during the summer months while the cress was flowering, and at its least valuable as a food. Between the world wars, watercress farming gave a decent livelihood for a number of people in the Midlands and south of England.

In folk medicine, watercress was valued as a tonic after the winter and as a remedy and preventative for scurvy. Its nourishing properties were well known. When the Macleods of Harris massacred many of the Macdonalds of Eigg in the sixteenth century, and left the survivors to starve, one old woman called after them, 'If I get shell-fish and dulse for my portion, tender watercress and a drink from the limpid well of Tolain, my need is served and I shall not want.'

The plant was sometimes used to cool fevers and, in the Scottish Highlands, to help women conceive. Mr C— of Norton Subcourse told in 1989 how, in the water meadows of Norfolk, people would still take a bruised sprig of watercress and rub it onto inflamed eyelids. A similar application was recorded by William Kingsbury, an early-eighteenth-century horseman from Norfolk:

> For weak Eyes such as Inflamation in A Cristain [Christian] take watter Crases and pulverise them in a mortar then Squeeze them close and dress your eyes with the Same.

In Ireland the plant was used for a very wide variety of ailments, including this unusual example:

> 'For a hurt sustained by someone doing manual work such as an over-tired arm, apply a bunch of watercress to skin and lay a slice of bread softened with hot water on afflicted part. Bandage and leave overnight. Hurt will disappear.'

Mrs E. P—, Co. Londonderry (2002)

In official medicine too, the plant was a renowned antiscorbutic. Salmon in 1693 observes that watercresses 'cure the scurvy, for which they are a Specifick. The green are better than the dry.' He also recommends watercress for dropsy and as 'an opener of all obstructions'. Culpeper in 1653 suggests using watercress for cleaning ulcers and clearing spots; he pronounced, 'Those that would live in health may use it if they please; if they will not, I cannot help it.' In later centuries, 'Spring juices' made from watercress, SCURVYGRASS, BROOKLIME and Seville oranges were popular. Watercress is now known to have a high vitamin C content as well as being rich in iodine and iron. It is truly a healthful salad plant and all those spring juices and tonics must once have made a great deal of difference to people's health. Present-day medical herbalists still recommend it as a tonic.

The pretty green leaves of watercress have featured in some unusual garnishes. In Ireland, it was used as a decoration on top of blancmange made from carrageen, a type of SEAWEED, and in the early twentieth century it was also used to decorate the Christmas pudding, in lieu of a sprig of holly.

Water Cress Soup

Wash and dry 2 good bunches of Water Cress, picking out the yellowish leaves. Plunge the stems and leaves into boiling salted water to scald for a moment, then strain it and chop it finely. Put a piece of butter into a saucepan and when it boils add the chopped Cress and turn it about with a wooden spoon for 5 minutes over a slow burner. Stir in a little water if necessary to keep it from burning. Cook 1 tablespoonful of tapioca in 1 pint of water till clear, then add 1 pint of milk and beat them together before adding the Water Cress. Season with salt and pepper to taste. Beat up the yolk of an egg in the soup tureen and add a lump of butter. Before pouring the soup, stir in a small cupful of cream, then pour it over the egg, stirring well to prevent curdling.

Audrey Wynne Hatfield, *Pleasures of Herbs* (1964)

White Bryony
(*Bryonia dioica*)

They take likewise the roots of mandrake, or, as I rather suppose, the roots of
briony, which simple folk take for the true mandrake, and make thereof an ugly
image, by which they represent the person on whom they intend to exercise
their witchcraft ...

William Coles, *The Art of Simpling* (1656)

Among the famous leaves of Southwell
Cathedral, carved in stone in the fourteenth century, are some that strongly
resemble bryony. It would have been
familiar to many as a hedgerow plant
weaving its way through shrubbery and
trees. This pretty climbing plant has long
tendrils that are coiled like springs, allowing
the plant to sway in the wind without damage. The five-petalled flowers are
pale yellowish-green and unnoticeable as a result, but they are quite beautiful
and worth examining more closely.

The plant is a member of the Cucurbitaceae family, which includes many
edible plants such as cucumbers and melons. However, this plant is quite
different: it is poisonous and bears bright red berries; the root is highly toxic
too. Despite the understandable caution surrounding poisonous plants,
country people have nevertheless found various uses for it.

Bryony root was at one time known as 'mandrake root' and in East Anglia
it was often passed off as the 'true' mandrake of the herbals, a Mediterranean
plant much prized for its magical and aphrodisiac qualities. Both plants have
long, sometimes divided taproots; that of the mandrake supposedly resembles the human form. Famously, the true mandrake is said to shriek when
uprooted, a story repeated in 1597 by Gerard among others. White bryony

is by far the safer bet in this respect. Bryony roots were sold as counterfeit mandrake, a deceit well worth practising since true mandrake root fetched very high prices. Pechey in 1694 tells us that: 'Juglers and Fortune-tellers make wonderful Monsters of this Root, which, when they have hid in the Sand for some Days, they dig up for Mandrakes; and by the Imposture these Knaves imposte on our Common People.' As recently as the 1920s, there was a fake mandrake made from bryony root displayed in a chemist's shop window in Sussex.

Mrs D. P— of Essex told in 1989 how, in East Anglia, the bright red, shiny berries would be crushed and rubbed on chilblains. However, in Hampshire this practice did not prevail, probably because there was a superstition that the juice from the berries could cause sores or 'tetters' if it touched the skin. The berries were therefore known in that county as 'tetter-berries'. The root was included in a liniment for treating rheumatism; a safer version of this remedy was simply to carry a piece of the root in the pocket. In the nine-teenth century, the plant was 'sometimes applied by the peasantry to bruises, and especially to black eyes, though never a very safe application'. A remnant of the old beliefs surrounding mandrake remained in East Anglia for many years where a tea, prepared from the white bryony root, was given to promote fertility.

The bryony is an example of a strange phenomenon in plant folklore, that of gender pairing, in which unrelated plants are paired as 'male' and 'female'. White bryony was regarded as 'female', BLACK BRYONY as 'male'. And so, traditionally, any remedy prepared would have to take this into account. The male of a pair could only treat a woman, and vice versa. One of the country names in Lincolnshire for white bryony is 'womandrake', in contrast to mandrake.

White bryony root was used in horse medicine, but exactly how is hard to determine. There is a great deal of secrecy surrounding horseman's lore, and this is no exception. It has been suggested that the root was fed to horses to improve the shine on their coat, but it may have had other applications too. The early-eighteenth-century notebook from Norfolk of a horseman, William Kingsbury, gives the following clue:

> For Driving of Horses take a Briany [sic] Root and Dry it to powder give them a small Quantity at A time if they be Stone Horses ... it will make them follow you.

The plant was used in official medicine as a drastic purge and, in medi-aeval England, for treating leprosy. Pechey in 1694 tells us that it 'is proper for diseases of the spleen, liver and womb', and is also good for asthma. By the eighteenth century, the plant was being prescribed more cautiously: Pierre Pomet tells us, 'The root of this plant is so violent, that the peasants call it the Mad Nip.'

Modern-day herbalists use white bryony with great care, for treating bronchitic complaints and rheumatism. Ongoing research suggests that the plant has strong antiviral properties, and there is some evidence that it may have some effect against tumours too. It might very well prove to be of value in the pharmacology of the future.

White Deadnettle
(*Lamium album*)

And there with whorls encircling grand
Of white and purple-tinted red,
The harmless Nettle's helmèd head;
Less apt with fragrance to delight
The smell than please the curious sight.

Bishop Mant (Bishop of Andrim 1823–1849)

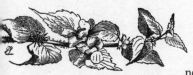

This plant is questionably native, but very widespread in the British Isles. Although unrelated to the stinging nettle, it grows in similar situations and the two are often found together. This has given rise to a lovely story: the fairies became cross at their shoes being continually stolen by centipedes, so they decided to hide them among the stinging nettles. (They first had to cast a spell so that they would not get stung when they went to retrieve their shoes.) Pick a piece of deadnettle and turn it upside-down: in every white flower, you will see two black pairs of fairy shoes, neatly hidden.

The plant has other hidden powers. In folk medicine, it has been utilized until the recent past in treating arthritis; at least one elderly lady gathered it regularly up to the 1980s and drank an infusion of the flowering tops, and found relief from her pain. In addition, deadnettle has been used for skin complaints, including deep cuts and eczema, as well as heavy periods and sore feet.

In official medicine, the plant has been used to treat the King's evil (scrofula), gout, dysentery and bleeding. Pechey in 1694 states that: 'One handful of the Herb, beaten up with Hog's lard, and applied to the King's-Evil-Swellings in the Neck or Throat, discusses them.' In the nineteenth century, an infusion of the flowers was also found to be a good remedy for treating 'whites' (leucorrhoea). Today's herbalists prescribe white deadnettle for heavy and painful periods and diarrhoea. Externally, a lotion of the flowering tops is administered for piles and varicose veins.

As a food source, a sweetmeat and a tonic, the white deadnettle was extremely valuable. The flowers would be baked with sugar in the sixteenth century, as was commonly done with roses, and a distillation of the flowers was used, in Gerard's words, 'to make the heart merry, to make a good colour in the face, and to refresh the vitall spirits'. The plant was eaten readily in the nineteenth century, being 'wholesome and palatable when boiled'. Today the young, tender flowering tops, washed and lightly steamed with butter, make a pleasant vegetable, and are made even tastier by adding chopped spring onions. A wine is still made from the flowers in Yorkshire, where the plant is sometimes called 'day nettle'.

Even the garden can benefit from white deadnettle; it makes an excellent contribution to the compost heap.

White Horehound
(*Marrubium vulgare*)

Pale hore-hound, which he holds of most especiall use.

Michael Drayton (1563–1631), *Polyolbion*

This softly hairy, untidy plant of hedgerows and wasteland has the square stems characteristic of the mint family, to which it belongs. The whitish, small flowers are borne in tight clusters in the axils of the rather small, oval, toothed leaves. White horehound is native to Britain, but is not a common plant and completely absent from the north of Scotland. It has an aromatic scent and a strange flavour and is one of the five bitter herbs eaten by Jews at Passover.

In folk medicine, the plant has been used above all to treat coughs and colds. As recently as the 1920s, bunches of the herb were dried and kept until needed and the plant was often cultivated in the garden for medicinal use. Preparations made from horehound were numerous; a candy for coughs, bronchitis and asthma was extremely popular. No doubt the refreshing horehound beer was a very palatable way of taking the herb, but its properties as a tonic and medicine were paramount. The same applied to horehound wine, famous for its pleasant and medicinal qualities. The stalks and leaves would be boiled with maize, and ginger and sugar added. It was then bottled and corked and kept for use as needed. Horehound tea was an easier tonic to prepare:

'Dandelion, blackcurrant leaves and hary hound [horehound] boiled together and strained make a spring medicine.'

Miss G—, Attleborough (*c.*1930)

The plant was used similarly in official medicine. Gerard in 1597 tells us that a 'Syrup made from the fresh greene leaves of the horehound, and sugar ... doth wonderfully, and above credit, ease such as have been long sicke of any consumption of the lungs.' Horehound syrup was still included in the British Pharmaceutical Codex of 1949. Present-day medical herbalists continue to use horehound for treating coughs and other respiratory complaints.

Recipe for horehound candy

Gather the horehound when it is in full flower, wash well, and cut the stem into inch-long pieces. You use the entire herb, stem, leaves and flowers. Add enough water to cover the herb and bring to the boil. Simmer for at least two hours, keeping the lid on the pan but adding fresh boiling water from time to time to keep up the quantity. Strain, squeezing thoroughly to get out all the juice. Put that juice into the preserving pan, measure, and to each pint of juice add a pound of sugar, brown if you can get it. Bring to the boil and boil, removing any scum that rises, until it has become quite thick. Have ready a baking tin lined with greased paper, pour in the syrup and allow to get cold. Using a greased knife cut into squares and store in airtight tins.

Mary Thorne Quelch, *Herbs and How to Know Them* (1946)

White Water Lily
(*Nymphaea alba*)

Yellow Water Lily
(*Nuphar lutea*)

And floating water-lilies, broad and bright,
Which lit the oak that overhung the hedge
With moonlight beams of their own watery light;

Percy Bysshe Shelley (1803–1882), *The Question*

Everything about the water lily is beautiful and striking. It sits serenely on the water, whether in lakes, canals or clean ponds, where its large leaves ('pads') provide platforms for insects and frogs. The flowers are among some of the largest in our native flora and are sweetly scented. It is not hard to imagine why there was a legend in the Scottish Highlands that fairies used white water lilies for enchantment. There was also a belief, which lasted well into the Victorian Age, that the blooms disappear under the surface of the water during the night.

Now folds the lily all her sweetness up,
And slips into the bosom of the lake:

Alfred, Lord Tennyson, *The Princess* (1847), VII

In fact the flowers simply close up and are so well camouflaged by their green sepals that they are almost invisible until the morning sun prompts them to open again, as the poem suggests.

There are several thirteenth-century sculptures of the flowers and leaves of the yellow water lily; the one in Lincoln Cathedral is particularly famous. The yellow water lily has as one of its country names 'brandy bottle', which may refer to the shape of the seed capsule or to the scent of the flowers, which is reminiscent of wine dregs.

Water lilies have been the source of some very interesting remedies. The seeds and roots were used in Elizabethan times to induce chastity. Pechey in 1694 describes the water lily as effective in 'lessening venery [the pursuit of sexual gratification]' and 'nocturnal pollutions'. The plant was also used by herbalists as a general sedative; in Culpeper's words, 'the syrup helpeth much to procure rest, and to settle the brains of frantic persons' – the unchaste, perhaps. Another unusual use was popular in the eighteenth century, when yellow-water-lily roots were effective and specific deterrents of cockroaches and crickets.

Also in official medicine, the roots were boiled in vinegar and applied as corn plasters, and the seeds of the white water lily served to treat headaches. An eighteenth-century manuscript includes a note about their effectiveness, to which the author adds, 'which my son use in France'. This then was a remedy that was actually used, rather than simply written down.

Kemsey in 1838 recommended the seeds and roots of lilies, both white and yellow, to 'stay fluxes' and the leaves and flowers to 'abate inflammation'. Today, medical herbalists prescribe white water lily for discharges, boils and abscesses as well as sore throat, kidney pain and catarrh. The plant is also found to be beneficial for insomnia and anxiety – 'the brains of frantic persons'. Perhaps surprisingly, recent research suggests that it really does diminish sexual drive, explaining why Pechey advises it.

We have few dependable records of the application of water lilies in folk medicine, but they were important sources of dyes. In the Scottish Highlands, black, dark brown and dark blue dyes for wool were obtained from both types of water lily. In addition, there was a demand for medicinal use. No doubt many plants were also taken from the wild for transplantation into gardens. Harvesting the roots from their deep mud was an incredibly difficult task and special rafts were constructed from which the lilies could be hooked out of the water, dragging the roots with them.

Wild Carrot
(*Daucus carota*)

The autumn carrot I'd give thee
My love, wert thou mine own.

'Croon of the shellfish gathering', recorded Alexander Carmichael,
Carmina Gadelica, vol. V (1940)

This plant is common on waysides and hedgerows throughout Britain, growing especially on chalky ground. It is easily distinguished from other members of its family (Apiaceae, formerly Umbelliferae) by the shape of its fruiting seed-head. This has a very characteristic, nest-like appearance: concave in the middle, with the seeds pressed tightly together. (One of the plant's country names is 'bird's nest'.) This form is created by the flowerstalks bending inwards after pollination; when the fruits ripen, the umbel flattens out again and the burred fruits are readily dispersed by passing animals. The whole plant is mildly aromatic and smells, as one would expect, faintly of carrot.

The cultivated carrot was developed from an eastern subspecies, rather than from our wild one. The taproots of the wild carrot are white rather than orange, but are just as edible and were an important source of food in times of famine. In the Outer Hebrides, children regard a forked carrot as particularly lucky, and when they find one they rub it on their head, reciting:

Fork joyful, joyful, joyful,
Fork of great carrot to me.

Carrot seed was a hop substitute in brewing and imparted a good flavour to the ale. Roasted carrot has served as a coffee substitute. The oil obtained from its seeds is still a source of flavouring for alcoholic drinks.

In Scotland, the wild carrot was a symbol of fertility; in the nineteenth century (and probably earlier), a ceremony would be held on the feast of St Michael, on 29 September. Wild carrots were dug by the women in preparation for the feast and tied with red, three-ply thread. These were given by women to men on the feast day as tokens of affection. Gerard in 1597 rather coyly refers to the carrot as 'serving for love matters' and adds that the wild species is more effective than the cultivated one.

Carrot seed has been utilized in folk medicine in an infusion to treat dropsy and kidney complaints, while the root has been mashed and applied as a poultice to burns and sores. In Scotland, this poultice was especially valued to treat cancerous sores and, according to Thomas Pennant in the eighteenth century, 'Even the faculty admit the salutary effect of the carrot-poultice in sweetening the intolerable foetor [smell] of the cancer.' Carrot poultices were clearly most effective and were still in favour in Suffolk country medicine in the early years of the twentieth century.

Wild-carrot seed was used in the same ways in official medicine – consistently so, right through to the nineteenth century. Pechey in 1694 quotes an instance that bears testimony to the effectiveness of the wild carrot seed in one of its most important applications:

> Mr Boyle, in his Book of the Usefulness of Natural Philosophy, says, That discoursing once with an eminently learned and experience'd Physician of the Anti-nephritical Virtue of the Seed of this Carrot, fermented in Small Ale, he smilingly told him, That he found its efficacy but too great; for, having prescrib'd it to some of his rich Patients, who were wont frequently to have recourse to him for the Stone [large urinary stones]; after the Use of this Drink for a pretty while, he seldom heard of them any more.

Kemsey in 1838 summarizes the value of carrots: 'The seed is good for the dropsy, and those whose bellies are swollen with wind. The leaves being applied, with honey, to running sores cleanses them.'

Today's medical herbalists value carrot as a detoxifier and source of vitamin C. It is prescribed too for kidney stones and flatulence, just as our forbears did. Carrots are rich in carotene, which is converted by the liver to vitamin A and improves night vision. Wild carrot is now known to contain chemicals called porphyrins, which increase the production of sex hormones by the pituitary gland; Gerard evidently was right when he said that the carrot serves in love matters.

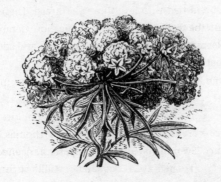

Wild Cherry
(*Prunus avium*)

Loveliest of trees, the cherry now
Is hung with bloom along the bough,
And stands about the woodland ride
Wearing white for Eastertide.

A. E. Housman, *A Shropshire Lad* (1896), II, 1–4

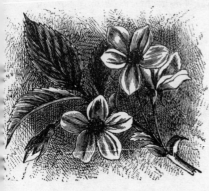

The wild cherry, or gean as it is known in Scotland, is still to be found scattered in woodland throughout Britain. The delicate, white, drooping flowers have a sweet, almond-like scent, unlike their garden counterparts. It is known as the 'merry tree' in Shetland, but despite this lovely appellation North-Country people considered it unlucky to use its blossom as decoration in a church for a wedding.

In folk medicine, the bark was used as a gargle for sore throat, coughs and colds. Sometimes the bark was mixed with that of sloe and plum. An astringent drink was made in the Scottish Highlands from the stalks of the cherries. A similar drink was made from the sap, which also provided a gum sometimes chewed by children for pleasure. The fruits – very sweet if picked at the right time – often flavoured rather more unhealthy drinks, such as whisky. We are not the only creatures to appreciate them. Pechey in 1694 notes that: 'The Livers of Sparrows grow very big at Cherry-time.'

As is the case with CRAB APPLES, in official medicine it would have been the cultivated variety that was preferred. Gerard in 1597 actually warned against the use of sweet wild cherries, saying with some certainty that they engender 'ill bloud, by reason whereof they do not onely breede wormes in the belly, but troublesome agues, and often pestilential fevers: and therefore in well governed common wealthes it is carefully provided, that they should not be sold in markets in the plague time'. Culpeper in 1653 recommended cherry gum (type unstated) dissolved in wine for sore throats, for gravel and stone (urinary stones), and for sharpening the appetite and the eyesight. In the seventeenth- and eighteenth-century Gunton Household Book, there is a recipe for treating sore nipples during nursing, consisting of applying the gum of cherry trees dissolved in water.

Tincture of wild cherry was still listed in the British Pharmaceutical Codex of 1949. Today's medical herbalists prescribe extracts of cherry for treating coughs, but these are usually obtained from related North American species.

Our other native species of cherry, the bird cherry (*Prunus padus*), produces hard, almost black fruit. The tree was known in Scotland as 'hagberry'. It was regarded as the witch's tree in northeast Scotland, and in those parts was never used in any way, at least by humans. On the other hand, it seems to have been regarded in Wester Ross as protective against evil; a walker carrying a bird-cherry stick would not get lost in the mist. Both types of cherry could be used in this piece of twentieth-century folklore, where the tree was used to foretell how long a person would live:

'"Cuckoo cherry tree
Come down and tell to me
How many years I have to live."

Then each child shakes one of the cherry tree branches and the number of cherries that fall tell him or her how many years he will live. A true saying heard when I was a child sixty years ago.'

Mrs J. S—, Essex (1991)

Willow
(*Salix* species)

The feathers of the willow
Are half of them grown yellow
  Above the swelling stream ...

Richard Watson Dixon (1833–1900), *Willow*

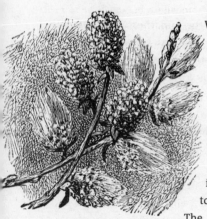

Willow, 'sally' and 'sallow' are all names for a widely distributed tree that has been exploited in innumerable ways for domestic and medicinal use. There are many species and hybrids of willow that are native to Britain, and for the most part they have been used interchangeably.

Willow was used in a number of ways in folk medicine. In Cornwall, it served to staunch bleeding and clear dandruff. The ashes of burnt willow dissolved in vinegar provided a remedy for corns and warts. Willow also acted as a painkiller. Within living memory, people in Lincolnshire chewed willow bark for headaches, especially for a hangover. Willow-bark tea was used for fever and, in the Fens when malaria was rife, it must have been a godsend. Watery places are of course the willow's preferred habitat and malarial fevers were still common in those areas right up to the nineteenth century.

Official medicine had also known for centuries about willow's effectiveness in bringing down fevers. In 1597 Gerard recommends this extravagant use of the tree: 'The greene boughs with the leaves may very well be brought into chambers and set about the beds of those that be sicke of fevers, for they doe mightily coole the heate of the aire, which thing is a wonderfull refreshing to the sicke Patients.'

Willow was also administered for a number of other ailments, gout in particular; Culpeper, for example, recommended it in 1653 for staunching bleeding and for corns and warts. Salmon in 1693 echoes these applications and adds that a cataplasm of leaves applied to the soles of the feet is good for a fever. Then in the middle of the eighteenth century, an Oxfordshire parson, Reverend Edmund Stone, singled out the use of willow for fevers and drew it to the attention of the medical profession. From then on, it became a widely approved remedy. Kemsey in 1838 describes willow as 'apparently more serviceable in phthisic and hectic fever than the cinchona bark, and, in some cases, of intermittents [malaria]'. Until then cinchona bark, the source of quinine, was the most effective remedy for fevers. In that very same year, salicylic acid was isolated from willow bark and in 1860 was synthesized in the laboratory for the first time. Aspirin was then developed from salicylic acid at the end of the nineteenth century.

This progress, important though it was, does not represent the end of the story. Today's medical herbalists still prescribe willow bark for fevers, headache and painful joints. It is found that the bark produces pain relief without many of the unwanted side effects of aspirin, such as irritation of the gut lining. Time and again, we learn that the effects of a plant extract are often very different from those of a single, isolated 'active ingredient'. Clearly, much more research is needed.

Willow actually has a sinister reputation in folklore. It is said in Somerset to follow one on a dark night, muttering to itself. In Scotland, willow wands were used in black magic and the word 'wicca' (witchcraft) is thought to derive from 'wicker'. The tree is also associated with sadness, and traditionally anyone forsaken in love wore a willow garland. Shakespeare alludes to this association in *Othello* (IV, iii, 25–30):

> My mother had a maid called Barbara;
> She was in love; and he she lov'd prov'd mad,
> And did forsake her. She had a song of 'willow';
> An old thing 'twas, but it express'd her fortune,
> And she died singing it. That song to-night
> Will not go from my mind ...

The wood of willow has been put to use in numerous ways. White willow (*Salix alba*) produces the finest cricket bats in the world, and its toughness and lightness make it perfect for artificial limbs and even polo balls. This fast-growing tree is still cultivated commercially along ditches and planted along riverbanks, its stems woven into a living lattice, to stabilize them. The slender branches (withies) have been used in basketmaking since at least the sixth century. In the Scottish Highlands, willows were important in domestic economy as a source of baskets, beehives, creels, lobster pots, twine and many other items – so much so that the expression 'It's time to be steeping the withies' became a way of saying that it is time to depart and get on with life's business.

The extreme flexibility of willow, especially when cut into thin strips, led to a cottage industry in Victorian England. Richard Jefferies commented that 'There were willow looms in the village, and to show their dexterity the weavers sometimes made a shirt of willow – of course only as a curiosity.' Living willow hedges, garden seats and sculptures have recently become fashionable in our gardens. Next time you sit on a seat of willow, think of the amazing favours this tree has done for us.

Wood Sorrel
(*Oxalis acetosella*)

The Apothecaries and Herbarists call it Alleluya, or Cuckowes meate, because either the Cuckow feedeth thereon or by reason when it springeth forth and floureth the Cuckow singeth most, at which time also Alleluya was wont to be sung in Churches.

John Gerard, *The Herball, or Generall Historie of Plantes* (1597)

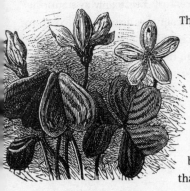

This pretty, creeping plant of damp woodland has bright yellow-green, three-lobed leaves and pale pink, drooping flowers with delicate purple veining. It blooms between Easter and Whitsun. The leaves fold up like little umbrellas at night and when the weather is changing, which has earned the plant the name of 'sleeping beauty' in Dorset. Pechey observed in 1694 that it had a further value as a weather forecaster: ''Tis observ'd, that when it bears a great many Flowers, the Year will be very rainy; but dry when there is a few.'

Wood sorrel was sometimes claimed to be 'shamrock' on account of its strong resemblance to the legendary plant that St Patrick employed to explain the Trinity, and no doubt wood sorrel was also credited with religious significance.

The leaves are pleasantly bitter and refreshing and are often nibbled by children. It can be eaten in moderation but it should not be eaten in excessively large amounts because of its high oxalate content. Wood sorrel was however popular as a salad ingredient and cooking herb until the introduction in Henry VIII's time of French sorrel (*Rumex scutatus*), which has large, fleshy leaves and a good flavour.

Wood sorrel has played a role in folk medicine, although infrequently, in a number of ways. In Scotland, an infusion of the plant quenched thirst during a fever and in a poultice it treated scrophula (glandular tuberculosis). It soothed bruises in Devon – the plant was boiled, cooled and then applied to the bruise – and in Ireland it was utilized to treat diarrhoea.

In official medicine, a jam called 'Conserva Ligulae', made from wood-sorrel leaves, sugar and orange peel, provided the basis of a cooling drink for feverish patients. Gerard in 1597 recommended wood sorrel made into a green sauce for 'them that have sicke and feeble stomackes; for it strengtheneth the stomacke, procureth appetite, and of all Sorrell sauces is the best, not onely in vertue, but also in the pleasantnesse of his taste'. He also, like Culpeper after him, advised it for fevers and mouth ulcers.

Unrelated sorrels have tended to be lumped together by many of the herbalists, including in the nineteenth century Kemsey, who states that 'Sorrell, Wood and Garden ... is used in all hot diseases, to cool any inflammation and heat of blood, and is cordial to the heart.' Despite this, the medicinal role of the plant declined in the twentieth century and it is little favoured by today's medical herbalists.

Woody Nightshade
(*Solanum dulcamara*)

Thou seem'st a crouching thing of fear;
But when the shedding woods grow sere,
Thy glittering clusters then appear –
Solanum dulcamara.

James Rigg, *To the Woody Nightshade, or Bittersweet* (1897)

This woody climber is a member of the family (Solanaceae) that includes tomatoes, potatoes and the deadly nightshade (*Atropa belladonna*). Like its relatives, woody nightshade is poisonous (as are the leaves of potatoes and tomatoes), although not as toxic as the deadly nightshade. Culpeper in 1653 wisely suggests, 'Have a care you mistake not the deadly Nightshade for this; if you know it not, you may let them both alone, and take no harm.' The berries and stems when eaten taste bitter at first, then the taste changes to sweet, hence its common name of 'bittersweet'. The entire plant is poisonous and eating the berries can prove fatal. The twigs once provided a tobacco substitute in Cumberland; they would be chewed rather than made into a tobacco. Perhaps the hint of danger added to the fun of chewing it.

The plant's sprays of purple flowers are borne in drooping clusters at the ends of its branches. Each flower is a thing of beauty: the five-pointed petals surround a ring of green and white sham-nectaries, which enclose a bright yellow cone, formed from the fused stamens. Pollen is shed through holes in the ends of the ripe stamens. The green and shiny berries ripen to a rich red, and birds eat them greedily. The seeds pass through the birds, leaving them unharmed, and so are disseminated. If the plant were not a weed, it would surely be grown in gardens for its ornamental qualities; in fact, a variant (*Solanum dulcamara* 'Variegatum') is grown as a garden plant.

In folk and official medicine, the plant has been used as a narcotic to aid sleep. One of Tutankhamen's coffins had on it a wreath, formed by threading dried woody-nightshade berries onto strips of date palm. Perhaps they were intended to ease his pain, or to keep him sweetly asleep. Salmon in 1693 confirms its reputation as a sedative, telling us that an extract of nightshade is 'soporiferous and operates much like Opium ... being given by a wise hand'.

This was not the only role for this plant. Chilblains and whitlows were treated with its juice in folk medicine, a remedy still in vogue in the 1940s. In Norfolk, the dried berries were threaded and worn as necklaces to help infant teething; presumably the fumes from the berries were considered helpful, or else these were worn as protection against the powers of evil. Infants were considered to be very vulnerable when teething. More boldly, in the Isle of Man the plant was boiled in beer as a tonic and to treat inward bruising: not a recommendation that would be made today.

Gerard in 1597 advocates the plant for external bruising: the juice is good 'for them that have fallen from high places, and have been thereby bruised'. Culpeper in 1653 advises it to cool inflammations. Also in the seventeenth century, Pechey recommends the juice of the plant for treating dropsy and jaundice, and a cataplasm of the leaves applied externally to inflammations and swellings while Salmon in 1693 tells us that it is employed mainly externally as an ointment or cataplasm, for pain and fevers. However, Kemsey in 1838 states that bittersweet 'has been found useful in asthma, dropsy, rheumatism and diseases of the skin', and that the dried leaves should be taken in milk.

Modern herbalists still use the plant with caution, to treat skin conditions, bronchitis and asthma as well as rheumatic conditions. Because it is toxic in excess, the plant should only be used under professional guidance.

Wormwood
(*Artemisia absinthium*)

While wormwood hath seed, get a bundle or twain,
To save against March, to make flea to refrain,
Where chamber is swept, and wormwood is strewn,
No flea, for his life, dare abide to be known.

Thomas Tusser, *Five Hundred Pointes of Good Husbandrie* (1557)

This fragrant, silvery weed was once grown in cottage gardens for domestic use. Now it is naturalized throughout England and Wales as a weed of wasteland and field edges, although it is uncommon in Scotland. It is particularly abundant in Wales, where it was and is employed in folk medicine as a tonic as well as a worm-killer. In England, too, wormwood tea was taken as a tonic and an aid to digestion. The plant was also used to destroy fleas and lice, strewn on floors and placed among clothing and bedding and, in the eighteenth century, it was even used to spray greenfly. A Suffolk man recalls the application of wormwood as an insect repellent:

'A retired rector came to live in the village some years ago, he being interested in the countryside and often came to see me. So one day I took him a rooted plant of wormwood. This he planted quite near his back door, and was quite convinced this kept his house free from flies. This, as you know, was used in the past to rid houses of fleas, and other pests.'

Mr M. G. R—, Lakenheath (1990)

Wormwood's extreme bitterness (*absinthium* means 'without sweetness') made it a valuable substance for weaning a child off the breast. In *Romeo and Juliet* (I, iii, 25–33), the nurse recalls weaning the infant Juliet:

And she was wean'd – I never shall forget it –
Of all the days of the year, upon that day;

For I had then laid wormwood to my dug,
Sitting in the sun under the dove-house wall ...
When it did taste the wormwood on the nipple
Of my dug, and felt it bitter, pretty fool,
To see it tetchy, and fall out with the dug!

This custom was taken, along with the plant, to seventeenth-century New England.

Wormwood was utilized in much the same way in official medicine as in domestic practice. Pechey in 1694 recommends it for strengthening the stomach and expelling worms as well as for jaundice, dropsy, fevers and for treating 'Tumors of the Kernels of the Throat'. In the eighteenth century, it came into vogue as a remedy for gout as well. In the nineteenth century, it was still being prescribed by Kemsey for dropsy, gout, intermittent fevers and scurvy, as well as for killing worms.

Today's medical herbalists use it mainly as a powerful digestive remedy, for stimulating bile secretion and easing wind. We now know that wormwood contains an array of ingredients, some of which stimulate digestive secretions, while others are anti-inflammatory and yet others strongly insecticidal.

Wormwood has strange and magical associations. In the Middle Ages, it was believed that a wreath made from it and thrown into a Midsummer Eve's fire would protect the thrower for an entire year. The herb was used in relatively recent times in Somerset to fend off the evil eye and, in Devon too, it was considered a powerful herb against witches. Perhaps because of its power against evil, dreaming of wormwood is said to be a good omen.

Oil of wormwood provided the basis of the now notorious liqueur absinthe, which was very popular in nineteenth-century France. One of wormwood's constituents, thujone, is a brain stimulant and, although safe in small amounts, is toxic in high doses. This fact, together with the liqueur's addictive nature, led to a ban on absinthe in the early twentieth century.

On a positive note, the related species *Artemisia annua*, which has been employed for thousands of years in China to treat malarial fevers, is showing great promise as a treatment of otherwise drug-resistant malaria.

Woundwort
(*Stachys sylvatica*)

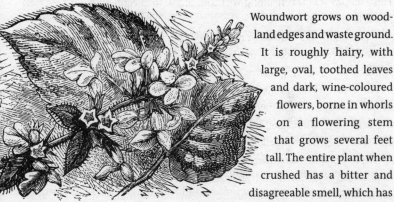

Woundwort grows on woodland edges and waste ground. It is roughly hairy, with large, oval, toothed leaves and dark, wine-coloured flowers, borne in whorls on a flowering stem that grows several feet tall. The entire plant when crushed has a bitter and disagreeable smell, which has led to a country saying that toads, with their unpleasant image, especially like to shelter under it. Woundwort's strong smell does not however repel the long-tongued flies and bees that sip the nectar in its flower-bases. Unlikely though it seems, during the nineteenth century both the tuberous roots and the shoots were cooked and eaten as a vegetable.

As its common name suggests, woundwort has been an important wound-healer, and one that folk medicine passed on to the medical profession. Gerard, the sixteenth-century surgeon, was walking one day in Kent and witnessed a man cutting himself badly with a scythe, 'wherein he made a wound to the bones, & withal very large and wide'. Gerard offered to help but the man refused his assistance, saying that he himself knew what to do. He gathered woundwort and poulticed the injury and Gerard was impressed with how effectively the bleeding stopped. Over the course of a few days, the wound healed. Gerard went on to use the plant in his own practice, but evidently his professional pride must have been hurt by the rejection of his aid; he christened the plant 'clown's woundwort', a slightly scathing name, which it keeps to this day.

One of Gerard's successes with this herb concerned a shoemaker's servant in Holborn who tried to kill himself with a dagger; 'which mortall wounds by God's permission and the virtues of this herbe I perfectly cured within twenty daies'. Woundwort has continued to be used in folk medicine for treating not only wounds but also boils and carbuncles.

Fifty years after Gerard's experiences, Culpeper says in 1653 of the plant that: 'A syrup made from the juice of it, is inferior to none for inward wounds, ruptures of veins, bloody flux, vessels broken, spitting, urining, or vomiting blood.' Its reputation had clearly been established. Pechey in 1694 gives an additional role for the herb: 'A Syrup made from it, is', he says, 'an excellent Remedy for Hoarsness.'

Medical herbalists in the nineteenth and early twentieth centuries continued to use woundwort as a wound-healer, and for gout and vertigo. Although not widely used today by British medical herbalists, it is still sometimes used as healing ointment for wounds, and internally for diar-rhoea and cramps. Among a whole host of interesting compounds contained in the plant, at least one, betonicine, is known to be haemostatic (stops blood flow). So we are beginning to understand how the plant acts as a wound-healer.

Yarrow

(*Achillea millefolium*)

I will pluck the yarrow fair,
That more benign shall be my face,
That more warm shall be my lips,
That more chaste shall be my speech,
Be my speech the beams of the sun,
Be my lips the sap of the strawberry.

May I be an isle in the sea,
May I be a star in the waning of the moon,
May I be a staff to the weak,
Wound can I every man,
Wound can no man me.

Alexander Carmichael, *Carmina Gadelic*a (1900–1971)

This Gaelic incantation shows the great respect in which this common plant was held. It was well known to our Anglo-Saxon forbears and has a long and venerable reputation. Even as recently as the twentieth century, it was considered lucky to attach a sprig of yarrow to a child's cot and that this would ensure a long and healthy life. Because it is so recognizable and therefore not liable to be confused with other plants, its social history can be traced quite easily. Its distinctive and beautiful, fern-like leaves are soft to the touch and its white or pale pink flowers are borne on surprisingly tough stems, making them very hard to pick. The entire plant is gently aromatic.

Yarrow's fine reputation is due to its powerful wound-healing properties. Achilles is said to have discovered it and used it to heal those wounded in battle, hence its generic name *Achillea*. The Gaelic name for yarrow translates as 'plant that staunches bleeding'. A popular way of utilizing yarrow was to turn it into an ointment:

> 'My late father, who was born in 1900 and was the third of nine children, told me of an ointment made by his mother to treat all cuts, grazes and injuries that had drawn blood. She would take yarrow plants – the whole plant including the flowers as well as the roots – and wash them well. They were then chopped up finely and boiled to a pulp in a little water, pushed through a sieve and the resulting paste then mixed into purified lard. This ointment was used on the many cuts and grazes suffered by her large family, and my father said that they all healed up cleanly and quickly. People used to come to the house and ask for some of the ointment regularly.'

Mrs. A. A—, Norfolk (1989)

The plant's other uses were very varied in folk medicine. Fevers were treated with yarrow tea; Orkney islanders drank the tea for melancholy. In Essex too, 'yarrow tea was used to cure depression especially if a little gin was added'. Chewing yarrow leaves was an excellent way of taking in its goodness and, in the Outer Hebridean islands, this was done to freshen the breath. A single yarrow leaf chewed can also bring remarkable relief from heavy periods.

In official medicine too, yarrow has been used as a wound herb. 'A Cataplasm of the Leaves closes up Wounds, stops their Bleeding, and keeps them from Inflammation,' reported Salmon in 1693. The fresh leaves were also recommended for toothache and the seventeenth- and eighteenth-century Gunton Household Book described a cake containing shredded yarrow, egg yolks, sugar and flour, to be baked for those who had consumption.

Despite these many uses, in the course of the eighteenth century the herb was officially dropped from the pharmacopoeia. Luckily, it continued to be used both in folk medicine and in official medical herbalism. Today's medical herbalists recommend it for cleaning wounds, regulating menstrual bleeding and treating feverish colds. Ongoing pharmacological studies of the plant confirm its anti-inflammatory and sedative properties, as well as the ability of the plant to reduce the clotting time of blood.

A plant regarded as having medicinal potency often generated a great deal of subsequent folklore about its supernatural power. Yarrow was no exception and it was used in numerous, inventive ways in love divination. It was said that yarrow leaves thrust up the nose would provoke nosebleed and relieve migraine, and this medicinal use was embroidered upon. Bleeding caused by pushing a sprig of yarrow up the nose is a sign of requited love, and the enquirer must recite this rhyme at the same time:

Yarroway, yarroway, bear a white blow
If my love love me, my nose will bleed now.

Alternatively, an ounce of yarrow sewn up in flannel could be placed under a girl's pillow; after repeating the following words, she will dream of her future husband:

Thou pretty herb of Venus' tree,
Thy true name it is yarrow;
Now who my bosom friend must be,
Pray tell me thou tomorrow.

If a girl is too shy to reveal her feelings for a man, she should wear a sprig of yarrow and get as close to him as possible. When she returns home, the sprig should be placed in a drawer. If it is still fresh the next day, her love will be returned.

In Gloucestershire, yarrow is called 'seven-year's love' and a sprig is enclosed in the bridal bouquet to ensure that it lives up to its name. Should the ageing process affect a person's ability to catch a mate, then the Welsh had a handy solution – yarrow was used to darken grey hair and thereby restore a youthful appearance.

Yellow Flag Iris
(*Iris pseudacorus*)

The marsh seemed lit up with these bright lamps of gold under the shadowy willows and dark alders.

Richard Jefferies, quoted G. Clarke Nutall, *Wild Flowers as they Grow*, vol. III, p. 25

This rather majestic plant grows at the edges of ponds and in other damp places. Its bright yellow, sweet-smelling flowers brighten a shady corner; hence the names 'fleur-de-luce' and 'fleur-de-lis', meaning 'flower of the light'. Other country names include 'segg', derived from the Anglo-Saxon for 'short sword' and clearly a reference to its spiky, upright leaves.

These leaves have proved to be extraordinarily versatile, with some important commercial uses. They were sometimes added to bulk out the reeds used for thatching in Orkney and the Scottish tweed industry extracted a valuable, bright green dye from them. The rhizomes and roots were productive too, yielding dark blue, grey and black dyes. Pechey tells us in 1694 that: 'The Highlanders in Scotland make excellent ink with this Root, infus'd, or a little boyl'd in Water twenty four Hours, by rubbing a white, rough Stone upon a knife, or a piece of good Steel in it, for some Hours.'

Scottish children played an imaginative game with iris leaves. A slit was made in a leaf and the tip of it threaded through it to form a 'seggie boat' that could be sailed on the water. Like other leaves of this shape, the leaf may be placed between straightened thumbs to produce a loud squeak when blown through – a game that has given the plant a local name of 'cheeper'. A strange belief came out of Orkney – it was said that chewing the leaves of wild iris would strike you dumb.

Medicinally, yellow flag iris seems to have been rather versatile. In folk medicine, the root was used as a violent purge, although this practice seemed to stop in the eighteenth century. The root was also chewed, to relieve tooth-ache and ulcers. An unusual remedy for toothache was to pour or sniff the juice of the iris into the nostrils. In the nineteenth century, a cosmetic use for the flowers was discovered. This tradition continued in twentieth-century Norfolk where Billy M—, a local man, was renowned for an ointment for freckles, spots and other skin complaints, which he made from iris root, oak apples, vinegar and wine.

In official medicine, Gerard in 1597 recommends the root for treating bruises. Culpeper suggests the root for fluxes, and the flowers for swellings and ulcers. In the nineteenth century the plant was still being used in similar ways and C. Pierpoint Johnson describes the plant as cathartic, in that it excites sneezing and helps headaches. He added that a slice of the rhizome held between the teeth was considered good for toothache. Kemsey in 1838 tells of an ointment used for ulcers which in his day was called 'Noli me Tangere'. This was also used as a hot fomentation on swellings.

Thereafter the role of yellow flag iris declined. Although nineteenth- and early-twentieth-century medical herbalists used it for treating leucorrhoea [vaginal discharge] and painful periods, it is little used today in British herbalism. It certainly needs to be treated with caution: taken internally in high doses it can cause uncontrolled vomiting and diarrhoea.

Yellow Loosestrife
(*Lysimachia vulgaris*)

Yellow Lysimachies, to give sweet rest,
To the faint shepherd, killing, where it comes,
All busy gnats and every fly that hums.

Collins, *The Faithful Shepherdess*

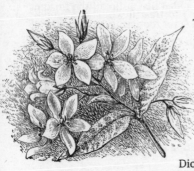

This tall and elegant plant with beautiful, yellow, starry flowers grows by marshes, ditches and rivers, and is sometimes planted in gardens. Yellow loosestrife is unrelated to PURPLE LOOSESTRIFE and is in fact a member of the PRIMROSE family. The name loosestrife is said to have been given to this plant by Dioscorides in the first century AD because the plant has the power to calm a horse and an ox yoked to the same plough and make them work together more effectively.

Sixteen centuries later, Culpeper repeated Dioscorides' assertion that: 'The smoak hereof being bruised, drives away flies and gnats, which in the night time molest people inhabiting near marshes, and in the fenny countries.' This property may hold the key to understanding the plant's name; if it was used to repel the maddening gnats and flies that bother working horses and oxen, then it may indeed have quietened them.

It seems that the plant has not figured significantly in folk medicine. There is some small evidence of its use. Doris E. Coates, the author of a book on cottage housekeeping in the early years of the twentieth century, recalls helping to gather the plant in the wild, for treating diarrhoea; this remedy is recorded by Roy Vickery as being used by gypsies.

In official medicine, loosestrife appears to have been much more widely prescribed. Culpeper in 1653 gives this account of its virtues:

This herb is good for all manner of bleeding ... and all fluxes of the belly ... it is a singular good wound-herb for green wounds, to stay the bleeding and close together the lips of the wound, if the herb be bruised, and the juice only applied.

By the nineteenth century, yellow loosestrife is described by Kemsey in 1838 as being 'good for fluxes of the belly, green wounds and sore mouths'.

A close relative of yellow loosestrife, the pretty creeping Jenny or money-wort (*Lysimachia nummularia*) was known to Gerard and later herbalists as 'herb twopence'. Pechey in 1694 describes it vividly: 'It has many long, slender Branches, that creep on the Ground, with two Leaves at each Joint, opposite to one another; they are almost as round as a Penny.' Like yellow loosestrife, it was used as a wound-healer and to treat fluxes and whooping cough.

Today's medical herbalists recommend yellow loosestrife for similar complaints: diarrhoea and dysentery, as well as bleeding both internal and external. It is also employed to cleanse wounds and as a mouthwash to help heal mouth ulcers and sore gums.

Yellow Toadflax
(*Linaria vulgaris*)

This pretty wild cousin of the garden snapdragon may or may not be native to Britain, but it is known to have been present at least since the sixteenth century. Its bi-coloured, yellow and orange flowers and typically narrow, flax-like leaves are very distinctive; among its country names are 'eggs and bacon' and 'eggs and butter'. The name of toadflax may have sprung from the flowers' resemblance to baby toads. A more picturesque name for the plant comes from Somerset, where it is called 'fairy's lanterns'.

There are records of several different roles for the plant in folk medicine. It was effective against warts and was combined with YARROW as a poultice for treating wounds. In Scotland, it was boiled in milk as a remedy for jaundice and also served to kill fleas. Botanist John Ray, writing in the seventeenth century, claimed that 'many people place this herb under the bare soles of their feet, and between the toes and heels to drive off quartan [malarial] fever'. But by the nineteenth century, it had a single use – the juice was applied as a cosmetic.

In official medicine, toadflax treatments are more numerous and widespread. All the herbalists recommended it for jaundice. Gerard in 1597 described it as good for diseases of the liver and spleen. Culpeper in 1653 praised it for dropsy, eye inflammation, spots and ulcers as well as being a miracle cure for ailing poultry: 'In Sussex we call it Gallwort, and lay it in our chickens' water to cure them of the gall; it relieves them when they are drooping.' Also Pechey tells us in 1694 that an ointment made from the shoots and flowers, and lard mixed with an egg yolk, will 'take off the Pain of the Piles'.

Modern herbalists occasionally prescribe the herb to treat constipation, jaundice, piles and skin diseases. It seems to be used more in continental Europe than in Britain. In Sweden, a fly poison is made from the flowers infused in milk, while in Germany a yellow dye has been obtained from the flowers.

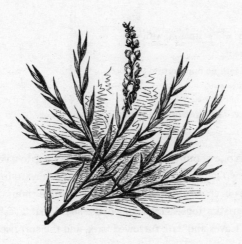

Yew

(*Taxus baccata*)

My shroud of white, stuck all with yew,
  O, prepare it!
My part of death no one so true
  Did share it.

Shakespeare, *Twelfth Night*, II, iv, 54–57

The yew tree is one of our few native conifers. It can live to a very great age; the oldest known living yew tree in Britain, in a churchyard in Fortingall in Perthshire, has been estimated to be more than three thousand years old. These characteristics, together with the dense shade that it casts, the beauty of its shining leaves and dark furrowed bark, and the surprise of its bright red berries like tiny lanterns, all combine to give the tree a dark and mysterious image. It was regarded as a sacred tree by the Druids, and was planted by them in their most holy places.

Individual yew trees have become legendary and justly venerated as much for their immense girth as their antiquity. A famous Derbyshire yew has been credited with inspiring the nursery rhyme 'Rock-a-bye-baby', after eighteenth-century charcoal burners hollowed out a bough to serve as a cradle. The ancient yew at Fortingall has many legends surrounding it and another in Devon is associated with fertility rites, as well as having the power to grant wishes.

Yew is often planted in churchyards, and a number of theories have arisen to explain this. The yew's longevity and the fact that it is evergreen have lent it enduring significance as a symbol of immortality. Others have suggested that yew wood was so valuable that it had to be 'conserved' in churchyards. Another possibility is that yew was actively associated with burials, possibly being used like FEVERFEW in modern times to preserve the corpse from putrefaction. According to one nineteenth-century writer, Samuel Rootsey, an infusion of yew leaves was used to bathe corpses, which preserved them for many weeks. Perhaps this explains the tradition of sewing yew sprigs into a shroud, referred to by Shakespeare's jester in his song (see previous page).

Yew berries are famously poisonous both to livestock and humans but that has not stopped children playing games with them. In several areas including Norfolk, there are people alive today who remember a game rather like Russian roulette. One child picked a berry and put it into his mouth while others tried to make him swallow it, with the conviction that he would die if he did. This game has been played at least since Gerard's time. In his herbal of 1597, he states: 'divers of my schoole fellows and likewise myself did eate our fils of the berries of this tree ... without any hurt at all'. The outer fleshy coating of the berry is actually very palatable, and birds eat it as well as children, without harm. It is the seed that is toxic and to be avoided, although probably more than one is needed to cause a fatality.

Yew has been little used in folk or official medicine. As Parkinson says in 1629, the yew is 'both a shadow and an ornament, in being always greene, and to deck up Houses in Winter: but ancient Writers have ever reckoned it to be dangerous at the least, if not deadly'. With some caution probably, country people devised a few, but very few, remedies. The liquid in which yew twigs had been steeped was taken for kidney trouble in Lincolnshire and there is a single record of the use of yew as an abortifacient. In Ireland, it was used to treat ringworm. Tiny quantities of dried yew were fed to horses in Wales to improve the shine of their coats and boost their appetites; 'But it could be real *deadly*, if you gave 'em too much.' Not surprisingly, it is not favoured by modern medical herbalists.

Yew has inspired a multitude of practical uses and associated folklore. Yew magic and ritual is endlessly fascinating. It has been said that dreaming of yew trees foretells the death of an aged person, and yew can lead a person to lost objects if used as a dowsing rod, perhaps a reminder of the ancient use of the wood to make magic wands.

Famously, yew wood was also used to make archers' bows; its generic name *Taxus* possibly being derived from the Greek word *taxon*, meaning 'a bow'. This in turn produced the adjective 'toxic'. Yew wood is very attractive and was much sought after in furniture-making. The traditional rod of office in the Scottish Highlands was made of yew, as were shuttles for spinning in Scotland – its strength no doubt came into play here.

In recent years, pharmacologists have found that a substance called taxol, derived from yew, can inhibit cell division. This discovery led to research into its use against cancers and clinical trials began in 1983; as a result, taxol is now important in the orthodox medical treatment of some ovarian and breast cancers. Drugs developed from yew are also utilized in the treatment of some other cancers. Although taxol is mainly obtained from the Pacific yew (*Taxus brevifolia*), some varieties of our native species contain it too. Clippings from yew hedges throughout Britain have been used in research projects. Yew may eventually be able to confer the gift, if not of immortality, at least of longer life.

Source Notes

Please note:

Full details of the principal sources, such as author's name, title, and so on, are given below, but abridged in the main listings for individual plant entries. For any other source, full details are given for the first mention in a particular entry, but abridged for the remainder of that entry. In each plant entry, the sources are given in the order of the text to which they refer.

PRINCIPAL SOURCES Allen, David E. and Hatfield, Gabrielle, *Medicinal Plants in Folk Tradition: An Ethnobotany of Britain and Ireland* (Timber Press, 2004). Beith, Mary, *Healing Threads: Traditional Medicines of the Highlands and Islands* (Polygon, 1995). Carmichael, Alexander, *Carmina Gadelica: Hymns and Incantations Collected in the Highlands and Islands of Scotland in the Last Century*, 6 vols in Gaelic and English (Edinburgh 1900–1971); English-only edn (Floris, 1992). Chevallier, Andrew, *The Encyclopedia of Medicinal Plants* (Dorling Kindersley, 1996). Culpeper, Nicholas, *The English Physitian* (London, 1652). Became generally known as *Culpeper's Complete Herbal* (modern edition: Wordsworth Reference, 1995). Darwin, Tess, *The Scots Herbal: The Plant Lore of Scotland* (Mercat Press, 1996). Essex Age Concern Essays: written in response to a competition organized by Age Concern (1991) and now kept at the Essex Records Office. Gerard, John, *The Herball; or, Generall Historie of Plantes* (John Norton, London, 1597); *Gerard's Herbal: The History of Plants*, ed. Marcus Woodward (Senate, 1994). Gunton Household Book: this manuscript kitchen book, kept successively by several ladies of the Harbord family who lived on the Gunton Estate, is thought to span the second half of the seventeenth century and the early years of the eighteenth. A few of the recipes in the collection are attributed to Sir Thomas Brown, famous physician and friend of the family. The manuscript is kept in the Church of St Peter Mancroft, Norwich (microfiche copy in the Norfolk Records Office). Hill, Sir John, *The Family Herbal* (C. Brightly and T. Kinnersley, *c*.1820). Kemsey, William, *The British Herbal: or, A Practical Treatise on the Use and Application of the Common Herbs of Great Britain* (Bristol, 1838). Parkinson, John, *Paradisi in Sole Paradisus Terrestris* (London, 1629); facsimile edn (Dover Publications, 1976 and 1991). Parkinson, John, *Theatrum Botanicum* (London, 1640). Pechey, John, *The Compleat Herbal of Physical Plants* (London, 1694). Quelch, Mary Thorne, *Herbal Remedies and Recipes* (Faber and Faber, 1945). Quelch, Mary Thorne, *Herbs for Daily Use* (Faber and Faber, 1941). Quelch, Mary Thorne, *Herbs and How to Know Them* (Faber and Faber, 1946). Salmon, William, *The Compleat English Physician* (London, 1693). Vickery, Roy, *A Dictionary of Plant-lore* (Oxford University Press, 1995).

AGRIMONY Brownlow, Margaret E., 'Herbs and the Fragrant Garden' (Herb Farm, 1957), quoted in Watts, Donald C., *Elsevier's Dictionary of Plant Names and their Origins* (Elsevier, 2000). Genders, Roy, *The Scented Wild Flowers of Britain* (Collins, 1971). Grigson, Geoffrey, *The Englishman's Flora* (Phoenix House, 1955). Darwin (1996). Hooper, James, *Magical and Medicinal Plants: Descriptive Notes on some British Plants used in Witchcraft and Medicine*, pamphlet (Norwich Castle Museum, 1915). Gerard (1597). Salmon (1693). Gunton Household Book. Kemsey (1838). Copy of anonymous twentieth-century pamphlet, loaned by Mr W. T— of Otley, Yorkshire. Chevallier (1996). Allen and Hatfield (2004). Mr F. C. W— of Norwich, pers. com. collected by author (1990). Quelch (1946). Watts, Donald C. (2000). **ALDER** Vickery (1995). Darwin (1996). Chevallier (1996). Freethy, Ron, *From Agar to Zenry* (Crowood Press, 1985). Milliken, W. and Bridgewater, S., *Flora Celtica: Plants and People in Scotland* (Birlinn, 2004). Darwin (1996). Grigson, Geoffrey, *The Englishman's Flora* (Phoenix House, 1955). Allen and Hatfield (2004). Vickery (1995). Hill, Sir John (*c*.1820). George Chapman notebook

(Gressenhall Country Life Museum, Norfolk, 1823).
Culpeper (1652). Cullum, Sir John, handwritten notes
in *Flora Anglica* (1762); in West Suffolk Records Office.
Scottish Records Office, GD1/384/26. Pechey (1694).
Woodforde, James, *Ansford Diary*, ed. Winstanley, R. I.
(Parson Woodforde Society, 1985), vol. III (1766–68).
Chevallier (1996). Grigson, Geoffrey (1955). Freethy,
Ron (1985). Darwin, Tess (1996). Gerard (1597). Grieve,
Mrs M., *A Modern Herbal*, ed. Leyel, Mrs C. F.
(Jonathan Cape, 1931). Johnson, C. Pierpoint, *The
Useful Plants of Great Britain*, illus. Sowerby, John E.
(Kent & Co., 1862). Britten, James and Holland, Robert,
A Dictionary of English Plant Names (English Dialect
Society, 1886). **ALEXANDERS** Quelch (1941) Grieve,
Mrs M., *A Modern Herbal*, ed. Leyel, Mrs C. F.
(Jonathan Cape, 1931). Parkinson (1629). Quelch (1941).
Allen and Hatfield (2004). Martin, Martin, *A
Description of the Western Isles of Scotland*, 2nd edn
(A. Bell, 1716), quoted in Beith (1995). Culpeper (1652).
Pechey (1694). Moncrief, John, *The Poor Man's
Physician, or the Receits of the Famous John Moncrief
of Tippermalloch*, 3rd edn (Edinburgh, 1731). Cullum,
Sir John, handwritten notes in *Flora Anglica* (1762); in
West Suffolk Records Office. Johnson, C. Pierpoint, *The
Useful Plants of Great Britain*, illus. Sowerby, John E.
(Kent & Co., 1862). **ASH** Moerman, Daniel E., *Native
American Ethnobotany* (Timber Press, 1998). Lafont,
Ann-Marie, *Devon's Heritage: A Herbal Folklore*
(Badger Books, 1984). Darwin (1996). Vickery (1995).
Ffennell, M. C., *Folk-lore 9* (Folklore Society, 1898).
Taylor, Dr Mark R., 'Magic, witchcraft, charm-cures
and customs in East Anglia', data for a never-
published book, collected largely by correspondence,
while he was Regional Medical Officer in Norwich
1920–27 (Norfolk Record Office, MS 4322, 57x1).
Culpeper (1652). Pechey (1694). Scottish Records
Office, GD18 2125. Gunton Household Book. Norfolk
Records Office, 26354. Kemsey (1838). Chevallier
(1996). Johnson, A. T. and Smith, H. A., *Plant Names
Simplified*, 2nd edn (Hamlyn, 1972). Darwin (1996).
Mason, James, 'The Folk-lore of British Plants', *Dublin
University Magazine*, vol. 82 (1873). Lafont, Ann-Marie
(1984). Halliwell, James Orchard, *Popular Rhymes and
Nursery Tales* (John Russell Smith, 1849). Hamerton,
Philip Gilbert, *Landscape* (1885). Quoted in Phythian,
J. Ernest, *Trees in Nature, Myth and Art* (Methuen,
1907). **BETONY** Old-English medical manuscript,
Stockholm Library (c.1400), reproduced in *Anglia*, vol.
18 (1896). Lafont, Ann-Marie, *Devon's Heritage: A
Herbal Folklore* (Badger Books, 1984). Johnson, A. T.
and Smith, H. A., *Plant Names Simplified*, 2nd edn
(Hamlyn, 1972). Beith (1995). Martin, Martin, *A
Description of the Western Isles of Scotland*, 2nd edn
(A. Bell, 1716). Allen, Andrew, *A Dictionary of Sussex
Folk Medicine* (Countryside Books, 1995). Allen and
Hatfield (2004). Grigson, Geoffrey, *The Englishman's
Flora* (Phoenix House, 1955). Bardswell, Frances Anne,
The Herb Garden (A&C Black, 1911). Coates, Doris E.,
*Tuppeny Rice and Treacle: Cottage Housekeeping
(1900–1920)* (Reader's Union, 1976). Mr A. R—,
Northampton, pers. com. collected by author (1985).
Culpeper (1652). Gerard (1597). Pechey (1694). Johnson,
C. Pierpoint, *The Useful Plants of Great Britain*, illus.

Sowerby, John E. (Kent & Co., 1862). Chevallier (1996).
BILBERRY Lafont, Ann-Marie, *Devon's Heritage: A
Herbal Folklore* (Badger Books, 1984). Vickery (1995).
Threlkeld, Caleb, 'Synopsis *Stirpium Hibernicarum*'
(1726), quoted in Britten, James and Holland, Robert,
A Dictionary of English Plant Names (English Dialect
Society, 1886). Darwin (1996). Neill, Patrick, 'Remarks
Made in a Tour Through Some of the Shetland
Islands in 1804, 1806', quoted in Darwin (1996).
Lightfoot, John, *Flora Scotica*, 2 vols (Benjamin White,
1777). Hutchinson, Peggy, *More Home-made Wine
Secrets* (W. Foulsham & Co., c.1945). Darwin (1996).
Allen and Hatfield (2004). Beith (1995). Freethy, Ron,
From Agar to Zenry (Crowood Press, 1985). Culpeper
(1652). Pechey (1694). Hill, Sir John (c.1820). Chevallier
(1996). Mabberley, D. J., *The Plant-Book* (Cambridge
University Press, 1987). Canter P. H. and Ernst, E.,
'Anthocyanosides of *Vaccinium myrtillus* (bilberry) for
night vision – a systematic review of placebo-
controlled trial.', *Surv. Ophthalmol*, vol. 49, pt 1, pp.
38–50 (2004). **BIRCH** Scottish ballad, quoted in Dyer,
T. F. Thiselton, *The Folk-lore of Plants* (London, 1889);
facsimile reprint (Llanerch Press, 1994). Radford, E.
and Radford, M. A., *Encyclopaedia of Superstitions*,
edited and revised by Hole, Christina (Hutchinson,
1974). Gunton Household Book. Johnson, C. Pierpoint,
The Useful Plants of Great Britain, illus. Sowerby, John
E. (Kent & Co., 1862). Darwin (1996). Allen and
Hatfield (2004). Pechey (1694). Chevallier (1996).
Lightfoot, John, *Flora Scotica*, 2 vols (Benjamin White,
1777). Gerard (1597). Coles, William, *Adam in Eden*
(London, 1657), quoted in Britten, James and Holland,
Robert, *A Dictionary of English Plant Names* (English
Dialect Society, 1886). **BIRD'S-FOOT TREFOIL** Poem
from Rigg, James, *Wild Flower Lyrics and other Poems*
(Alexander Gardner, 1897). Grigson, Geoffrey, *The
Englishman's Flora* (Phoenix House, 1955). Allen and
Hatfield (2004). Tongue, Ruth L., *Somerset Folklore*,
ed. Briggs, K. M. (Folklore Society, 1965). Culpeper
(1652). Salmon (1693). Britten, James and Holland,
Robert, MSS, quoted in Vickery (1995). **BISTORT**
Grieve, Mrs M., *A Modern Herbal*, ed. Leyel, Mrs C. F.
(Jonathan Cape, 1931). Mabey, Richard, *Food for Free*
(Fontana, 1972). Chevallier (1996). Quelch (1941).
Johnson, C. Pierpoint, *The Useful Plants of Great
Britain*, illus. Sowerby, John E. (Kent & Co., 1862).
Grigson, Geoffrey, *The Englishman's Flora* (Phoenix
House, 1955). Mabberley, D. J., *The Plant-Book*
(Cambridge University Press, 1987). Culpeper (1652).
Pechey (1694). Kemsey (1838). Allen and Hatfield
(2004). Mr R. W—, Norwich, pers. correspondence
collected by author (1990). **BITTER VETCH** Allen and
Hatfield (2004). Martin, Martin, *A Description of the
Western Isles of Scotland* (A. Bell, 1703). Lightfoot,
John, *Flora Scotica*, 2 vols. (Benjamin White, 1777).
Gerard (1597). Pechey (1694). MacFarlane, Angus,
'Gaelic Names of Plants: study of their uses and lore',
Transactions of the Gaelic Society of Inverness, vol. 32
(1922–24), quoted in Beith (1995). **BLACK BRYONY**
Grigson, Geoffrey, *The Englishman's Flora* (Phoenix
House, 1955). Wren, R. C., *Potter's New Cyclopaedia of
Botanical Drugs and Preparations*, revised by
Williamson, Elizabeth M. and Evans, Fred J. (C. W.

Daniel Company, 1988). Salmon (1693). Culpeper (1652). Watts, Donald C., *Elsevier's Dictionary of Plant Names and their Origins* (Elsevier, 2000). Bryant, Charles, *Flora Dietetica* (Benjamin White, 1783). Mabberley, D. J., *The Plant-Book* (Cambridge University Press, 1987). **BLACKTHORN** Vickery (1995). Milliken, W. and Bridgewater, S., *Flora Celtica: Plants and People in Scotland* (Birlinn, 2004). MacLeod, F., *Where the Forest Murmurs* (1906), quoted in Milliken, W. and Bridgewater, S., *Flora Celtica: Plants and People in Scotland* (Birlinn, 2004). Mason, James, 'The Folklore of British Plants', *Dublin University Magazine*, vol. 82 (1873). Vickery (1995). Lafont, Ann-Marie, *Devon's Heritage: A Herbal Folklore* (Badger Books, 1984). Mabberley, D. J., *The Plant-Book* (Cambridge University Press, 1987). Bloomfield, Robert, 'The Farmer's Boy', quoted in Pratt, Anne (1898). Pratt, Anne, *Wild Flowers*, 2 vols (Society for Promoting Christian Knowledge, 1898). Nuttall, G. Clarke, *Wild Flowers as They Grow*, 5 vols (Waverley Book Company, c.1920). Quelch, Mary Thorne (1941). Marshall, Sybil, *Under the Hawthorn* (J. M. Dent & Sons, 1981). Buckley, Anthony D., 'Unofficial Healing in Ulster', *Ulster Folklife*, vol. 26 (1980). Allen and Hatfield (2004). Gerard (1597). Miles, Archie, *Silva: The Tree in Britain* (Ebury Press, 1999). Johnson, C. Pierpoint, *The Useful Plants of Great Britain*, illus. Sowerby, John E. (Kent & Co., 1862). **BLUEBELL** Rackham, Oliver, *The History of the Countryside* (J. M. Dent & Sons, 1987). Gerard (1597). Dyer, T. F. Thiselton, *The Folk-lore of Plants* (London, 1889); facsimile reprint (Llanerch Press, 1994). Lafont, Ann-Marie, *Devon's Heritage: A Herbal Folklore* (Badger Books, 1984). Allen and Hatfield (2004). Parkinson (1629). Milliken, W. and Bridgewater, S., *Flora Celtica: Plants and People in Scotland* (Birlinn, 2004). **BOG MYRTLE** Grigson, Geoffrey, *The Englishman's Flora* (Phoenix House, 1955). Vickery (1995). *Independent*, August 1994. Darwin (1996). Beith (1995). Rorie, David, *Folk Traditions and Folk Medicine in Scotland: the Writings of David Rorie*, ed. David Buchan (Canongate Academic, 1994). Allen and Hatfield (2004). Milliken, W. and Bridgewater, S., *Flora Celtica: Plants and People in Scotland* (Birlinn, 2004). Wren, R. C., *Potter's New Cyclopaedia of Botanical Drugs and Preparations*, revised by Williamson, Elizabeth M. and Evans, Fred J. (C. W. Daniel Company, 1988). Grigson, Geoffrey, *The Englishman's Flora* (Phoenix House, 1955). Mabberley, D. J., *The Plant-Book* (Cambridge University Press, 1987). Darwin (1996). Milliken, W. and Bridgewater, S., *Flora Celtica: Plants and People in Scotland* (Birlinn, 2004). **BOGBEAN** Poem from Rigg, James, *Wild Flower Lyrics and other Poems* (Alexander Gardner, 1897). Kemsey (1838). Gerard (1597). Johnson, A. T. and Smith, H. A., *Plant Names Simplified*, 2nd edn (Hamlyn, 1972). Allen and Hatfield (2004). McGlinchey, Charles, *The Last of the Name*, ed. Brian Friel (Blackstaff Press, 1986). Milliken, W. and Bridgewater, S., *Flora Celtica: Plants and People in Scotland* (Birlinn, 2004). Vickery (1995). Pechey (1694). Darwin (1996). Kemsey (1838). Chevallier (1996). **BRAMBLE OR BLACKBERRY** Poem from Rigg, James, *Wild Flower Lyrics and other Poems* (Alexander

Gardner, 1897). Milliken, W. and Bridgewater, S., *Flora Celtica: Plants and People in Scotland* (Birlinn, 2004). Britten, James and Holland, Robert, *A Dictionary of English Plant Names* (English Dialect Society, 1886). Tusser, Thomas, 'February's Abstract', quoted in Nuttall, G. Clarke, *Wild Flowers as They Grow*, 5 vols (Waverley Book Company, c.1920). Lafont, Ann-Marie, *Devon's Heritage: A Herbal Folklore* (Badger Books, 1984). Allen and Hatfield (2004). Gerard (1597). Chevallier (1996). Watts, Donald C., *Elsevier's Dictionary of Plant Names and their Origins* (Elsevier, 2000). Patrick, W. A., *A popular description of the indigenous plans of Lanarkshire with an introduction to botany and a glossary of botanical terms* (Daniel Lizars, 1831), quoted in Milliken and Bridgewater (2004). Milliken, W. and Bridgewater, S. (2004). Salmon (1693). Hutchinson, Peggy, *More Home-made Wine Secrets* (W. Foulsham & Co., c.1945). Darwin (1996). Lafont, Ann-Marie, *Devon's Heritage: A Herbal Folklore* (Badger Books, 1984). **BROOKLIME** Johnson, A. T. and Smith, H. A., *Plant Names Simplified*, 2nd edn (Hamlyn, 1972). Allen and Hatfield (2004). Pechey (1694). Parkinson (1640). Ó Clara, Padraig, 'The Big Mrs Pearson', *Cork Holly Bough* (Christmas 1978). Pyne, K. Lawther, letter; copy of original in Wellcome Library. Kemsey (1838). Wren, R. C., *Potter's New Cyclopaedia of Botanical Drugs and Preparations*, 8th edn (Health Science Press, 1975). **BROOM** Gerard (1597). Grieve, Mrs M., *A Modern Herbal*, ed. Leyel, Mrs C. F. (Jonathan Cape, 1931). Milliken, W. and Bridgewater, S., *Flora Celtica: Plants and People in Scotland* (Birlinn, 2004). Moloney, Michael F., *Irish Ethnobotany and the Evolution of Medicine in Ireland* (M. H. Gill and Son, 1919). Freethy, Ron, *From Agar to Zenry* (Crowood Press, 1985). Salmon (1693). Wren, R. C., *Potter's New Cyclopaedia of Botanical Drugs and Preparations*, 8th edn (Health Science Press, 1975). Chevallier (1996). **BUCKTHORN, ALDER BUCKTHORN** Watts, Donald C., *Elsevier's Dictionary of Plant Names and their Origins* (Elsevier, 2000). Step, Edward, *Wayside and Woodland Trees* (Frederick Warne, n.d.). Dodoens, Rembert, *A Niewe Herbal, or Historie of Plantes*, trans. Henry Lyte (London, 1578), quoted Quelch (1941). Salmon (1693). Quelch (1945). Hill, Sir John (c.1820). Chevallier (1996). Pechey (1694). Johnson, C. Pierpoint, *The Useful Plants of Great Britain*. illus. Sowerby, John E. (Kent & Co., 1862). Vickery (1995). Step, Edward (n.d.). Watts, Donald C., *Elsevier's Dictionary of Plant Names and their Origins* (Elsevier, 2000). **BUGLE** Estienne, Charles, *Maison Rustique*, (c.1569); trans. Surflet, R., *Countrie Farm* (1600). Watts, Donald C., *Elsevier's Dictionary of Plant Names and their Origins* (Elsevier, 2000). Pechey (1694). Allen and Hatfield (2004). Gerard (1597). Culpeper (1652). Kemsey (1838). Chevallier (1996). **BUGLOSS** Watts, Donald C., *Elsevier's Dictionary of Plant Names and their Origins* (Elsevier, 2000). Culpeper (1652). Gerard (1597). Johnson, C. Pierpoint, *The Useful Plants of Great Britain*. illus. Sowerby, John E. (Kent & Co., 1862). Johnson, A. T. and Smith, H. A., *Plant Names Simplified*, 2nd edn (Hamlyn, 1972). Sidwell, Keith, *Reading Medieval Latin* (Cambridge University Press, 1995). Tongue, Ruth L., *Somerset*

Folklore, ed. Briggs, K. M. (Folklore Society, 1965). Wren, R. C., *Potter's New Cyclopaedia of Botanical Drugs and Preparations*, revised by Williamson, Elizabeth M. and Evans, Fred J. (C. W. Daniel Company, 1988). Chevallier (1996). **BURDOCK** Darwin (1996). Norfolk Records Office, MC 54/91. Allen and Hatfield (2004). Parkinson (1640). Chevallier (1996). Quelch (1946). 'Tradition – A Pint of the Unusual', *Waitrose Food and Drink* (November 2005); also on www. waitrose.com. Salmon (1693). **BUTCHER'S BROOM** Mabberley, D. J., *The Plant-Book* (Cambridge University Press, 1987). Lafont, Ann-Marie, *Devon's Heritage: A Herbal Folklore* (Badger Books, 1984). Culpeper (1652). Pechey (1694). Salmon (1693). Chevallier (1996). Lafont, Ann-Marie (1984). **BUTTERBUR** Dodoens, Rembert, *A Niewe Herball, or Historie of Plantes*, trans. Henry Lyte (London, 1578), quoted in Grieve, Mrs M., *A Modern Herbal*, ed. Leyel, Mrs C. F. (Jonathan Cape, 1931). Gerard (1597). Vickery (1995). Allen and Hatfield (2004). Gerard (1597). Norfolk Records Office, MC54/91. Salmon (1693). Kemsey (1838). Chevallier (1996). Halliwell, James Orchard, *Popular Rhymes and Nursery Tales* (John Russell Smith, 1849). Carmichael (1900–71). **BUTTERCUP** Gerard (1597). Thornton, Robert John, *A New Family Herbal* (Richard Taylor & Co., 1810), quoted in Grieve, Mrs M., *A Modern Herbal*, ed. Leyel, Mrs C. F. (Jonathan Cape, 1931). Pechey (1694). Beith (1995). *Farmhouse Fare: Country Recipes Collected by Farmer's Weekly* (Countrywise Books, 1973). E. M—, Co. Tyrone, letter to Vickery, Roy (1986). Allen and Hatfield (2004). Grieve, Mrs M., *A Modern Herbal*, ed. Leyel, Mrs C. F. (Jonathan Cape, 1931). Grigson, Geoffrey, *The Englishman's Flora* (Phoenix House, 1955). **BUTTERWORT** Watts, Donald C., *Elsevier's Dictionary of Plant Names and their Origins* (Elsevier, 2000). Johnson, A. T. and Smith, H. A., *Plant Names Simplified*, 2nd edn (Hamlyn, 1972). Darwin (1996). Vickery (1995). Beith (1995). Torrey, Bradford, *A Florida Sketchbook* (Boston, 1894), quoted in Coffey, Timothy, *The History and Folklore of North American Wildflowers* (Facts on File, New York, 1993). Britten, James and Holland, Robert, *A Dictionary of English Plant Names* (English Dialect Society, 1886). Allen and Hatfield (2004). Freethy, Ron, *From Agar to Zenry* (Crowood Press, 1985). Pechey (1694). **CENTAURY** Allen and Hatfield (2004). Grieve, Mrs M., *A Modern Herbal*, ed. Leyel, Mrs C. F. (Jonathan Cape, 1931). Dyer, T. F. Thiselton, *The Folk-lore of Plants* (London, 1889); facsimile reprint (Llanerch Press, 1994). Beith (1995). Hutchinson, Peggy, *More Home-made Wine Secrets* (W. Foulsham & Co., c.1945). Hill, Sir John (c.1820). Quelch (1941). D. K —, Suffolk, privately owned MS. Culpeper (1652). Salmon (1693). Kemsey (1838). Chevallier (1996). **CHAMOMILE** Watts, Donald C., *Elsevier's Dictionary of Plant Names and their Origins* (Elsevier, 2000). Anon, Lay of the Nine Healing Herbs (n.d.); a fragment of a Saxon manuscript – the Lacnunga – written originally in the Wessex dialect and translated repeatedly over the years. Allen and Hatfield (2004). Mrs L. P—, Suffolk, pers. com. collected by author (1989). Trevelyan, Marie, *Folk-lore and Folk-stories of Wales* (Elliot Stock, 1909). Culpeper

(1652). Pechey (1694). Salmon (1693). Gunton Household Book. Chevallier (1996). Marshall, Sybil, *Under the Hawthorn* (J. M. Dent & Sons, 1981). Bardswell, Frances Anne, *The Herb Garden* (A&C Black, 1911). **CHICKWEED** Dyer, T. F. Thiselton, *The Folk-lore of Plants* (London, 1889); facsimile reprint (Llanerch Press, 1994). Withering, W., *A Botanical Arrangement of the Vegetables Naturally Growing in Great Britain* (Birmingham, 1776). Martin, Martin, *A Description of the Western Isles of Scotland* (A. Bell, 1703), 4th edn (Eneas Mackay, 1934). Vickery (1995). Allen and Hatfield (2004). Gerard (1597). Pechey (1694). Salmon (1693). Gunton Household Book. Kemsey (1838). Chevallier (1996). **CHICORY** Pechey (1694). Smith, Sir James, quoted in Grieve, Mrs M., *A Modern Herbal*, ed. Leyel, Mrs C. F. (Jonathan Cape, 1931). Harland, Elizabeth M., *No Halt at Sunset: the Diary of a Country Housewife* (London, 1951). Vickery (1995). Parkinson (1640). Pechey (1694). Lady Clerk of Penicuik. Notes taken from Moncrief, John *The Poor Man's Physician, or the Receits of the Famous John Moncrief of Tippermalloch*, 3rd edn (Edinburgh, 1731); in Scottish Records Office GD18–2130. Chevallier (1996). Hutchinson, Peggy, *More Home-made Wine Secrets* (W. Foulsham & Co., c.1945). **CLUBMOSSES** Fairweather, Barbara, *Highland Plant Lore* (Glencoe and North Lorn Folk Museum, n.d., c.1980). Grieve, Mrs M., *A Modern Herbal*, ed. Leyel, Mrs C. F. (Jonathan Cape, 1931). Mabberley, D. J., *The Plant-Book* (Cambridge University Press, 1987). Darwin (1996). Dyer, T. F. Thiselton, *The Folk-lore of Plants* (London, 1889); facsimile reprint (Llanerch Press, 1994). Beith (1995). Henderson, D. M. and Dickson, J. H., *A Naturalist in the Highlands: James Robertson, His Life and Travels in Scotland 1767–1771* (Scottish Academic Press, 1994). Leete, E., *The Alkaloids*, vol. I (John Wiley, 1983). Gerard (1597). Salmon (1693). Chevallier (1996). **COLTSFOOT** Quelch (1941). Darwin (1996). Allen and Hatfield (2004). Scottish Records Office, GD18/2142. Hutchinson, Peggy, *More Home-made Wine Secrets* (W. Foulsham & Co., c.1945). Gerard (1597). Quelch (1941). Chevallier (1996). Milliken, W. and Bridgewater, S., *Flora Celtica: Plants and People in Scotland* (Birlinn, 2004). **COMFREY** Baker, George, *Jewell of Health* (1567), quoted in Grieve, Mrs M., *A Modern Herbal*, ed. Leyel, Mrs C. F. (Jonathan Cape, 1931). Culpeper (1652). Salmon (1693). Withering, William, *A Systematic Arrangement of British Plants*, 5th edn (Scott, Webster and Geary, 1841). Johnson, C. Pierpoint, *The Useful Plants of Great Britain*, illus. Sowerby, John E. (Kent & Co., 1862). Mrs M. T—, Staffordshire, pers. com. collected by author (2002). H. G—, Manchester, pers. com. collected by author (1985). Allen and Hatfield (2004). Grieve, Mrs M., *A Modern Herbal*, ed. Leyel, Mrs C. F. (Jonathan Cape, 1931). Hutchinson, Peggy, *More Home-made Wine Secrets* (W. Foulsham & Co., c.1945). **CORN MARIGOLD** Poem from Rigg, James, *Wild Flower Lyrics and other Poems* (Alexander Gardner, 1897). Parkinson (1640). Grigson, Geoffrey, *The Englishman's Flora* (Phoenix House, 1955). Vickery (1995). Milliken, W. and Bridgewater, S., *Flora Celtica: Plants and People in Scotland* (Birlinn, 2004). Vickery (1995). **CORNFLOWER** Hatfield, Gabrielle, *Country*

Remedies: Traditional East Anglian Plant Remedies in the Twentieth Century (Boydell Press, 1994). Gunton Household Book. Gerard (1597). Culpeper (1652). Pechey (1694). Hill, Sir John (c.1820). Chevallier (1996). Grieve, Mrs M., *A Modern Herbal*, ed. Leyel, Mrs C. F. (Jonathan Cape, 1931). Norfolk Records Office, GD 1/384/26. **COUCH GRASS** L. W—, Norwich, pers. com. collected by author (1990). Record no. M42, English Folklore Survey MSS (1960s); in University College London Library. Gerard (1597). Salmon (1693). Culpeper (1652). Kemsey (1838). Chevallier (1996). Withering, William, quoted in Grieve, Mrs M., *A Modern Herbal*, ed. Leyel, Mrs C. F. (Jonathan Cape, 1931). Burgess, J. T., *Old English Wild Flowers* (Frederick Warne, 1868). Moloney, Michael F., *Irish Ethnobotany and the Evolution of Medicine in Ireland* (M. H. Gill and Son, 1919). Hatfield, Audrey Wynne, *How to Enjoy your Weeds* (Frederick Muller, 1969). **COW PARSLEY** Pechey (1694). Allen and Hatfield (2004). Darwin (1996). Milliken, W. and Bridgewater, S., *Flora Celtica: Plants and People in Scotland* (Birlinn, 2004). **COWSLIP** Plues, Margaret, *Rambles in Search of Wild Flowers*, 4th edn (George Bell, 1892). Farley's recipe for cowslip wine, printed in Burnett, M. A., *Plantae Utiliores*, 2 vols (Whittaker, 1842). Burgess, J. T., *Old English Wild Flowers* (Frederick Warne, 1868). Allen and Hatfield (2004). Wilde, Lady (Jane), *Ancient Cures, Charms, and Usages of Ireland* (London, 1898). Salmon (1693). Pechey (1694). Wren, R. C., *Potter's New Cyclopaedia of Botanical Drugs and Preparations*, 8th edn (Health Science Press, 1975). Chevallier (1996). Genders, Roy, *The Scented Wild Flowers of Britain* (Collins, London, 1971). **CRAB APPLE** Vickery (1995). Horwood, A. R., *A New British Flora* (1921), quoted in Higgins, Rodney, 'The Plant-Lore of Courtship and Marriage', in *Plant-Lore Studies*, ed. Vickery, Roy (Folklore Society, 1984). Britten, James and Holland, Robert, *A Dictionary of English Plant Names* (English Dialect Society, 1886). Withering, William, *A Botanical Arrangement of British Plants*, 2nd edn (M. Swinney, 1787–92). Moloney, Michael F., *Irish Ethnobotany and the Evolution of Medicine in Ireland* (M. H. Gill and Son, 1919). Milliken, W. and Bridgewater, S., *Flora Celtica: Plants and People in Scotland* (Birlinn, 2004). Black, William George, *Folk-Medicine: A Chapter in the History of Culture* (Folklore Society, 1883); reprint (Burt Franklin, 1970). Allen and Hatfield (2004). MS notes from Mundford Primary School, Norfolk (1980s). Salmon (1693). Pechey (1694). Parkinson (1629). Hill, Sir John (c.1820). Mabey, Richard, *Plants with a Purpose: A Guide to the Everyday Uses of Wild Plants* (Collins, 1977). Johnson, C. Pierpoint, *The Useful Plants of Great Britain*, illus. Sowerby, John E. (Kent & Co., 1862). **CUCKOO PINT** Watts, Donald C., *Elsevier's Dictionary of Plant Names and their Origins* (Elsevier, 2000). Vickery (1995). Grigson, Geoffrey, *The Englishman's Flora* (Phoenix House, 1955). Turner, William, *The Names of Herbes* (1548), ed. Britten, James (English Dialect Society, 1881). Vickery (1995). Porter, Enid M., *Cambridgeshire Customs and Folklore* (Routledge, 1969), quoted in Vickery (1995). Tongue, Ruth L., *Somerset Folklore*, ed. Briggs, K. M. (Folklore Society, 1965). Allen and Hatfield (2004). Dyer, T. F.

Thiselton, *The Folk-lore of Plants* (London, 1889); facsimile reprint (Llanerch Press, 1994). Culpeper (1652). Pechey (1694). Moncrief, John, *The Poor Man's Physician, or the Receits of the Famous John Moncrief of Tippermalloch*, 3rd edn (Edinburgh, 1731). Johnson, C. Pierpoint, *The Useful Plants of Great Britain*, illus. Sowerby, John E. (Kent & Co., 1862). Gerard (1597). Vickery (1995). **CUDWEED** Mascal, Leonard, *Government of Cattle* (1662), quoted in Grigson, Geoffrey, *The Englishman's Flora* (Phoenix House, 1955). de l'Obel, Matthias, *Plantarum seu Stirpium Historia* (Plantin, 1576). Pechey (1694). Fairweather, Barbara, *Highland Plant Lore* (Glencoe and North Lorn Folk Museum, c.1980). Gerard (1597). Culpeper (1652). Pechey (1694). Hill, Sir John (c.1820). Chevallier (1996). **DAFFODIL** Dyer, T. F. Thiselton, *The Folk-lore of Plants* (London, 1889); facsimile reprint (Llanerch Press, 1994). Lafont, Ann-Marie, *Devon's Heritage: A Herbal Folklore* (Badger Books, 1984). Genders, Roy, *The Scented Wild Flowers of Britain* (Collins, 1971). Tongue, Ruth L., *Somerset Folklore*, ed. Briggs, K. M. (Folklore Society, 1965). Vickery (1995). Parkinson (1629). Gerard (1597). Pechey (1694). Ernst, Edzard, ed., *Herbal Medicine: A Concise Overview for Professionals* (Butterworth-Heinemann, 2000). **DAISY** Lafont, Ann-Marie, *Devon's Heritage: A Herbal Folklore* (Badger Books, 1984). Gerard (1597). Allen and Hatfield (2004). Rawlence, E. A., 'Folk-lore and superstitions still obtaining in Dorset', *Proceedings of the Dorset Natural History and Antiquarian Field Club*, vol. 35, pp. 81–87 (Dorset, 1914). Hatfield, Audrey Wynne, *How to Enjoy your Weeds* (Frederick Muller, 1969). **DANDELION** Gerard (1597). Watts, Donald C., *Elsevier's Dictionary of Plant Names and their Origins* (Elsevier, 2000). Hennels, C. E., 'The Wild Herb Men', *East Anglian Magazine* (December 1972). Taylor, Dr Mark R., 'Magic, witchcraft, charm-cures and customs in East Anglia', data for a never-published book, collected largely by correspondence, while Regional Medical Officer in Norwich 1920–27 (Norfolk Record Office, MS 4322, 57x1). Allen and Hatfield (2004). Culpeper (1652). Kemsey (1838). Chevallier (1996). Allen and Hatfield (2004). **DEADLY NIGHTSHADE** Poem from Rigg, James, *Wild Flower Lyrics and other Poems* (Alexander Gardner, 1897). Britten, James and Holland, Robert, *A Dictionary of English Plant Names* (English Dialect Society, 1886). Darwin (1996). Salmon (1693). Gerard (1597), quoted in Nuttall, G. Clarke, *Wild Flowers as They Grow*, 5 vols (Waverley Book Company, c.1920). Burnett, M. A., *Plantae Utiliores*, 2 vols (Whittaker, 1842). Edlin, H. L., *British Plants and their Uses* (Batsford, 1951). Chevallier (1996). **DEVIL'S BIT** Culpeper (1652). Kemsey (1838). Allen and Hatfield (2004). Fairweather, Barbara, *Highland Plant Lore* (Glencoe and North Lorn Folk Museum, c.1980). Milliken, W. and Bridgewater, S., *Flora Celtica: Plants and People in Scotland* (Birlinn, 2004). Grigson, Geoffrey, *The Englishman's Flora* (Phoenix House, 1955). **DOCK** Darwin (1996). Milliken, W. and Bridgewater, S., *Flora Celtica: Plants and People in Scotland* (Birlinn, 2004). Vickery (1995). Beith (1995). Mr F. H—, Bedfordshire, pers. com. collected by author (1985). Mrs G. R. F—, Norfolk, pers. com.

collected by author (1989). Allen and Hatfield (2004). Mrs D. M. P—, Sussex, pers. com. collected by author (1996). Milliken, W. and Bridgewater, S., *Flora Celtica: Plants and People in Scotland* (Birlinn, 2004). Pechey (1694). Chevallier (1996). Darwin (1996). **DOG ROSE** Genders, Roy, *The Scented Wild Flowers of Britain* (Collins, 1971). Hastings, Laura and Prendergast, Hew, 'Naked Ladies and the Hunt for Health', MAFF [Ministry of Agriculture, Fisheries and Food] Bulletin (January 1995). Quelch (1945). Allen and Hatfield (2004). Taylor, Dr Mark R., 'Magic, witchcraft, charm-cures and customs in East Anglia', data for a never-published book, collected largely by correspondence, while Regional Medical Officer in Norwich 1920–27 (Norfolk Record Office, MS 4322, 57x1). Watts, Donald C., *Elsevier's Dictionary of Plant Names and their Origins* (Elsevier, 2000). Pechey (1694). Anon, *A Compendious Body of Physick: the Common-place Book of a late able Physician*, 3rd edn, printed in *Family Magazine*, pt II (J. Osborn, 1747). Moncrief, John, *The Poor Man's Physician, or the Receits of the Famous John Moncrief of Tippermalloch*, 3rd edn (Edinburgh, 1731). Kemsey (1838). Chevallier (1996). Grieve, Mrs M., *A Modern Herbal*, ed. Leyel, Mrs C. F. (Jonathan Cape, 1931). Lafont, Ann-Marie, *Devon's Heritage: A Herbal Folklore* (Badger Books, 1984). **EARLY PURPLE ORCHID** Britten, James and Holland, Robert, *A Dictionary of English Plant Names* (English Dialect Society, 1886). Grigson, Geoffrey, *The Englishman's Flora* (Phoenix House, 1955). Genders, Roy, *The Scented Wild Flowers of Britain* (Collins, 1971). Darwin (1996). Bryant, Charles, *Flora Dietetica* (Benjamin White, 1783). Johnson (1862), quoted in Fairweather, Barbara, *Highland Plant Lore* (Glencoe and North Lorn Folk Museum, c.1980). Grieve, Mrs M., *A Modern Herbal*, ed. Leyel, Mrs C. F. (Jonathan Cape, 1931). Fairweather, Barbara, *Highland Plant Lore* (Glencoe and North Lorn Folk Museum, c.1980). Beith (1995). Pechey (1694). Culpeper (1652). Withering, William, quoted in Grigson, Geoffrey, *The Englishman's Flora* (Phoenix House, 1955). Wren, R. C., *Potter's New Cyclopaedia of Botanical Drugs and Preparations*, 8th edn (Health Science Press, 1975). Leyel, Mrs C. F., *Elixirs of Life* (Faber and Faber, 1987). **EARTHNUT** Moloney, Michael F., *Irish Ethnobotany and the Evolution of Medicine in Ireland* (M. H. Gill and Son, 1919). Milliken, W. and Bridgewater, S., *Flora Celtica: Plants and People in Scotland* (Birlinn, 2004). Logan, James, 'The Scottish Gael' (1831), quoted in Darwin (1996). Bryant, Charles, *Flora Dietetica* (Benjamin White, 1783). Rackham, Oliver, *The History of the Countryside* (J. M. Dent & Sons, 1987). Pechey (1694). Allen and Hatfield (2004). Fargher, D. C., *The Manx Have a Word for It*, pt 5, 'Manx Gaelic Names of Flora' (privately published, Port Erin, 1969). Plues, Margaret, *Rambles in Search of Wild Flowers* (George Bell, 1892). Burgess, J. T. *Old English Wild Flowers* (Frederick Warne, 1868). **ELDER** Poem from Lady Nairne, quoted in McNeill, F. Marian, *The Scots Kitchen* (Blackie & Son, 1929). Rackham, Oliver, *The History of the Countryside* (J. M. Dent & Sons, 1987). Sharkey, Olive, *Old Days, Old Ways* (O'Brien Press, 1985). Quelch (1941). Radbill, Samuel X., 'Whooping Cough in Fact

and Fancy', *Bulletin of History of Medicine*, vol. 13 (The Johns Hopkins University Press, 1943). Hartland, Edwin Sidney, *County Folklore: Gloucestershire*, printed extracts, no.1, vol. 37 (Folklore Society, 1895). Allen and Hatfield (2004). Milliken, W. and Bridgewater, S., *Flora Celtica: Plants and People in Scotland* (Birlinn, 2004). Essex Age Concern Essay (1991). Vickery, Roy, own MSS. Gerard (1597). Culpeper (1652). Pechey (1694). Chevallier (1996). Milliken, W. and Bridgewater, S., *Flora Celtica: Plants and People in Scotland* (Birlinn, 2004). Mrs E. D—, Taunton, Somerset, pers. com. collected by author (1985). Recipe for elder syrup in early-twentieth century notebook owned by S. W—, Norwich. **ELECAMPANE** Mediaeval saying quoted in Chevallier (1996). Mabberley, D. J., *The Plant-Book* (Cambridge University Press, 1987). Genders, Roy, *The Scented Wild Flowers of Britain* (Collins, 1971). Britten, James and Holland, Robert, *A Dictionary of English Plant Names* (English Dialect Society, 1886). Allen and Hatfield (2004). Norfolk Records Office, MC43/6. Taylor, Dr Mark R., 'Magic, witchcraft, charm-cures and customs in East Anglia', data for a never-published book, collected largely by correspondence, while Regional Medical Officer in Norwich 1920–27 (Norfolk Record Office, MS 4322, 57x1). Newall, Carol A., Anderson, Linda A. and Phillipson, J. David, *Herbal Medicines: A Guide for Health Professionals* (Pharmaceutical Press, 1996). Gerard (1597). Culpeper (1652). Gunton Household Book. Fernie, W. T., *Herbal Simples Approved for Modern Uses of Cure*, 3rd edn (Bristol, 1914). Kemsey (1838). Chevallier (1996). Genders, Roy, *The Scented Wild Flowers of Britain* (Collins, 1971). Cantrell C. L., Abate L., Fronczek F. R, Franzblau S. G, Quijano L. and Fischer N. H., 'Antimycobacterial eudesmanolides from *Inula helenium* and *Rudbeckia subtomentosa*', *Planta Med* (May 1999). Allen and Hatfield (2004). William Kingsbury's Notebook, Sprowston, Norfolk (1710); in Gressenhall Museum, G.7.983. Allen, Andrew, *A Dictionary of Sussex Folk Medicine* (Countryside Books, 1995). de Baïracli-Levy, Juliette, *Wanderers in the New Forest* (London, 1958). **ELM** Vickery (1995). Johnson, C. Pierpoint, *The Useful Plants of Great Britain*, illus. Sowerby, John E. (Kent & Co., 1862). Milliken, W. and Bridgewater, S., *Flora Celtica: Plants and People in Scotland* (Birlinn, 2004). Evans, George Ewart, *The Pattern Under the Plough* (Faber and Faber, 1966). Johnston, George, *The Natural History of the Eastern Borders* (Van Voorst, 1853). Williams, Alfred, *Round about the Upper Thames* (Duckworth, 1922). Allen and Hatfield (2004). Britten, James and Holland, Robert, *A Dictionary of English Plant Names* (English Dialect Society, 1886). Gerard (1597). Culpeper (1652). Pechey (1694). Kemsey (1838). Chevallier (1996). Moerman, Daniel E., *Native American Ethnobotany* (Timber Press, 1998). **EYEBRIGHT** Dyer, T. F. Thiselton, *The Folk-lore of Plants* (London, 1889); facsimile reprint (Llanerch Press, 1994). Coates, Doris E., *Tuppeny Rice and Treacle: Cottage Housekeeping (1900–1920)* (Reader's Union, 1976). Allen and Hatfield (2004). Milliken, W. and Bridgewater, S., *Flora Celtica: Plants and People in Scotland* (Birlinn, 2004). Culpeper (1652). Pechey (1694). Grieve, Mrs M., *A*

Modern Herbal, ed. Leyel, Mrs C. F. (Jonathan Cape, 1931). Lightfoot, John, *Flora Scotica*, 2 vols (Benjamin White, 1777). Chevallier (1996). **FAIRY FLAX** Freethy, Ron, *From Agar to Zenry* (Crowood Press, 1985). Milliken, W. and Bridgewater, S., *Flora Celtica: Plants and People in Scotland* (Birlinn, 2004). Carmichael (1900–71). Robertson, James, MS (1768) in National Antiquities Museum, quoted in Beith (1995). Vickery (1995). Fairweather, Barbara, *Highland Plant Lore* (Glencoe and North Lorn Folk Museum, *c.*1980). Moloney, Michael F., *Irish Ethnobotany and the Evolution of Medicine in Ireland* (M. H. Gill and Son, 1919). Pechey (1694). Chevallier (1996). **FAT HEN, GOOD KING HENRY** Johnson, A. T. and Smith, H. A., *Plant Names Simplified*, 2nd edn (Hamlyn, 1972). Watts, Donald C., *Elsevier's Dictionary of Plant Names and their Origins* (Elsevier, 2000). Porter, Enid M., *The Folklore of East Anglia* (Batsford, 1974). Allen and Hatfield (2004). Bryant, Charles, *Flora Dietetica* (Benjamin White, 1783). Gerard (1597). Pechey (1694). Hatfield, Audrey Wynne, *How to Enjoy your Weeds* (Frederick Muller, 1969). Watts, Donald C. (2000). Hatfield, Audrey Wynne (1969). **FERNS** Allen, David E., *The Victorian Fern Craze: A History of Pteridomania* (Hutchinson, 1969). Mason, James, 'The Folk-lore of British Plants', *Dublin University Magazine*, vol. 82, (1873). Radford, E. and Radford, M. A., *Encyclopaedia of Superstitions*, edited and revised by Hole, Christina (Hutchinson, 1974). Dyer, T. F. Thiselton, *The Folk-lore of Plants* (London, 1889); facsimile reprint (Llanerch Press, 1994). Frith, Roger, 'Old Remedies and Charms of Essex', *East Anglian Magazine* (June 1965). **ADDER'S TONGUE FERN** Britten, James and Holland, Robert, *A Dictionary of English Plant Names* (English Dialect Society, 1886). Grieve, Mrs M., *A Modern Herbal*, ed. Leyel, Mrs C. F. (Jonathan Cape, 1931). de Baïracli-Levy, Juliette, *Wanderers in the New Forest* (London, 1958). Dyer, T. F. Thiselton, *The Folk-lore of Plants* (London, 1889); facsimile reprint (Llanerch Press, 1994). **BRACKEN** Watts, Donald C., *Elsevier's Dictionary of Plant Names and their Origins* (Elsevier, 2000). Pechey (1694). Johnson, C. Pierpoint, *The Useful Plants of Great Britain*, illus. Sowerby, John E. (Kent & Co., 1862). Vickery (1995). Chevallier (1996). **MALE FERN** Pechey (1694). Kemsey (1838). Chevallier (1996). Pechey (1694). Salmon (1693). **ROYAL FERN** Beith (1995). Allen and Hatfield (2004). Milliken, W. and Bridgewater, S., *Flora Celtica: Plants and People in Scotland* (Birlinn, 2004). Britten, James and Holland, Robert, *A Dictionary of English Plant Names* (English Dialect Society, 1886). Barnum (1996). Pechey (1694). Carmichael (1900–71). **FEVERFEW** Johnson, A. T. and Smith, H. A., *Plant Names Simplified*, 2nd edn (Hamlyn, 1972). Mr F. C. W—, Norwich, pers. com. collected by author (1990). Pechey (1694). Gerard (1597). Culpeper (1652). Pechey (1694). Kemsey (1838). Taylor, Dr Mark R., 'Magic, witchcraft, charm-cures and customs in East Anglia', data for a never-published book, collected largely by correspondence, while Regional Medical Officer in Norwich 1920–27 (Norfolk Record Office, MS 4322, 57x1). Mrs F. S—, Cley, pers. com. collected by author (1988). Milliken, W. and Bridgewater, S., *Flora Celtica: Plants and People in*

Scotland (Birlinn, 2004). Pechey (1694). **FIGWORT** Allen and Hatfield (2004). Carmichael (1900–71). Mrs D. P—, Little Totham, pers. com. collected by author (1988). Lafont, Ann-Marie, *Devon's Heritage: A Herbal Folklore* (Badger Books, 1984). Marshall, Sybil, *Fenland Chronicle* (Cambridge University Press, 1967). Culpeper (1652). Pechey (1694). Porter, Roy, ed., *The Cambridge Illustrated History of Medicine* (Cambridge University Press, 1996). Chevallier (1996). **FORGET-ME-NOT** Nuttall, G. Clarke, *Wild Flowers as They Grow*, 5 vols (Waverley Book Company, *c.*1920). Strickland, Miss Agnes, *Lives of the Queens of England* (George Bell & Sons, 1840), quoted in Burgess, J. T., *Old English Wild Flowers* (Frederick Warne, 1868). Grigson, Geoffrey, *The Englishman's Flora* (Phoenix House, 1955). Gerard (1597). Johnson, C. Pierpoint, *The Useful Plants of Great Britain*, illus. Sowerby, John E. (Kent & Co., 1862). Milliken, W. and Bridgewater, S., *Flora Celtica: Plants and People in Scotland* (Birlinn, 2004). **FOXGLOVE** Allen, D. E., own MS. Porter, Roy, ed., *The Cambridge Illustrated History of Medicine* (Cambridge University Press, 1996). Gerard, John, quoted Wren, R. C., *Potter's New Cyclopaedia of Botanical Drugs and Preparations*, 8th edn (Health Science Press, 1975). Salmon (1693). Kemsey (1838). Allen and Hatfield (2004). Beith (1995). Milliken, W. and Bridgewater, S., *Flora Celtica: Plants and People in Scotland* (Birlinn, 2004). Beith (1995). Mrs E. D—, Somerset, pers. com. collected by author (1985). Allen and Hatfield (2004). **FUMITORY** Old-English medical manuscript, Stockholm Library (*c.*1400), quoted in Grigson, Geoffrey, *The Englishman's Flora* (Phoenix House, 1955). Marshall, Sybil, *Under the Hawthorn* (J. M. Dent & Sons, 1981). Nuttall, G. Clarke, *Wild Flowers as They Grow*, 5 vols (Waverley Book Company, *c.*1920). Culpeper (1652). Hill, Sir John (*c.*1820). Kemsey (1838). Quelch (1941). Grieve, Mrs M., *A Modern Herbal*, ed. Leyel, Mrs C. F. (Jonathan Cape, 1931). Vickery (1995). Allen and Hatfield (2004). **GARLIC** Letter from Mrs Campbell (1778), quoted in Lochead, Marion, *The Scots Household in the Eighteenth Century* (Moray Press, 1948). Harvey, John H., 'Vegetables in the Middle Ages', *Garden History*, vol. 12, pt 2 (1984). Taylor, Dr Mark R., 'Magic, witchcraft, charm-cures and customs in East Anglia', data for a never-published book, collected largely by correspondence, while Regional Medical Officer in Norwich 1920–27 (Norfolk Record Office, MS 4322, 57x1). Essex Age Concern Essay (1991). Culpeper (1652). Pechey (1694). Kemsey (1838). Grieve, Mrs M., *A Modern Herbal*, ed. Leyel, Mrs C. F. (Jonathan Cape, 1931). Newall, Carol A., Anderson, Linda A. and Phillipson, J. David, *Herbal Medicines: A Guide for Health Professionals* (Pharmaceutical Press, 1996). Chevallier (1996). **GOAT'S BEARD** Bishop Mant, quoted in Dyer, T. F. Thiselton, *The Folk-lore of Plants* (London, 1889); facsimile reprint (Llanerch Press, 1994). Vickery (1995). Gerard (1597). Pechey (1694). Fairweather, Barbara, *Highland Plant Lore* (Glencoe and North Lorn Folk Museum, *c.*1980). Chevallier (1996). **GOLDENROD** Eastman, Elaine Goodale, quoted in Jill Duchess of Hamilton, Penny Hart & John Simmons, *English Plants for your Garden* (Frances Lincoln, 2000). Pratt, Anne, *Wild Flowers*, 2 vols

(Society for Promoting Christian Knowledge, 1898). Dyer, T. F. Thiselton, *The Folk-lore of Plants* (London, 1889); facsimile reprint (Llanerch Press, 1994). Vickery (1995). Martin, Martin, *A Description of the Western Isles of Scotland* (A. Bell, 1703). Coates, Doris E., *Tuppeny Rice and Treacle: Cottage Housekeeping (1900–1920)* (Reader's Union, 1976). Record no. M106, English Folklore Survey MSS (1960s); in University College London Library. Vickery (1995). Allen and Hatfield (2004). Moloney, Michael F., *Irish Ethnobotany and the Evolution of Medicine in Ireland* (M. H. Gill and Son, 1919). Gerard (1597). Culpeper (1652). Pechey (1694). Kemsey (1838). Chevallier (1996). **GOOSEGRASS** Britten, James and Holland, Robert, *A Dictionary of English Plant Names* (English Dialect Society, 1886). Johnson, A. T. and Smith, H. A., *Plant Names Simplified*, 2nd edn (Hamlyn, 1972). Milliken, W. and Bridgewater, S., *Flora Celtica: Plants and People in Scotland* (Birlinn, 2004). Sharkey, Olive, *Old Days, Old Ways* (O'Brien Press, 1985). Gerard (1597). Allen and Hatfield (2004). Wren, R. C., *Potter's New Cyclopaedia of Botanical Drugs and Preparations*, 8th edn (Health Science Press, 1975). Chevallier (1996). **GORSE** Milliken, W. and Bridgewater, S., *Flora Celtica: Plants and People in Scotland* (Birlinn, 2004). Fairweather, Barbara, *Highland Plant Lore* (Glencoe and North Lorn Folk Museum, c.1980). Darwin (1996). Sharkey, Olive, *Old Days, Old Ways* (O'Brien Press, 1985). Grieve, Mrs M., *A Modern Herbal*, ed. Leyel, Mrs C. F. (Jonathan Cape, 1931). Lafont, Ann-Marie, *Devon's Heritage: A Herbal Folklore* (Badger Books, 1984). Darwin (1996). Milliken, W. and Bridgewater, S., (2004). Emerson, P. H., *Pictures of East Anglian Life* (Sampson Low, 1887). Jones, Anne E., 'Folk Medicine in Living Memory in Wales', *Folk Life*, vol. 18 (1980). Sekers, Simone, *The Country Housewife* (Hodder and Stoughton, 1983). Lucas, A. T., *Furze: A Survey and History of its Uses in Ireland* (The Stationery Office, London, 1960). Allen and Hatfield (2004). Gerard (1597). Culpeper (1652) **GREATER CELANDINE** Pechey (1694). Lafont, Ann-Marie, *Devon's Heritage: A Herbal Folklore* (Badger Books, 1984). Taylor, Dr Mark R., 'Magic, witchcraft, charm-cures and customs in East Anglia', data for a never-published book, collected largely by correspondence, while Regional Medical Officer in Norwich 1920–27 (Norfolk Record Office, MS 4322, 57x1). Grieve, Mrs M., *A Modern Herbal*, ed. Leyel, Mrs C. F. (Jonathan Cape, 1931). Mrs D. L—, Denver Mill, pers. com. collected by author (2002). Gerard (1597). Salmon (1693). Culpeper (1652). Kemsey (1838). Ernst, E. and Schmidt, B., *Cancer*, vol. 5, pt 69 (July 2005). **GREATER PLANTAIN** Anon, Lay of the Nine Healing Herbs (n.d.); a fragment of a Saxon manuscript – the Lacnunga – written originally in the Wessex dialect and translated repeatedly over the years, quoted in Grigson, Geoffrey, *The Englishman's Flora* (Phoenix House, 1955). Wheelwright, Edith Grey, *The Physick Garden* (Jonathan Cape, 1934). Vickery (1995). Allen and Hatfield (2004). Mrs M. B—, Yarmouth, pers. com. collected by author (1988). Gerard (1597). Salmon (1693). Pechey (1694). Kemsey (1838). Chevallier (1996). **GROUND ELDER** Gerard (1597). Britten, James and Holland, Robert, *A*

Dictionary of English Plant Names (English Dialect Society, 1886). Kemsey (1838). Milliken, W. and Bridgewater, S., *Flora Celtica: Plants and People in Scotland* (Birlinn, 2004). Essex Age Concern Essay (1991). Mrs W—, Stanton, pers. com. collected by author (1987). **GROUND IVY** Roxburghe Ballads, quoted in Genders, Roy, *The Scented Wild Flowers of Britain* (Collins, 1971). Dyer, T. F. Thiselton, *The Folk-lore of Plants* (London, 1889); facsimile reprint (Llanerch Press, 1994). Plues, Margaret, *Rambles in Search of Wild Flowers*, 4th edn (George Bell, 1892). Taylor, Dr Mark R., 'Magic, witchcraft, charm-cures and customs in East Anglia', data for a never-published book, collected largely by correspondence, while Regional Medical Officer in Norwich 1920–27 (Norfolk Record Office, MS 4322, 57x1). Darwin (1996). Lafont, Ann-Marie, *Devon's Heritage: A Herbal Folklore* (Badger Books, 1984). Hatfield, Audrey Wynne, *How to Enjoy your Weeds* (Frederick Muller, 1969). Mrs D. P—, Little Totham, pers. com. collected by author (1989). Gerard (1597). Salmon (1693). Kemsey (1838). Wren, R. C., *Potter's New Cyclopaedia of Botanical Drugs and Preparations*, 8th edn (Health Science Press, 1975). Chevallier (1996). **GROUNDSEL** Bullein, William, *The Booke of Simples* (1562), quoted in Grigson, Geoffrey, *The Englishman's Flora* (Phoenix House, 1955). Haggard, Lilias Rider, ed., *I Walked by Night: by the King of the Norfolk Poachers* (Boydell Press, 1974). Howkins, Chris, *Valuable Garden Weeds* (Chris Howkins, 1991). Lafont, Ann-Marie, *Devon's Heritage: A Herbal Folklore* (Badger Books, 1984). Culpeper (1652). Vickery (1995). Mr F. C. W—, Norwich, pers. com. collected by author (1988). Milliken, W. and Bridgewater, S., *Flora Celtica: Plants and People in Scotland* (Birlinn, 2004). Darwin (1996). Allen and Hatfield (2004). Gerard (1597). Salmon (1693). Mrs H. S—, Norfolk, pers. com. collected by author (1988). **HAREBELL** Britten, James and Holland, Robert, *A Dictionary of English Plant Names* (English Dialect Society, 1886). Vickery (1995). Plues, Margaret, *Rambles in Search of Wild Flowers*, 4th edn (George Bell, 1892). Gregor, Walter, 'Notes on the Folk-lore of the North-east of Scotland', quoted in Britten, James and Holland, Robert, *A Dictionary of English Plant Names* (English Dialect Society, 1886). Mason, James, 'The Folk-lore of British Plants', *Dublin University Magazine*, vol. 82 (1873). **HAWTHORN** Grigson, Geoffrey, *The Englishman's Flora* (Phoenix House, 1955). Page, Robin, *The Country Way of Love* (Penguin, 1983). Vickery (1995). Milliken, W. and Bridgewater, S., *Flora Celtica: Plants and People in Scotland* (Birlinn, 2004). de la Mare, Walter, 'The hawthorn hath a deathly smell', from *The Listeners* (1914), quoted in Genders, Roy, *The Scented Wild Flowers of Britain* (Collins, 1971). Vickery (1995). Mrs A. B—, Cheshire, pers. com. collected by author (2002). British Medical Journal (1875), vol. 35. Hatfield, Gabrielle, *Memory, Wisdom and Healing* (Sutton, 1999). Milliken, W. and Bridgewater, S., *Flora Celtica: Plants and People in Scotland* (Birlinn, 2004). Beith (1995). Westropp, Thomas, 'A Folklore Survey of County Clare', *Folk-Lore* 22 (Folklore Society, 1911). Lafont, Ann-Marie, *Devon's Heritage: A Herbal Folklore* (Badger Books, 1984).

Allen and Hatfield (2004). Culpeper (1652). Salmon (1693). Gunton Household Book. Chevallier (1996). Ernst, Edzard, ed., *Herbal Medicine: A Concise Overview for Professionals* (Butterworth-Heinemann, 2000). **HAZEL** Rackham, Oliver, *The History of the Countryside* (J. M. Dent & Sons, 1987). Milliken, W. and Bridgewater, S., *Flora Celtica: Plants and People in Scotland* (Birlinn, 2004). Pechey (1694). Britten, James and Holland, Robert, *A Dictionary of English Plant Names* (English Dialect Society, 1886). Darwin (1996). Gerard (1597). Darwin (1996). Salmon (1693). Allen and Hatfield (2004). Grigson, Geoffrey, *The Englishman's Flora* (Phoenix House, 1955). Vickery (1995). Porter, Enid M., *The Folklore of East Anglia* (Batsford, 1974). Milliken, W. and Bridgewater, S., *Flora Celtica: Plants and People in Scotland* (Birlinn, 2004). Dyer, T. F. Thiselton, *The Folk-lore of Plants* (London, 1889); facsimile reprint (Llanerch Press, 1994). Tongue, Ruth L., *Somerset Folklore*, ed. Briggs, K. M. (Folklore Society, 1965). Radford, E. and Radford, M. A., *Encyclopaedia of Superstitions*, edited and revised by Hole, Christina (Hutchinson, 1974). Milliken, W. and Bridgewater, S. (2004). Vickery (1995). **HEARTSEASE** Darwin (1996). Parkinson (1640). Britten, James and Holland, Robert, *A Dictionary of English Plant Names* (English Dialect Society, 1886). Gerard (1597). Moncrief, John, *The Poor Man's Physician, or the Receits of the Famous John Moncrief of Tippermalloch*, 3rd edn (Edinburgh, 1731). Chevallier (1996). **HEATHS AND HEATHERS** Howitt, Mary, quoted in Hulme, Frederick Edward, *Familiar Wild Flowers*, 6 vols (Cassell & Co., c.1910). Milliken, W. and Bridgewater, S., *Flora Celtica: Plants and People in Scotland* (Birlinn, 2004). Darwin (1996). Beith (1995). Milliken, W. and Bridgewater, S. (2004). Freethy, Ron, *From Agar to Zenry* (Crowood Press, 1985). Chevallier (1996). Milliken, W. and Bridgewater, S. (2004). Burgess, J. T., *Old English Wild Flowers* (Frederick Warne, 1868). Darwin (1996). **HELLEBORE** Poem by Burton, Robert, quoted in Grieve, Mrs M., *A Modern Herbal*, ed. Leyel, Mrs C. F. (Jonathan Cape, 1931). White, Gilbert, quoted in Grigson, Geoffrey, *The Englishman's Flora* (Phoenix House, 1955). Culpeper (1652). Gerard (1597). Culpeper (1652). Curtis, William, *Flora Londinensis*, 3 vols (Henry G. Bohn, 1777–98). Chevallier (1996). Bracken, Henry, *Farriery Improved*, 2nd edn (London, 1789). Taylor, Dr Mark R., 'Magic, witchcraft, charm-cures and customs in East Anglia', data for a never-published book, collected largely by correspondence, while Regional Medical Officer in Norwich 1920–27 (Norfolk Record Office, MS 4322, 57x1). William Kingsbury's Notebook, Sprowston, Norfolk (1710); in Gressenhall Museum, G.7.983. Mrs B—, Brundall, Norfolk, pers. com. collected by author (1889). **HENBANE** Wheelwright, Edith Grey, *The Physick Garden* (Jonathan Cape, 1934). Genders, Roy, *The Scented Wild Flowers of Britain* (Collins, 1971). Chevallier (1996). Thomas, Keith, *Religion and the Decline of Magic* (Penguin, 1973). Johnson, C. Pierpoint, *The Useful Plants of Great Britain*, illus. Sowerby, John E. (Kent & Co., 1862). Darwin (1996). Gerard (1597). Culpeper (1652). Pechey (1694). Kemsey (1838). William Kingsbury's Notebook, Sprowston,

Norfolk (1710); in Gressenhall Museum, G.7.983. Gerard (1597). Mr C—, quoted in English Folklore Survey MSS (1960s); in University College London Library. Darwin (1996). Allen and Hatfield (2004). Whitlock, Ralph, *Wiltshire Folklore and Legends* (Robert Hale, 1992). Wheelwright, Edith Grey, *The Physick Garden* (Jonathan Cape, 1934). Chevallier (1996). **HERB BENNET OR WOOD AVENS** Anon., *Ortus Sanitatis*, a medieval herbal (1491), quoted in Britten, James and Holland, Robert, *A Dictionary of English Plant Names* (English Dialect Society, 1886). Pratt, Anne, *Wild Flowers*, 2 vols (Society for Promoting Christian Knowledge, 1898). Quelch (1946). Hutchinson, Peggy, *More Home-made Wine Secrets* (W. Foulsham & Co., c.1945). Pechey (1694). Gerard (1597). Moncrief, John, *The Poor Man's Physician, or the Receits of the Famous John Moncrief of Tippermalloch*, 3rd edn (Edinburgh, 1731). English Folklore Survey MSS (1960s); in University College London Library. Vickery (1995). **HERB ROBERT** Milliken, W. and Bridgewater, S., *Flora Celtica: Plants and People in Scotland* (Birlinn, 2004). Tongue, Ruth L., *Somerset Folklore*, ed. Briggs, K. M. (Folklore Society, 1965). Allen and Hatfield (2004). Pechey (1694). Kemsey (1838). Chevallier (1996). **HOGWEED** Mrs M. P—, Somerset, pers. com. collected by author (2002). Taylor, J. E., *Flowers: their Origins, Shapes, Perfumes, and Colours*, 4th edn (W. H. Allen, c.1890). Statistical Account of Scotland, quoted in Britten, James and Holland, Robert, *A Dictionary of English Plant Names* (English Dialect Society, 1886). Allen and Hatfield (2004). Gerard (1597). Culpeper (1652). Pechey (1694). Sowerby, J., *English Botany* (George Bell & Sons, 1899), quoted Grigson, Geoffrey, *The Englishman's Flora* (Phoenix House, 1955). **HOLLY** Irish saying, quoted in McGlinchey, Charles, *The Last of the Name*, ed. Friel, Brian (Blackstaff Press, 1986). Dyer, T. F. Thiselton, *The Folk-lore of Plants* (London, 1889); facsimile reprint (Llanerch Press, 1994). Mason, James, 'The Folk-lore of British Plants', *Dublin University Magazine*, vol. 82, (1873). Tongue, Ruth L., *Somerset Folklore*, ed. Briggs, K. M. (Folklore Society, 1965). Milliken, W. and Bridgewater, S. (2004). Britten, James and Holland, Robert, *A Dictionary of English Plant Names* (English Dialect Society, 1886). Vickery (1995). Milliken, W. and Bridgewater, S. (2004). Allen and Hatfield (2004). Tongue, Ruth L. (1965). Allen and Hatfield (2004). Lafont, Ann-Marie, *Devon's Heritage: A Herbal Folklore* (Badger Books, 1984). Dyer, T. F. Thiselton (1889). Culpeper (1652). Pechey (1694). Chevallier (1996). Miles, Archie, *Silva: The Tree in Britain* (Ebury Press, 1999). **HONEYSUCKLE OR WOODBINE** Parkinson (1629). Lankester, Phebe, *Wild Flowers Worth Notice* (Routledge, 1905). Milliken, W. and Bridgewater, S., *Flora Celtica: Plants and People in Scotland* (Birlinn, 2004). Beith (1995). Vickery (1995). Pechey (1694). Kemsey (1838). Wren, R. C., *Potter's New Cyclopaedia of Botanical Drugs and Preparations*, 8th edn (Health Science Press, 1975). **HORSETAIL** Mabey, Richard, *Flora Britannica* (Sinclair Stevenson, 1996). Turner, William, *Libellus de re Herbaria nova* (London, 1538). Bown, Deni, *The Royal Horticultural Society Encyclopedia of Herbs and their Uses* (Dorling

Kindersley, 1995). Hatfield, Audrey Wynne, *How to Enjoy your Weeds* (Frederick Muller, 1969). Chevallier (1996). Fairweather, Barbara, *Highland Plant Lore* (Glencoe and North Lorn Folk Museum, c.1980). Darwin (1996). Parkinson quoted in Wren, R. C., *Potter's New Cyclopaedia of Botanical Drugs and Preparations*, 8th edn (Health Science Press, 1975). Fairweather, Barbara, *Highland Plant Lore* (Glencoe and North Lorn Folk Museum, c.1980). Allen and Hatfield (2004). Barton, Benjamin H. and Castle, Thomas, *The British Flora Medica or History of the Medicinal Plants of Great Britain* (E. Cox, 1837). Culpeper (1652). Pechey (1694). Chevallier (1996). Crellin, John K. and Philpott, Jane, *A Reference Guide to Medicinal Plants* (Duke University Press, 1990). **HOUSELEEK** Hill, Thomas, *Natural and Artificial Conclusions* (1670), quoted in Quelch (1946). Vickery (1995). Dyer, T. F. Thiselton, *The Folk-lore of Plants* (London, 1889); facsimile reprint (Llanerch Press, 1994). Allen and Hatfield (2004). Gerard (1597). Pechey (1694). Kemsey (1838). Culpeper (1652). Norfolk Records Office, MC 43/9. Chevallier (1996). **IVY** Giles Fletcher poem from Quiller-Couch, Sir Arthur, ed., *The Oxford Book of English Verse* (Oxford University Press, 1939). Darwin (1996). McNeil, quoted Milliken, W. and Bridgewater, S., *Flora Celtica: Plants and People in Scotland* (Birlinn, 2004). Lupton, J., *A Thousand Notable Things* (1660), quoted in Radford, E. and Radford, M. A., *Encyclopaedia of Superstitions*, edited and revised by Hole, Christina (Hutchinson, 1974). MS notes from Mundford Primary School, Norfolk (1980s). Jones, Anne E., 'Folk Medicine in Living Memory in Wales', *Folk Life*, vol. 18 (1980). Mr and Mrs S—, Devon, pers. com. collected by author (2002). Mr A—, Ayrshire, pers. com. collected by author (1989). Fairweather, Barbara, *Highland Plant Lore* (Glencoe and North Lorn Folk Museum, c.1980). Allen and Hatfield (2004). Mason, James, 'The Folk-lore of British Plants', *Dublin University Magazine*, vol. 82 (1873). Gerard (1597). Culpeper (1652). Tongue, Ruth L., *Somerset Folklore*, ed. Briggs, K. M. (Folklore Society, 1965). Salmon (1693). Kemsey (1838). Jones, Anne E. (1980). Mrs S—, Guernsey, pers. com. collected by author (2001). Lafont, Ann-Marie, *Devon's Heritage: A Herbal Folklore* (Badger Books, 1984). Vickery (1995). **JACK-BY-THE-HEDGE** Genders, Roy, *The Scented Wild Flowers of Britain* (Collins, 1971). Gerard (1597). Turner, William, *The Names of Herbes* (1548), quoted in Watts, Donald C., *Elsevier's Dictionary of Plant Names and their Origins* (Elsevier, 2000). Burgess, J. T., *Old English Wild Flowers* (Frederick Warne, 1868). Watts, Donald C. (2000). Britten, James and Holland, Robert, *A Dictionary of English Plant Names* (English Dialect Society, 1886). Allen and Hatfield (2004). Tongue, Ruth L., *Somerset Folklore*, ed. Briggs, K. M. (Folklore Society, 1965). D. P—, Little Totham, pers. com. collected by author (1989). Hulme, Frederick Edward, *Familiar Wild Flowers*, 6 vols (Cassell & Co., c.1910). Gerard (1597). Salmon (1693). Pechey (1694). Culpeper (1652). Kemsey (1838). **JUNIPER** 'The Queen's Maries' is a traditional ballad, of which there are many variants; this version is in Quiller-Couch, Sir Arthur, ed., *The Oxford Book of English Verse* (Oxford

University Press, 1939). Wallace, W., *East Anglian Magazine* (December 1975). Evans, George Ewart, *The Pattern Under the Plough* (Faber and Faber, 1966). Pechey (1694). Allen and Hatfield (2004). Beith (1995). Mrs D. C—, Norwich, pers. com. collected by author (1990). Salmon (1693). Grigson, Geoffrey, *The Englishman's Flora* (Phoenix House, 1955). Chevallier (1996). Darwin (1996). Johnson, C. Pierpoint, *The Useful Plants of Great Britain*, illus. Sowerby, John E. (Kent & Co., 1862). Essex Age Concern Essay (1991). Ellis, William, *Modern Husbandman* (1750), vol. VII, pt ii, p. 142, quoted in Britten, James and Holland, Robert, *A Dictionary of English Plant Names* (English Dialect Society, 1886). Gerard (1597). Milliken, W. and Bridgewater, S., *Flora Celtica: Plants and People in Scotland* (Birlinn, 2004). **KINGCUP OR MARSH MARIGOLD** Johnson, A. T. and Smith, H. A., *Plant Names Simplified*, 2nd edn (Hamlyn, 1972). Grigson, Geoffrey, *The Englishman's Flora* (Phoenix House, 1955). Vickery (1995). Darwin (1996). Allen and Hatfield (2004). Turner, William, quoted in Johnson, C. Pierpoint, *The Useful Plants of Great Britain*, illus. Sowerby, John E. (Kent & Co., 1862). Withering, Dr, quoted in Lankester, Phebe, *Wild Flowers Worth Notice* (Routledge, 1905). Johnson, C. Pierpoint, (1862). Grieve, Mrs M., *A Modern Herbal*, ed. Leyel, Mrs C. F. (Jonathan Cape, 1931). Milliken, W. and Bridgewater, S., *Flora Celtica: Plants and People in Scotland* (Birlinn, 2004). Nuttall, G. Clarke, *Wild Flowers as They Grow*, 5 vols (Waverley Book Company, c.1920). **KNAPWEED** Britten, James and Holland, Robert, *A Dictionary of English Plant Names* (English Dialect Society, 1886). Allen and Hatfield (2004). Culpeper (1652). Kemsey (1838). Page, Robin, *The Country Way of Love* (Penguin, 1983). **KNOTGRASS** Watts, Donald C., *Elsevier's Dictionary of Plant Names and their Origins* (Elsevier, 2000). Burgess, J. T., *Old English Wild Flowers* (Frederick Warne, 1868). Gerard (1597). Tongue, Ruth L., *Somerset Folklore*, ed. Briggs, K. M. (Folklore Society, 1965). Allen and Hatfield (2004). Culpeper (1652). Salmon (1693). Gunton Household Book. Kemsey (1838). Chevallier (1996). **LADY'S BEDSTRAW** Vickery (1995). Chaucer, Geoffrey, *The Merchant's Tale*, line 1784: from Cawley, A. C., ed., *Chaucer: Canterbury Tales* (J. M. Dent & Sons, 1958). Watts, Donald C., *Elsevier's Dictionary of Plant Names and their Origins* (Elsevier, 2000). Britten, James and Holland, Robert, *A Dictionary of English Plant Names* (English Dialect Society, 1886). Pechey (1694). Hill, Sir John (c.1820). Gerard (1597). Miller, Joseph, *Botanicum Officinale, or a Compendious Herbal* (1722), quoted in Wren, R. C., *Potter's New Cyclopaedia of Botanical Drugs and Preparations*, 8th edn (Health Science Press, 1975). Chevallier (1996). Gerard (1597). Vickery (1995). Howkins, Chris, *The Dairymaid's Flora* (Chris Howkins, 1994). Fairweather, Barbara, *Highland Plant Lore* (Glencoe and North Lorn Folk Museum, c.1980). Milliken, W. and Bridgewater, S., *Flora Celtica: Plants and People in Scotland* (Birlinn, 2004). **LADY'S MANTLE** Watts, Donald C., *Elsevier's Dictionary of Plant Names and their Origins* (Elsevier, 2000). Hulme, Frederick Edward, *Familiar Wild Flowers*, 6 vols (Cassell & Co., c.1910). Dyer, T. F. Thiselton, *The Folk-lore of Plants* (London, 1889); facsimile reprint (Llanerch Press, 1994). Grigson, Geoffrey, *The Englishman's Flora* (Phoenix House, 1955). Beith (1995). Allen and Hatfield (2004). Britten, James and Holland, Robert, *A Dictionary of English Plant Names* (English Dialect Society, 1886). Culpeper (1652). Pechey (1694). Kemsey (1838). Gerard (1597). Pechey (1694). Hill, Sir John (c.1820). Chevallier (1996). **LADY'S SMOCK** Fairweather, Barbara, *Highland Plant Lore* (Glencoe and North Lorn Folk Museum, c.1980). Allen and Hatfield (2004). Culpeper (1652). Nuttall, G. Clarke, *Wild Flowers as They Grow*, 5 vols (Waverley Book Company, c.1920). Johnson, C. Pierpoint, *The Useful Plants of Great Britain*, illus. Sowerby, John E. (Kent & Co., 1862). Hatfield, Gabrielle, *Encyclopedia of Folk Medicine: Old World and New World Traditions* (ABC Clio, 2004). Bown, Deni, *The Royal Horticultural Society Encyclopedia of Herbs and their Uses* (Dorling Kindersley, 1995). **LESSER CELANDINE** Burgess, J. T., *Old English Wild Flowers* (Frederick Warne, 1868). Vickery (1995). Lafont, Ann-Marie, *Devon's Heritage: A Herbal Folklore* (Badger Books, 1984). Grigson, Geoffrey, *The Englishman's Flora* (Phoenix House, 1955). Fairweather, Barbara, *Highland Plant Lore* (Glencoe and North Lorn Folk Museum, c.1980). Allen and Hatfield (2004). Vickery (1995). Gerard (1597). Culpeper (1652). Pechey (1694). Chevallier (1996). Newall, Carol A., Anderson, Linda A. and Phillipson, J. David, *Herbal Medicines: A Guide for Health Professionals* (Pharmaceutical Press, 1996). Wren, R. C., *Potter's New Cyclopaedia of Botanical Drugs and Preparations*, revised by Williamson, Elizabeth M. and Evans, Fred J. (C. W. Daniel Company, 1988). **LICHENS** Darwin (1996). Fairweather, Barbara, *Highland Plant Lore* (Glencoe and North Lorn Folk Museum, c.1980). Hooker, Sir W. J., *Flora Scotica* (Archibald Constable, 1821). Fairweather, Barbara (c.1980). Allen and Hatfield (2004). Withering, William, *A Botanical Arrangement of British Plants*, 2nd edn (M. Swinney, 1787–92). **DOG LICHEN** Salmon (1693). Culpeper (1652). **TREE LUNGWORT** Culpeper (1652). Pechey (1694). Kemsey (1838). Allen and Hatfield (2004). Chevallier (1996). **LILY OF THE VALLEY** Poem by Lawrence, John, quoted in Genders, Roy, *The Scented Wild Flowers of Britain* (Collins, 1971). Mason, James, 'The Folk-lore of British Plants', *Dublin University Magazine*, vol. 82 (1873). Nuttall, G. Clarke, *Wild Flowers as They Grow*, 5 vols (Waverley Book Company, c.1920). Bown, Deni, *The Royal Horticultural Society Encyclopedia of Herbs and their Uses* (Dorling Kindersley, 1995). Vickery (1995). Dyer, T. F. Thiselton, *The Folk-lore of Plants* (London, 1889); facsimile reprint (Llanerch Press, 1994). Vickery (1995). Allen and Hatfield (2004). Prince, Dennis, *Grandmother's Cures: An A–Z of Herbal Remedies* (Fontana, 1991). Gerard (1597). Culpeper (1652). Pratt, Anne, *Wild Flowers*, 2 vols (Society for Promoting Christian Knowledge, 1898). Freethy, Ron, *From Agar to Zenry* (Crowood Press, 1985). *The British Pharmacopoiea* (1949), published for the General Medical Council (Constable). Chevallier (1996). **LOUSEWORT** Dodoens, Rembert, *A Niewe Herball, or Historie of Plantes*, trans. Henry Lyte (London, 1578).

Gerard (1597). Freethy, Ron, *From Agar to Zenry* (Crowood Press, 1985). Darwin (1996). Allen and Hatfield (2004). McKay, Margaret M., ed., *The Rev. Dr John Walker's Report on the Hebrides of 1764 and 1771* (Edinburgh, 1980). Gerard (1597). Culpeper (1652). Kemsey (1838). **MALLOW** Grieve, Mrs M., *A Modern Herbal*, ed. Leyel, Mrs C. F. (Jonathan Cape, 1931). Quelch (1941). Lawson, A., *The Modern Farrier* (London, 1842). Pechey (1694). Salmon (1693). Kemsey (1838). Chevallier (1996). **MARJORAM** Poem by Skelton, John, in Quiller-Couch, Sir Arthur, ed., *The Oxford Book of English Verse* (Oxford University Press, 1939). Dyer, T. F. Thiselton, *The Folk-lore of Plants* (London, 1889); facsimile reprint (Llanerch Press, 1994). Bardswell, Frances Anne, *The Herb Garden* (A&C Black, 1911). Coates, Doris E., *Tuppeny Rice and Treacle: Cottage Housekeeping (1900–1920)* (Reader's Union, 1976). Gerard (1597), quoted in Hatfield, Audrey Wynne, *Pleasures of Herbs* (London Museum Press, 1964). Culpeper (1652). Chevallier (1996). Burgess, J. T., *Old English Wild Flowers* (Frederick Warne, 1868). Grieve, Mrs M., *A Modern Herbal*, ed. Leyel, Mrs C. F. (Jonathan Cape, 1931). Quelch (1946). William Kingsbury's Notebook, Sprowston, Norfolk (1710); in Gressenhall Museum, G.7.983. **MEADOWSWEET** Allen and Hatfield (2004). Aubrey, John, *Remaines of Gentilisme and Judaisme* (1686–87), Britten, J., ed. (London, 1881). Allen and Hatfield (2004). Coates, Doris E., *Tuppeny Rice and Treacle: Cottage Housekeeping (1900–1920)* (Reader's Union, 1976). Salmon (1693). Pechey (1694). Grieve, Mrs M., *A Modern Herbal*, ed. Leyel, Mrs C. F. (Jonathan Cape, 1931). Gerard (1597). Parkinson (1640). Gerard (1597). Vickery (1995). **MILKWORT** Grigson, Geoffrey, *The Englishman's Flora* (Phoenix House, 1955). Pratt, Anne, *Wild Flowers*, 2 vols (Society for Promoting Christian Knowledge, 1898), vol. I. Gerard (1597). Pechey (1694). Johnson, C. Pierpoint, *The Useful Plants of Great Britain*, illus. Sowerby, John E. (Kent & Co., 1862). Chevallier (1996). Carmichael (1990–71). Robertson, J., 'Journal' (1771), quoted in Milliken, W. and Bridgewater, S., *Flora Celtica: Plants and People in Scotland* (Birlinn, 2004). **MINT** *Edinburgh Evening Courant* (12 July 1753). Gerard (1597). Culpeper (1652). Kemsey (1838). Milliken, W. and Bridgewater, S., *Flora Celtica: Plants and People in Scotland* (Birlinn, 2004). Vickery (1995). Allen and Hatfield (2004). Record no. 100, English Folklore Survey MSS (1960s); in University College London Library. Taylor, Dr Mark R., 'Magic, witchcraft, charm-cures and customs in East Anglia', data for a never-published book, collected largely by correspondence, while Regional Medical Officer in Norwich 1920–27 (Norfolk Record Office, MS 4322, 57x1). Beith (1995). Darwin (1996). Vickery (1995). Scottish Records Office, GD1/384/26. Allen and Hatfield (2004). Darwin (1996). Tongue, Ruth L., *Somerset Folklore*, ed. Briggs, K. M. (Folklore Society, 1965). **MISTLETOE** Watts, Donald C., *Elsevier's Dictionary of Plant Names and their Origins* (Elsevier, 2000). Radford, E. and Radford, M. A., *Encyclopaedia of Superstitions*, edited and revised by Hole, Christina (Hutchinson, 1974). Pennant, Thomas (1774), quoted in Darwin (1996). *Notes and Queries 3* (London, 1869).

Beith (1995). Mrs D. W—, Colchester, pers. com. collected by author (1990). Culpeper (1652). Pechey (1694). Chevallier (1996). Wren, R. C., *Potter's New Cyclopaedia of Botanical Drugs and Preparations*, revised by Williamson, Elizabeth M. and Evans, Fred J. (C. W. Daniel Company, 1988). Ernst, Edzard, ed., *Herbal Medicine: A Concise Overview for Professionals* (Butterworth-Heinemann, 2000). **MONKSHOOD** Mabberley, D. J., *The Plant-Book* (Cambridge University Press, 1987). Grieve, Mrs M., *A Modern Herbal*, ed. Leyel, Mrs C. F. (Jonathan Cape, 1931). Vickery (1995). Mr F. C. W—, Norwich, pers. com collected by author (1988). Grigson, Geoffrey, *The Englishman's Flora* (Phoenix House, 1955). Johnson, A. T. and Smith, H. A., *Plant Names Simplified*, 2nd edn (Hamlyn, 1972). Gerard (1597). Burnett, M. A., *Plantae Utiliores*, 2 vols (Whittaker, 1842). Kemsey (1838). *The British Pharmacopoeia* (1914), published for the General Medical Council, (London). Wheelwright, Edith Grey, *The Physick Garden* (Jonathan Cape, 1934). Chevallier (1996). Wren, R. C., *Potter's New Cyclopaedia of Botanical Drugs and Preparations*, revised by Williamson, Elizabeth M. and Evans, Fred J. (C. W. Daniel Company, 1988). **MUGWORT** Proverb quoted in Black, William George, *Folk-Medicine: A Chapter in the History of Culture* (Folklore Society, 1883); reprint (Burt Franklin, 1970). Mr A. R—, Northampton, pers. com. collected by author (1985). Watts, Donald C., *Elsevier's Dictionary of Plant Names and their Origins* (Elsevier, 2000). Chevallier (1996). Gunton Household Book. Pechey (1694). Salmon (1693). Wren, R. C., *Potter's New Cyclopaedia of Botanical Drugs and Preparations*, revised by Williamson, Elizabeth M. and Evans, Fred J. (C. W. Daniel Company, 1988). Chevallier (1996). Pliny the Elder, quoted in Dyer, T. F. Thiselton, *The Folk-lore of Plants* (London, 1889); facsimile reprint (Llanerch Press, 1994). Cockayne, Revd Thomas Oswald, *Leechdoms, Wortcunning and Starcraft of Early England* (Holland Press, 1961). Tongue, Ruth L., *Somerset Folklore*, ed. Briggs, K. M. (Folklore Society, 1965). Grieve, Mrs M., *A Modern Herbal*, ed. Leyel, Mrs C. F. (Jonathan Cape, 1931). Allen, Andrew, *A Dictionary of Sussex Folk Medicine* (Countryside Books, 1995). Allen and Hatfield (2004). McGlinchey, Charles, *The Last of the Name*, ed. Brian Friel (Blackstaff Press, 1986). **MULLEIN** Johnson, C. Pierpoint, *The Useful Plants of Great Britain*, illus. Sowerby, John E. (Kent & Co., 1862). Bullein, William, *The Booke of Simples* (1562), quoted in Britten, James and Holland, Robert, *A Dictionary of English Plant Names* (English Dialect Society, 1886). Allen and Hatfield (2004). de Bäiracli Levy, Juliette, *The Illustrated Herbal Handbook*, 2nd edn (Faber and Faber, 1982). Pechey (1694). Moncrief, John, *The Poor Man's Physician, or the Receits of the Famous John Moncrief of Tippermalloch*, 3rd edn (Edinburgh, 1731). Kemsey (1838). Wren, R. C., *Potter's New Cyclopaedia of Botanical Drugs and Preparations*, revised by Williamson, Elizabeth M. and Evans, Fred J. (C. W. Daniel Company, 1988). Chevallier (1996). **NAVELWORT** Vickery (1995). Lafont, Ann-Marie, *Devon's Heritage: A Herbal Folklore* (Badger Books, 1984). Vickery, Roy, *A Dictionary of Plant-lore* (Oxford

University Press, 1995). Britten, James and Holland, Robert, *A Dictionary of English Plant Names* (English Dialect Society, 1886). Vickery (1995). Johnson, C. Pierpoint, *The Useful Plants of Great Britain*, illus. Sowerby, John E. (Kent & Co., 1862). Allen and Hatfield (2004). Pechey (1694). Kemsey (1838). Mrs M. M—, Wiltshire, pers. com. collected by author (1998). **NETTLE** Poem from Rigg, James, *Wild Flower Lyrics and other Poems* (Alexander Gardner, 1897). Culpeper (1652). Campbell, Thomas, *Letters from the South*, 2 vols (London, 1837), quoted in Grieve, Mrs M., *A Modern Herbal*, ed. Leyel, Mrs C. F. (Jonathan Cape, 1931). McNeill, F. Marian, *The Scots Kitchen* (Blackie & Son, 1929). Essex Age Concern Essay (1991). National Library of Scotland, MS 3774. Ernst, Edzard, ed., *Herbal Medicine: A Concise Overview for Professionals* (Butterworth-Heinemann, 2000). Randall, C., et al, *Journal of the Royal Society of Medicine*, vol. 93, issue 6 (2000). Bracken, Henry, *Farriery Improved*, 2nd edn (London, 1789). Allen and Hatfield (2004). Martin Martin, quoted in Milliken, W. and Bridgewater, S., *Flora Celtica: Plants and People in Scotland* (Birlinn, 2004). Salmon (1693). Pechey (1694). Kemsey (1838). Wren, R. C., *Potter's New Cyclopaedia of Botanical Drugs and Preparations*, 8th edn (Health Science Press, 1975). Ernst, Edzard, ed., *Herbal Medicine: A Concise Overview for Professionals* (Butterworth-Heinemann, 2000). **OAK** Tongue, Ruth L., *Somerset Folklore*, ed. Briggs, K. M. (Folklore Society, 1965). Dyer, T. F. Thiselton, *The Folk-lore of Plants* (London, 1889); facsimile reprint (Llanerch Press, 1994). Vickery (1995). Dyer, T. F. Thiselton (1994). Black, William George, *Folk-Medicine: A Chapter in the History of Culture* (Folklore Society, 1883); reprint (Burt Franklin, 1970). McGlinchey, Charles, *The Last of the Name*, ed. Brian Friel (Blackstaff Press, 1986). Allen and Hatfield (2004). Gerard (1597). Culpeper (1652). Pechey (1694). Gunton Household Book. D. K., Suffolk, privately owned MS. Wren, R. C., *Potter's New Cyclopaedia of Botanical Drugs and Preparations*, 8th edn (Health Science Press, 1975). Chevallier (1996). Milliken, W. and Bridgewater, S., *Flora Celtica: Plants and People in Scotland* (Birlinn, 2004). Darwin (1996). **ONION** Harrison, S. G., Masefield, G. B. and Wallis, Michael, *The Oxford Book of Food Plants* (Peerage Books, 1985). Beith (1995). Chevallier (1996). Dyer, T. F. Thiselton, *The Folk-lore of Plants* (London, 1889); facsimile reprint (Llanerch Press, 1994). Ethnomedica database (www.rbgkew.org.uk/ethnomedica), based at the Royal Botanic Gardens, Kew (*see also* Introduction). Mr M—, Wymondham, Norfolk, pers. com. collected by author (1987). Essex Age Concern Essay (1991). Mrs D. H—, Essex, pers. com. collected by author (1991). Vickery (1995). Wren, R. C., *Potter's New Cyclopaedia of Botanical Drugs and Preparations*, revised by Williamson, Elizabeth M. and Evans, Fred J. (C. W. Daniel Company, 1988). Gerard (1597). Pechey (1694). Kemsey (1838). Chevallier (1996). J. D—, Great Waltham, pers. com. collected by author (1991). **ORPINE** Vickery (1995). Culpeper (1652). Pechey (1694). Kemsey (1838). Allen and Hatfield (2004). Britten, James and Holland, Robert, *A Dictionary of English Plant Names* (English Dialect Society, 1886). Mrs E.

R—, Quy, Cambridgeshire, pers. com. collected by author (1990). Johnson, C. Pierpoint, *The Useful Plants of Great Britain*, illus. Sowerby, John E. (Kent & Co., 1862). Coffey, Timothy, *The History and Folklore of North American Wildflowers* (Facts on File, New York, 1993). **OX-EYE DAISY** Tongue, Ruth L., *Somerset Folklore*, ed. Briggs, K. M. (Folklore Society, 1965). Gerard (1597). Quelch (1946). Vickery (1995). Nuttall, G. Clarke, *Wild Flowers as They Grow*, 5 vols (Waverley Book Company, *c.*1920). Vickery (1995). Pratt, Anne, *Wild Flowers*, 2 vols (Society for Promoting Christian Knowledge, 1898). Allen and Hatfield (2004). Grieve, Mrs M., *A Modern Herbal*, ed. Leyel, Mrs C. F. (Jonathan Cape, 1931). Pechey (1694). Buchan, William, *Domestic Medicine*, 3rd edn (Edinburgh, 1774). Kemsey (1838). Wren, R. C., *Potter's New Cyclopaedia of Botanical Drugs and Preparations*, 8th edn (Health Science Press, 1975). **PELLITORY-OF-THE-WALL** Culpeper (1652). Salmon (1693). Vickery (1995). Allen and Hatfield (2004). Quelch (1941). Quelch (1946). Chevallier (1996). Britten, James and Holland, Robert, *A Dictionary of English Plant Names* (English Dialect Society, 1886). Vermeulen, Nico, *Encyclopaedia of Herbs* (Rebo Productions, 1998). Pratt, Anne, *Wild Flowers* (Society for Promoting Christian Knowledge, 1898). **PENNYROYAL** Quelch (1946). Gerard (1597). Pechey (1694). De Bäiracli Levy, Juliette, *The Illustrated Herbal Handbook*, 2nd edn (Faber and Faber, 1982). Allen and Hatfield (2004). Quelch (1941). Lafont, Ann-Marie, *Devon's Heritage: A Herbal Folklore* (Badger Books, 1984). Garrad, Larch S., 'Some Manx Plant-Lore' in *Plant Lore Studies*, ed. Vickery, Roy (Folklore Society, 1984). Gerard (1597). Pechey (1694). Kemsey (1838). Wren, R. C., *Potter's New Cyclopaedia of Botanical Drugs and Preparations*, 8th edn (Health Science Press, 1975). Chevallier (1996). Britten, James, and Holland, Robert, *A Dictionary of English Plant Names* (English Dialect Society, 1886). Grieve, Mrs M., *A Modern Herbal*, ed. Leyel, Mrs C. F. (Jonathan Cape, 1931). Riddle, John M., *Contraception and Abortion from the Ancient World to the Renaissance* (Harvard University Press, 1992). Nurse S., English Folklore Survey. Notes kept at University College London. **PERIWINKLE** Grieve, Mrs M., *A Modern Herbal*, ed. Leyel, Mrs C. F. (Jonathan Cape, 1931). Extract from Apuleius Platonicus's *Herbarium*, quoted in Hooper, James, *Magical and Medicinal Plants: Descriptive Notes on some British Plants used in Witchcraft and Medicine*, pamphlet (Norwich Castle Museum, 1915). Culpeper (1652). Vickery (1995). Allen and Hatfield (2004). Pechey (1694). Kemsey (1838). Coles, William, *Adam in Eden* (London, 1657). Allen and Hatfield (2004). Chevallier (1996). **PINE** Vickery (1995). Darwin (1996). Britten, James and Holland, Robert, *A Dictionary of English Plant Names* (English Dialect Society, 1886). Milliken, W. and Bridgewater, S., *Flora Celtica: Plants and People in Scotland* (Birlinn, 2004). Darwin (1996). Milliken, W. and Bridgewater, S. (2004). Essex Age Concern Essay (1991). Milliken, W. and Bridgewater, S. (2004). Allen and Hatfield (2004). Darwin (1996). Vickery (1995). Pechey (1694). *The British Pharmacopoeia* (1914), published for the General Medical Council (London). Chevallier (1996).

POPLAR Poem from Rigg, James, *Wild Flower Lyrics and other Poems* (Alexander Gardner, 1897). Johnson, A. T. and Smith, H. A., *Plant Names Simplified*, 2nd edn (Hamlyn, 1972). Rackham, Oliver, *The History of the Countryside* (J. M. Dent & Sons, 1987). Johns, C. A., *Forest Trees of Britain* (London, 1849), quoted Vickery (1995). Vickery (1995). Darwin (1996). Rorie, David, *Folk Tradition and Folk Medicine in Scotland: the Writings of David Rorie*, ed. Buchan, David (Canongate Academic, 1994). Gerard (1597), quoted in Wren, R. C., *Potter's New Cyclopaedia of Botanical Drugs and Preparations*, 8th edn (Health Science Press, 1975). Culpeper (1652). Pechey (1694). Moncrief, John, *The Poor Man's Physician, or the Receits of the Famous John Moncrief of Tippermalloch*, 3rd edn (Edinburgh, 1731). Tongue, Ruth L., *Somerset Folklore*, ed. Briggs, K. M. (Folklore Society, 1965). Chevallier (1996). Milliken, W. and Bridgewater, S., *Flora Celtica: Plants and People in Scotland* (Birlinn, 2004). Johnson, C. Pierpoint, *The Useful Plants of Great Britain*, illus. Sowerby, John E. (Kent & Co., 1862). **POPPY** Poem from Rigg, James, *Wild Flower Lyrics and other Poems* (Alexander Gardner, 1897). Mrs W—, Wicklewood, pers. com. collected by author (1987). Mr F. C. W—, Wigby, Norwich, pers. com. collected by author (1990). Mr J. A. L—, Norwich, pers. com. collected by author (1988). Burnett, M. A., *Plantae Utiliores*, 2 vols (Whittaker, 1842). Milliken, W. and Bridgewater, S., *Flora Celtica: Plants and People in Scotland* (Birlinn, 2004). Watts, Donald C., *Elsevier's Dictionary of Plant Names and their Origins* (Elsevier, 2000). Allen and Hatfield (2004). Gunton Household Book. Salmon (1693). Gerard (1597). Culpeper (1652). Wren, R. C., *Potter's New Cyclopaedia of Botanical Drugs and Preparations*, 8th edn (Health Science Press, 1975). Chevallier (1996). **PRIMROSE** Rackham, Oliver, *The History of the Countryside* (J. M. Dent & Sons, 1987). Garrad, Larch S., 'Some Manx Plant-Lore' in *Plant Lore Studies*, ed. Vickery, Roy (Folklore Society, 1984). Vickery (1995). 'A Plain Plantain', quoted in Grieve, Mrs M., *A Modern Herbal*, ed. Leyel, Mrs C. F. (Jonathan Cape, 1931). Vickery (1995). Freethy, Ron, *From Agar to Zenry* (Crowood Press, 1985). Milliken, W. and Bridgewater, S., *Flora Celtica: Plants and People in Scotland* (Birlinn, 2004). Sharkey, Olive, *Old Days, Old Ways* (O'Brien Press, 1985). Pechey (1694). Salmon (1693). Kemsey (1838). Lloyd, Gwynedd, ed., *Lotions and Potions: Recipes of Women's Institute Members and their Ancestors* (National Federation of Women's Institutes, 1955). **PUFFBALL FAMILY** Allen and Hatfield (2004). R. H., Eriswell, Suffolk, pers. com. collected by author (1990). Mr F. C. W—, Norwich, pers. com. collected by author (1988). Allen and Hatfield (2004). Mrs C. H—, London, pers. com. collected by author (2001). Parkinson (1640). Johnson, C. Pierpoint, *The Useful Plants of Great Britain*, illus. Sowerby, John E. (Kent & Co., 1862). Beith (1995). **PURPLE LOOSESTRIFE** Marshall, Sybil, *Fenland Chronicle* (Cambridge University Press, 1967). Allen and Hatfield (2004). Culpeper (1652). Kemsey (1838). Britten, James and Holland, Robert, *A Dictionary of English Plant Names* (English Dialect Society, 1886). Chevallier

(1996). Jill Duchess of Hamilton, Penny Hart & John Simmons, *English Plants for your Garden* (Frances Lincoln, 2000). **RAGWORT** Rigg, James, *Wild Flower Lyrics and other Poems* (Alexander Gardner, 1897). Fairweather, Barbara, *Highland Plant Lore* (Glencoe and North Lorn Folk Museum, c.1980). Darwin (1996). Martin, Martin, *A Description of the Western Isles of Scotland* (A. Bell, 1703). Hulme, Frederick Edward, *Familiar Wild Flowers*, 6 vols (Cassell & Co., c.1910). Allen and Hatfield (2004). Gerard (1597). Pechey (1694). Kemsey (1838). Wren, R. C., *Potter's New Cyclopaedia of Botanical Drugs and Preparations*, 8th edn (Health Science Press, 1975). Chevallier (1996). **RAMSON OR WILD GARLIC** Fairweather, Barbara, *Highland Plant Lore* (Glencoe and North Lorn Folk Museum, c.1980). Milliken, W. and Bridgewater, S., *Flora Celtica: Plants and People in Scotland* (Birlinn, 2004). Vickery (1995). Allen and Hatfield (2004). Gerard (1597). **RASPBERRY** Grigson, Geoffrey, *The Englishman's Flora* (Phoenix House, 1955). Darwin (1996). Lightfoot, John, *Flora Scotica*, 2 vols (Benjamin White, 1777). Allen and Hatfield (2004). Vickery (1995). Fairweather, Barbara, *Highland Plant Lore* (Glencoe and North Lorn Folk Museum, c.1980). Gerard (1597). Pechey (1694). Salmon (1693). Chevallier (1996). Dyer, T. F. Thiselton, *The Folk-lore of Plants* (London, 1889); facsimile reprint (Llanerch Press, 1994). Macself, A. J., ed., *The Woman's Treasury for Home and Garden* (Amateur Gardening Offices, c.1920). **RED CAMPION** Grigson, Geoffrey, *The Englishman's Flora* (Phoenix House, 1955). Vickery (1995). Gerard (1597). Greene, Robert, 'A Quip for an Upstart Courtier' (1592), quoted in Grigson, Geoffrey, *The Englishman's Flora* (Phoenix House, 1955). Culpeper (1652). Tongue, Ruth L., *Somerset Folklore*, ed. Briggs, K. M. (Folklore Society, 1965). Allen, Andrew, *A Dictionary of Sussex Folk Medicine* (Countryside Books, 1995). Hutchinson, Peggy, *More Home-made Wine Secrets* (W. Foulsham & Co., c.1945). Bryant, Charles, *Flora Dietetica* (Benjamin White, 1783). **RED CLOVER** Mason, James, 'The Folk-lore of British Plants', *Dublin University Magazine*, vol. 82, (1873). Dyer, T. F. Thiselton, *The Folk-lore of Plants* (London, 1889); facsimile reprint (Llanerch Press, 1994). Record no. FLS M174, English Folklore Survey MSS (1960s); in University College London Library. Anonymous pamphlet, from W. T., Otley, Yorkshire. Allen and Hatfield (2004). Freethy, Ron, *From Agar to Zenry* (Crowood Press, 1985). Gerard (1597). Culpeper (1652). Salmon (1693). Chevallier (1996). Milliken, W. and Bridgewater, S., *Flora Celtica: Plants and People in Scotland* (Birlinn, 2004). **RESTHARROW** Edlin, H. L., *British Plants and their Uses* (Batsford, 1951). Gerard (1597). Pechey (1694). Salmon (1693). Moloney, Michael F., *Irish Ethnobotany and the Evolution of Medicine in Ireland* (M. H. Gill and Son, 1919). Johnson, C. Pierpoint, *The Useful Plants of Great Britain*, illus. Sowerby, John E. (Kent & Co., 1862). Chevallier (1996). Parkinson (1640). **RIBWORT PLANTAIN** Grieve, Mrs M., *A Modern Herbal*, ed. Leyel, Mrs C. F. (Jonathan Cape, 1931). Beith (1995). Allen and Hatfield (2004). Salmon (1693). Chevallier (1996). Darwin (1996). Britten, James and Holland, Robert, *A Dictionary of English Plant Names*

(English Dialect Society, 1886). **ROSEBAY WILLOWHERB** Gerard (1597). Coffey, Timothy, *The History and Folklore of North American Wildflowers* (Facts on File, New York, 1993). Green, Thomas, *The Universal Herbal*, 2nd edn (London, 1824), quoted in Grieve, Mrs M., *A Modern Herbal*, ed. Leyel, Mrs C. F. (Jonathan Cape, 1931). Bryant, Charles, *Flora Dietetica* (Benjamin White, 1783). Quelch (1946). Parkinson (1629). Grieve, Mrs M., *A Modern Herbal*, ed. Leyel, Mrs C. F. (Jonathan Cape, 1931). Chevallier (1996). Coffey, Timothy, *The History and Folklore of North American Wildflowers* (Facts on File, New York, 1993). **ROWAN OR MOUNTAIN ASH** Traditional Scottish rhyme, quoted in Black, William George, *Folk-Medicine: A Chapter in the History of Culture* (Folklore Society, 1883); reprint (Burt Franklin, 1970). Watts, Donald C., *Elsevier's Dictionary of Plant Names and their Origins* (Elsevier, 2000). Tongue, Ruth L., *Somerset Folklore*, ed. Briggs, K. M. (Folklore Society, 1965). Lafont, Ann-Marie, *Devon's Heritage: A Herbal Folklore* (Badger Books, 1984). Darwin (1996). Vickery (1995). Lightfoot, John, *Flora Scotica*, 2 vols (Benjamin White, 1777). Lafont, Ann-Marie (1984). Allen and Hatfield (2004). Moloney, Michael F., *Irish Ethnobotany and the Evolution of Medicine in Ireland* (M. H. Gill and Son, 1919). Beith (1995). Williams, Anne. E., data collected in the survey 'Folk Medicine in Living Memory in Wales, 1977–89' for the Welsh Folk museum, Cardiff; MS in her possession. Pechey (1694). Wren, R. C., *Potter's New Cyclopaedia of Botanical Drugs and Preparations*, revised by Williamson, Elizabeth M. and Evans, Fred J. (C. W. Daniel Company, 1988). Chevallier (1996). Wren, R. C. (1988). Edlin, H. L., *British Plants and their Uses* (Batsford, 1951). **RUSH** Fairweather, Barbara, *Highland Plant Lore* (Glencoe and North Lorn Folk Museum, c.1980). Moloney, Michael F., *Irish Ethnobotany and the Evolution of Medicine in Ireland* (M. H. Gill and Son, 1919). Lafont, Ann-Marie, *Devon's Heritage: A Herbal Folklore* (Badger Books, 1984). Allen and Hatfield (2004). Culpeper (1652). Vickery (1995). Britten, James and Holland, Robert, *A Dictionary of English Plant Names* (English Dialect Society, 1886). **ST JOHN'S WORT** Alfred Lear Huxford poem, quoted in Pratt, Anne, *Wild Flowers*, 2 vols (Society for Promoting Christian Knowledge, 1898), vol. I. Genders, Roy, *The Scented Wild Flowers of Britain* (Collins, 1971). Banckes, Richard, *Herball* (1525), quoted in Grigson, Geoffrey, *The Englishman's Flora* (Phoenix House, 1955). Milliken, W. and Bridgewater, S., *Flora Celtica: Plants and People in Scotland* (Birlinn, 2004). Beith (1995). Moloney, Michael F., *Irish Ethnobotany and the Evolution of Medicine in Ireland* (M. H. Gill and Son, 1919). Allen and Hatfield (2004). Milliken, W. and Bridgewater, S. (2004). Gerard (1597). Salmon (1693). Scottish Records Office, GD10/911. Kemsey (1838). Wren, R. C., *Potter's New Cyclopaedia of Botanical Drugs and Preparations*, 8th edn (Health Science Press, 1975). Chevallier (1996). Ernst, Edzard, ed., *Herbal Medicine: A Concise Overview for Professionals* (Butterworth-Heinemann, 2000). **SCARLET PIMPERNEL** Darwin (1996). Culpeper (1652). Pechey (1694). Moncrief, John, *The Poor Man's*

Physician, or the Receits of the Famous John Moncrief of Tippermalloch, 3rd edn (Edinburgh, 1731). Gunton Household Book. Kemsey (1838). Wren, R. C., *Potter's New Cyclopaedia of Botanical Drugs and Preparations*, 8th edn (Health Science Press, 1975). Chevallier (1996). Allen and Hatfield (2004). Tongue, Ruth L., *Somerset Folklore*, ed. Briggs, K. M. (Folklore Society, 1965). Watts, Donald C., *Elsevier's Dictionary of Plant Names and their Origins* (Elsevier, 2000). 'Mother Bumby' rhyme, quoted in Halliwell, James Orchard, *Popular Rhymes and Nursery Tales* (John Russell Smith, 1849). **SCOTS LOVAGE** Martin, Martin, *A Description of the Western Isles of Scotland*, 2nd edn (A. Bell, 1716), quoted in Beith (1995). Darwin (1996). Culpeper (1652). Pechey (1694). Kemsey (1838). Maclean, Alistair, *Hebridean Altars: Some Studies of the Spirit of an Island Race* (Marya Press, 1937), quoted in Beith (1995). Chevallier (1996). **SCURVYGRASS** Allen, Andrew, *A Dictionary of Sussex Folk Medicine* (Countryside Books, 1995). Freethy, Ron, *From Agar to Zenry* (Crowood Press, 1985). Pechey (1694). Allen and Hatfield (2004). Martin, Martin, *A Description of the Western Isles of Scotland* (A. Bell, 1703). Fairweather, Barbara, *Highland Plant Lore* (Glencoe and North Lorn Folk Museum, c.1980). Beith (1995). Grigson, Geoffrey, *The Englishman's Flora* (Phoenix House, 1955). Gunton Household Book. Salmon (1693). Kemsey (1838). Chevallier (1996). **SEA HOLLY** Poem from Young, Andrew, quoted in Jill Duchess of Hamilton, Penny Hart & John Simmons, *English Plants for your Garden* (Frances Lincoln, 2000). Leyel, Mrs C. F., *Elixirs of Life* (Faber and Faber, 1987). *Essex Naturalist*, quoted in Allen and Hatfield (2004). Grigson, Geoffrey, *The Englishman's Flora* (Phoenix House, 1955). Gerard (1597). Culpeper (1652). Pechey (1694). Kemsey (1838). Chevallier (1996). Allen and Hatfield (2004). Grieve, Mrs M., *A Modern Herbal*, ed. Leyel, Mrs C. F. (Jonathan Cape, 1931). **SEAWEEDS** Darwin (1996). Johnson, C. Pierpoint, *The Useful Plants of Great Britain*, illus. Sowerby, John E. (Kent & Co., 1862). Darwin (1996). Milliken, W. and Bridgewater, S., *Flora Celtica: Plants and People in Scotland* (Birlinn, 2004). Ruby E—, Essex, pers. com. collected by author (1990). Darwin (1996). Moloney, Michael F., *Irish Ethnobotany and the Evolution of Medicine in Ireland* (M. H. Gill and Son, 1919). Eley, Geoffrey, *A Hundred and One Wild Plants for the Kitchen* (E. P. Publishing Ltd, 1977). Chevallier (1996). Neill, Patrick, *A Tour through some of the Islands of Orkney and Shetland* (A. Constable & John Murray, 1806), quoted in Darwin (1996). Allen and Hatfield (2004). Martin, Martin, *A Description of the Western Isles of Scotland* (A. Bell, 1703), quoted in Milliken, W. and Bridgewater, S., *Flora Celtica: Plants and People in Scotland* (Birlinn, 2004). Johnson, C. Pierpoint (1862). Darwin (1996). Johnson, C. Pierpoint (1862). McNeill, F. Marian, *The Scots Kitchen* (Blackie & Son, 1929). Allen and Hatfield (2004). Darwin (1996). McNeill, F. Marian (1929). Bryant, Charles, *Flora Dietetica* (Benjamin White, 1783). Mrs A. A—, Walcott, pers. com. collected by author (1987). Quelch (1941). Freethy, Ron, *From Agar to Zenry* (Crowood Press, 1985). Allen and Hatfield (2004). Pechey (1694). Johnson, C. Pierpoint

(1862). Quelch (1941). Grieve, Mrs M., *A Modern Herbal*, ed. Leyel, Mrs C. F. (Jonathan Cape, 1931). Chevallier (1996). Vickery (1995). **SELFHEAL** Watts, Donald C., *Elsevier's Dictionary of Plant Names and their Origins* (Elsevier, 2000). Mabey, Richard, *Flora Britannica* (Sinclair Stevenson, 1996). Coates, Doris E., *Tuppeny Rice and Treacle: Cottage Housekeeping (1900–1920)* (Reader's Union, 1976). Allen and Hatfield (2004). Moloney, Michael F., *Irish Ethnobotany and the Evolution of Medicine in Ireland* (M. H. Gill and Son, 1919). Vickery (1995). Gerard (1597). Culpeper (1652). Kemsey (1838). Chevallier (1996). **SHEPHERD'S PURSE** Poem from Rigg, James, *Wild Flower Lyrics and other Poems* (Alexander Gardner, 1897). Milliken, W. and Bridgewater, S., *Flora Celtica: Plants and People in Scotland* (Birlinn, 2004). Grigson, Geoffrey, *The Englishman's Flora* (Phoenix House, 1955). Watts, Donald C., *Elsevier's Dictionary of Plant Names and their Origins* (Elsevier, 2000). Pechey (1694). Norfolk Records Office, MC 1811/82. Vickery (1995). Burgess, J. T., *Old English Wild Flowers* (Frederick Warne, 1868). Gerard (1597). Culpeper (1652). Salmon (1693). Wren, R. C., *Potter's New Cyclopaedia of Botanical Drugs and Preparations*, 8th edn (Health Science Press, 1975). Chevallier (1996). Pratt, Anne, *Wild Flowers*, 2 vols (Society for Promoting Christian Knowledge, 1898). Quelch (1941). Coffey, Timothy, *The History and Folklore of North American Wildflowers* (Facts on File, New York, 1993). Milliken, W. and Bridgewater, S. (2004). Bown, Deni, *The Royal Horticultural Society Encyclopedia of Herbs and their Uses* (Dorling Kindersley, 1995). **SILVERWEED** Grigson, Geoffrey, *The Englishman's Flora* (Phoenix House, 1955). Gerard (1597). Black, William George, *Folk-Medicine: A Chapter in the History of Culture* (Folklore Society, 1883); reprint (Burt Franklin, 1970). Pechey (1694). Allen and Hatfield (2004). Salmon (1693). Chevallier (1996). Darwin (1996). Pechey (1694). **SORREL** Marshall, Sybil, *Fenland Chronicle* (Cambridge University Press, 1967). Hatfield, Audrey Wynne, *Pleasures of Herbs* (London Museum Press, 1964). Evelyn, John, 'Diary', quoted in Grigson, Geoffrey, *The Englishman's Flora* (Phoenix House, 1955). Allen and Hatfield (2004). Milliken, W. and Bridgewater, S., *Flora Celtica: Plants and People in Scotland* (Birlinn, 2004). Allen and Hatfield (2004). Mrs P. M—, Selkirk, pers. com. collected by author (2002). Salmon (1693). Anon, *A Compendious Body of Physick: the Common-place Book of a late able Physician*, 3rd edn, printed in *Family Magazine*, pt II (J. Osborn, 1747). Barrett, W. H. and R. P. Garrod, *East Anglian Folklore and Other Tales* (Routledge and Kegan Paul, 1976). Chevallier (1996). Milliken, W. and Bridgewater, S. (2004). Mrs P. R—, Selkirk, pers. com. collected by author (2002). **SOW THISTLE** Topsell, Edward, *Historie of Four-footed Beasts* (1607), quoted in Dyer, T. F. Thiselton, *The Folk-lore of Plants* (London, 1889); facsimile reprint (Llanerch Press, 1994). Allen and Hatfield (2004). Mr J. K—, Norfolk, pers. com. collected by author (1989). Culpeper (1652). Kemsey (1838). Hatfield, Audrey Wynne, *How to Enjoy your Weeds* (Frederick Muller, 1969). **SPEEDWELL, BIRD'S-EYE OR GERMANDER, HEATH**

SPEEDWELL Poem from Rigg, James, *Wild Flower Lyrics and other Poems* (Alexander Gardner, 1897). Grigson, Geoffrey, *The Englishman's Flora* (Phoenix House, 1955). Britten, James and Holland, Robert, *A Dictionary of English Plant Names* (English Dialect Society, 1886). Watts, Donald C., *Elsevier's Dictionary of Plant Names and their Origins* (Elsevier, 2000). Allen and Hatfield (2004). Fargher, D. C., *The Manx Have a Word for It*, pt 5, 'Manx Gaelic Names of Flora' (privately published, Port Erin, 1969). Salmon (1693). Kemsey (1838). Chevallier (1996). Corrigan, Desmond, 'The Scientific Basis of Folk Medicine: the Irish Dimension', *Plant Lore Studies*, ed. Vickery, Roy (Folklore Society, 1984). Wren, R. C., *Potter's New Cyclopaedia of Botanical Drugs and Preparations*, revised by Williamson, Elizabeth M. and Evans, Fred J. (C. W. Daniel Company, 1988). **SPURGE** Allen and Hatfield (2004). Millspaugh, Charles F., *American Medicinal Plants* (1892), quoted in Coffey, Timothy, *The History and Folklore of North American Wildflowers* (Facts on File, New York, 1993). Gerard (1597). Parkinson (1640). Chevallier (1996). Salmon (1693). Hatfield, Audrey Wynne, *How to Enjoy your Weeds* (Frederick Muller, 1969). Plues, Margaret, *Rambles in Search of Wild Flowers*, 4th edn (George Bell, 1892). **STONECROP** Evans, Revd R. W., quoted in Pratt, Anne, *Wild Flowers*, 2 vols (Society for Promoting Christian Knowledge, 1898), vol. I. Hulme, Frederick Edward, *Familiar Wild Flowers*, 6 vols (Cassell & Co., c.1910). Vickery (1995). Evelyn, John, 'Acetaria: A Discourse of Sallets' (London, 1699), quoted in Coffey, Timothy, *The History and Folklore of North American Wildflowers* (Facts on File, New York, 1993). Beith (1995). Allen and Hatfield (2004). Fairweather, Barbara, *Highland Plant Lore* (Glencoe and North Lorn Folk Museum, c.1980). Grieve, Mrs M., *A Modern Herbal*, ed. Leyel, Mrs C. F. (Jonathan Cape, 1931). Johnson, C. Pierpoint, *The Useful Plants of Great Britain*. illus. Sowerby, John E. (Kent & Co., 1862). Friend, H., *A Glossary of Devonshire Plant-names* (London, 1882), quoted in Vickery (1995). **STRAWBERRY, WILD** Butler, Dr William (1535–1618), quoted in Walton, Izaac, *The Compleat Angler* (London, 1653). Darwin (1996). Household Roll of the Countess of Leicester, quoted in Grieve, Mrs M., *A Modern Herbal*, ed. Leyel, Mrs C. F. (Jonathan Cape, 1931). Nuttall, G. Clarke, *Wild Flowers as They Grow*, 5 vols (Waverley Book Company, c.1920). Tusser, Thomas, *Five Hundred Pointes of Good Husbandrie* (London, 1557). Aubrey, John, *Natural History of Wiltshire* (London, 1685); ed. Britten, J. (1847). Fairweather, Barbara, *Highland Plant Lore* (Glencoe and North Lorn Folk Museum, c.1980). Deane, Tony and Shaw, Tony, *The Folklore of Cornwall* (Batsford, 1975). Gerard (1597). Parkinson (1629). Nuttall, G. Clarke, *Wild Flowers as They Grow*, 5 vols (Waverley Book Company, c.1920). Culpeper (1652). Gunton Household Book. Kemsey (1838). Chevallier (1996). Grieve, Mrs M., *A Modern Herbal*, ed. Leyel, Mrs C. F. (Jonathan Cape, 1931). **SUNDEW** Poem from Rigg, James, *Wild Flower Lyrics and other Poems* (Alexander Gardner, 1897). Garrad, Larch S., 'Some Manx Plant-Lore' in *Plant Lore Studies*, ed. Vickery, Roy (Folklore

Society, 1984). Milliken, W. and Bridgewater, S., *Flora Celtica: Plants and People in Scotland* (Birlinn, 2004). Darwin (1996). Allen and Hatfield (2004). Fairweather, Barbara, *Highland Plant Lore* (Glencoe and North Lorn Folk Museum, c.1980). Turner, William, *A New Herball* (London and Cologne, 1568). Gunton Household Book. Darwin (1996). Culpeper (1652). Pechey (1694). Chevallier (1996). Fairweather, Barbara (c.1980). Darwin (1996). **SWEET VIOLET** Poem from Fletcher, John, quoted in Quiller-Couch, Sir Arthur, ed., *The Oxford Book of English Verse* (Oxford University Press, 1939). Hatfield, Audrey Wynne, *Pleasures of Herbs* (London Museum Press, 1964). Gerard (1597). Hatfield, Audrey Wynne (1964). Culpeper (1652). Salmon (1693). Pechey (1694). Kemsey (1838). Chevallier (1996). Farnsworth, N. R., et al., 'Biological and Phytochemical Evaluation of Plants'. *Lloydia* 31 (1968), p. 246. Macself, A. J., ed., *The Woman's Treasury for Home and Garden* (Amateur Gardening Offices, c.1920). Quelch (1941). Lightfoot, John, *Flora Scotica*, 2 vols (Benjamin White, 1777), quoted in Darwin (1996). Allen and Hatfield (2004). Hughes, Anne, *The Diary of a Farmer's Wife 1796–7* (Penguin Books, 1981). Tongue, Ruth L., *Somerset Folklore*, ed. Briggs, K. M. (Folklore Society, 1965). Allen and Hatfield (2004). **TANSY** Boerhaave, Dr Hermann, quoted in Johnson, C. Pierpoint, *The Useful Plants of Great Britain*, illus. Sowerby, John E. (Kent & Co., 1862). Britten, James and Holland, Robert, *A Dictionary of English Plant Names* (English Dialect Society, 1886). Hulme, Frederick Edward, *Familiar Wild Flowers*, 6 vols (Cassell & Co., c.1910). Evans, George Ewart, *The Farm and the Village* (Faber and Faber, 1969). Mr F. C. W—, Norwich, pers. com. collected by author (1990). Taylor, Dr Mark R., 'Magic, witchcraft, charm-cures and customs in East Anglia', data for a never-published book, collected largely by correspondence, while Regional Medical Officer in Norwich 1920–27 (Norfolk Record Office, MS 4322, 57x1). Milliken, W. and Bridgewater, S., *Flora Celtica: Plants and People in Scotland* (Birlinn, 2004). Allen and Hatfield (2004). Porter, Enid M., *Cambridgeshire Customs and Folklore* (Routledge, 1969). Vesey-Fitzgerald (1944), quoted in Vickery (1995). Allen and Hatfield (2004). Milliken, W. and Bridgewater, S. (2004). Record no. NM1 52, English Folklore Survey MSS (1960s); in University College London Library. Mrs M. H—, Skipton, pers. com. collected by author (1980). Culpeper (1652). Kemsey (1838). Chevallier (1996). Gerard (1597). Norfolk Records Office, N.R.O. 26354. Pratt, Anne, *Wild Flowers*, 2 vols (Society for Promoting Christian Knowledge, 1898). Article by Westwood, Jennifer, *Flora, Facts and Fables*, ed. Corne, Grace, no. 20 (winter 1999). **TEASEL** Johnson, A. T. and Smith, H. A., *Plant Names Simplified*, 2nd edn (Hamlyn, 1972). Grieve, Mrs M., *A Modern Herbal*, ed. Leyel, Mrs C. F. (Jonathan Cape, 1931). Vickery (1995). Chevallier (1996). Gerard (1597). Allen and Hatfield (2004). Culpeper (1652). Pechey (1694). Chevallier (1996). Edlin, H. L., *British Plants and their Uses* (Batsford, 1951). **THISTLE** Poem by Dixon, Richard Watson, lines 7–9, from Quiller-Couch, Sir Arthur, ed., *The Oxford Book of English Verse* (Oxford University

Press, 1939). Fairweather, Barbara, *Highland Plant Lore* (Glencoe and North Lorn Folk Museum, *c.*1980). Gerard (1597). Coffey, Timothy, *The History and Folklore of North American Wildflowers* (Facts on File, New York, 1993). Jefferies, Richard, *Wild Life in a Southern County* (Nelson, n.d.). Prince, Dennis, *Grandmother's Cures: An A–Z of Herbal Remedies* (Fontana, 1991). Kemsey (1838). Salmon (1693). Grieve, Mrs M., *A Modern Herbal*, ed. Leyel, Mrs C. F. (Jonathan Cape, 1931). Chevallier (1996). Grieve, Mrs M. (1931). Allen and Hatfield (2004). **THYME** Armstrong, John, 'The Art of Preserving Health: A Poem', quoted in Black, William George, *Folk-Medicine: A Chapter in the History of Culture*, (Folklore Society, 1883); reprint (Burt Franklin, 1970). Quelch (1941). Dyer, T. F. Thiselton, *The Folk-lore of Plants* (London, 1889); facsimile reprint (Llanerch Press, 1994). Nuttall, G. Clarke, *Wild Flowers as They Grow*, 5 vols (Waverley Book Company, *c.*1920). Vickery (1995). Allen and Hatfield (2004). Dyer, T. F. Thiselton (Llanerch Press, 1994). Milliken, W. and Bridgewater, S., *Flora Celtica: Plants and People in Scotland* (Birlinn, 2004). Culpeper (1652). Pechey (1694). Johnson, C. Pierpoint, *The Useful Plants of Great Britain*, illus. Sowerby, John E. (Kent & Co., 1862). Chevallier (1996). Hutchinson, Peggy, *More Home-made Wine Secrets* (W. Foulsham & Co., *c.*1945). Beith (1995). Milliken, W. and Bridgewater, S. (2004). Darwin (1996). **TORMENTIL** Lightfoot, John, letter (1772), quoted in Darwin (1996). Moffat, Dr Brian, Midlothian, Scotland, pers. com. collected by author (1995). Vickery (1995). Freethy, Ron, *From Agar to Zenry* (Crowood Press, 1985). Darwin (1996). Allen and Hatfield (2004). Lightfoot, John, *Flora Scotica* (1777), quoted in Darwin (1996). Salmon (1693). Pechey (1694). Gerard (1597). Grieve, Mrs M., *A Modern Herbal*, ed. Leyel, Mrs C. F. (Jonathan Cape, 1931). Chevallier (1996). Grigson, Geoffrey, *The Englishman's Flora* (Phoenix House, 1955). Darwin (1996). Freethy, Ron (1985). Grieve, Mrs M. (1931). **TRAVELLER'S JOY** Gerard (1597). Johnson, A. T. and Smith, H. A., *Plant Names Simplified*, 2nd edn (Hamlyn, 1972). Vickery (1995). Johnson, C. Pierpoint, *The Useful Plants of Great Britain*, illus. Sowerby, John E. (Kent & Co., 1862). Hulme, Frederick Edward, *Familiar Wild Flowers*, 6 vols (Cassell & Co., *c.*1910). Vickery (1995). Tongue, Ruth L., *Somerset Folklore*, ed. Briggs, K. M. (Folklore Society, 1965). Gerard (1597). Johnson, C. Pierpoint (1862). Grieve, Mrs M., *A Modern Herbal*, ed. Leyel, Mrs C. F. (Jonathan Cape, 1931). Chevallier (1996). Freethy, Ron, *From Agar to Zenry* (Crowood Press, 1985). **VALERIAN** Coles, William, *Adam in Eden* (1657), quoted in Britten, James and Holland, Robert, *A Dictionary of English Plant Names* (English Dialect Society, 1886). Grieve, Mrs M., *A Modern Herbal*, ed. Leyel, Mrs C. F. (Jonathan Cape, 1931). Turner, William (1568), quoted in Grieve, Mrs M., *A Modern Herbal*, ed. Leyel, Mrs C. F. (Jonathan Cape, 1931). Allen and Hatfield (2004). Gerard (1597). Chaucer, Geoffrey, quoted in Watts, Donald C., *Elsevier's Dictionary of Plant Names and their Origins* (Elsevier, 2000). Culpeper (1652). Pechey (1694). Mr D. K—, Suffolk, own MS. Gunton Household Book. Colonna, Fabio,

Phytobasanos (Naples, 1592). Kemsey (1838). Grieve, Mrs M., *A Modern Herbal*, ed. Leyel, Mrs C. F. (Jonathan Cape, 1931). Ernst, Edzard, ed., *Herbal Medicine: A Concise Overview for Professionals* (Butterworth-Heinemann, 2000). Chevallier (1996). Mrs C. A—, Peebles-shire, pers. com. collected by author (1975). Burnett, M. A., *Plantae Utiliores*, 2 vols (Whittaker, 1842). **VERVAIN** Elizabethan MS, Chetham Library, Manchester, quoted in Burnett, M. A., *Plantae Utiliores*, 2 vols (Whittaker, 1842). Dyer, T. F. Thiselton, *The Folk-lore of Plants* (London, 1889); facsimile reprint (Llanerch Press, 1994). Black, William George, *Folk-Medicine: A Chapter in the History of Culture* (Folklore Society, 1883); reprint (Burt Franklin, 1970). Vickery (1995). Lafont, Ann-Marie, *Devon's Heritage: A Herbal Folklore* (Badger Books, 1984). Garrad, Larch S., 'Some Manx Plant-Lore' in *Plant Lore Studies*, ed. Vickery, Roy (Folklore Society, 1984). Watts, Donald C., *Elsevier's Dictionary of Plant Names and their Origins* (Elsevier, 2000). Allen and Hatfield (2004). Hatfield, Gabrielle, *Country Remedies: Traditional East Anglian Plant Remedies in the Twentieth Century* (Boydell Press, 1994). Old-English medical manuscript, Stockholm Library (*c.*1400), reproduced in *Anglia*, vol. 18 (1896), p. 325. Gerard (1597). Culpeper (1652). Pechey (1694). Moncrief, John, *The Poor Man's Physician, or the Receits of the Famous John Moncrief of Tippermalloch*, 3rd edn (Edinburgh, 1731). Gunton Household Book. Kemsey (1838). Chevallier (1996). Ernst, Edzard, ed., *Herbal Medicine: A Concise Overview for Professionals* (Butterworth-Heinemann, 2000). Scottish Records Office, GD1/384/26. **WATERCRESS** Poem from Rigg, James, *Wild Flower Lyrics and other Poems* (Alexander Gardner, 1897). Vickery (1995). Beith (1995). Darwin (1996). Mr C—, Norton Subcourse, pers. com. collected by author (1989). Allen and Hatfield (2004). William Kingsbury's Notebook, Sprowston, Norfolk (1710); in Gressenhall Museum, G.7.983. Mrs E. P—, Co. Londonderry, pers. com. collected by author (2002). Salmon (1693). Culpeper (1652). Johnson, C. Pierpoint, *The Useful Plants of Great Britain*, illus. Sowerby, John E. (Kent & Co., 1862). Chevallier (1996). Moloney, Michael F., *Irish Ethnobotany and the Evolution of Medicine in Ireland* (M. H. Gill and Son, 1919). Hatfield, Audrey Wynne, *Pleasures of Herbs* (London Museum Press, 1964). **WHITE BRYONY** Gerard (1597). Pechey (1694). Allen, Andrew, *A Dictionary of Sussex Folk Medicine* (Countryside Books, 1995). Mrs D. P—, Little Totham, pers. com. collected by author (1989). Britten, James and Holland, Robert, *A Dictionary of English Plant Names* (English Dialect Society, 1886). Allen and Hatfield (2004). Johnson, C. Pierpoint, *The Useful Plants of Great Britain*, illus. Sowerby, John E. (Kent & Co., 1862). Porter, Enid M., *The Folklore of East Anglia* (Batsford, 1974). Grigson, Geoffrey, *The Englishman's Flora* (Phoenix House, 1955). William Kingsbury's Notebook, Sprowston, Norfolk (1710); in Gressenhall Museum, G.7.983. Chevallier (1996). Pechey (1694). Pomet, Pierre, *A Compleat History of Druggs*, 3rd edn (Bonwicke, 1737), quoted in Watts, Donald C., *Elsevier's Dictionary of Plant Names and their Origins* (Elsevier, 2000). Chevallier (1996). Wren, R. C., *Potter's New*

Cyclopaedia of Botanical Drugs and Preparations, revised by Williamson, Elizabeth M. and Evans, Fred J. (C. W. Daniel Company, 1988). **WHITE DEADNETTLE** Verse by Bishop Mant, quoted in Plues, Margaret, *Rambles in Search of Wild Flowers*, 4th edn (George Bell, 1892). Allen and Hatfield (2004). Pechey (1694). Hill, Sir John (*c*.1820). Chevallier (1996). Gerard (1597). Johnson, C. Pierpoint, *The Useful Plants of Great Britain*, illus. Sowerby, John E. (Kent & Co., 1862). Hatfield, Audrey Wynne, *How to Enjoy your Weeds* (Frederick Muller, 1969). Hutchinson, Peggy, *More Home-made Wine Secrets* (W. Foulsham & Co., *c*.1945). **WHITE HOREHOUND** Poem by Drayton, Michael, quoted in Genders, Roy, *The Scented Wild Flowers of Britain* (Collins, 1971). Allen and Hatfield (2004). Miss G—, Attleborough (*c*.1930), quoted in Taylor, Dr Mark R., 'Magic, witchcraft, charm-cures and customs in East Anglia', data for a never-published book, collected largely by correspondence, while Regional Medical Officer in Norwich 1920–27 (Norfolk Record Office, MS 4322, 57X1). Gerard (1597). Quelch (1946). **WHITE WATER LILY, YELLOW WATER LILY** Darwin (1996). Grigson, Geoffrey, *The Englishman's Flora* (Phoenix House, 1955). Pechey (1694). Culpeper (1652). Withering, William, *A Botanical Arrangement of British Plants*, 2nd edn (M. Swinney, 1787–92). Darwin (1996). Scottish Records Office, GD10/911. Kemsey (1838). Chevallier (1996). Fairweather, Barbara, *Highland Plant Lore* (Glencoe and North Lorn Folk Museum, *c*.1980). Darwin (1996). **WILD CARROT** Milliken, W. and Bridgewater, S., *Flora Celtica: Plants and People in Scotland* (Birlinn, 2004). Beith (1995). Mabberley, D. J., *The Plant-Book* (Cambridge University Press, 1987). Darwin (1996). Gerard (1597). Allen and Hatfield (2004). Pennant, Thomas, *A Tour in Scotland and Voyage to the Hebrides* (1772), quoted in Beith (1995). Taylor, Dr Mark R., 'Magic, witchcraft, charm-cures and customs in East Anglia', data for a never-published book, collected largely by correspondence, while Regional Medical Officer in Norwich 1920–27 (Norfolk Record Office, MS 4322, 57X1). Pechey (1694). Kemsey (1838). Chevallier (1996). **WILD CHERRY** Genders, Roy, *The Scented Wild Flowers of Britain* (Collins, 1971). Darwin (1996). Vickery (1995). Hatfield, Gabrielle, *Country Remedies: Traditional East Anglian Plant Remedies in the Twentieth Century* (Boydell Press, 1994). Beith (1995). Pechey (1694). Gerard (1597). Culpeper (1652). Gunton Household Book. Chevallier (1996). Vickery (1995). Milliken, W. and Bridgewater, S., *Flora Celtica: Plants and People in Scotland* (Birlinn, 2004). Mrs J. S—, Essex, pers. com. collected by author (1991). **WILLOW** Poem by Dixon, Richard Watson, lines 1–3, quoted in Quiller-Couch, Sir Arthur, ed., *The Oxford Book of English Verse* (Oxford University Press, 1939). Freethy, Ron, *From Agar to Zenry* (Crowood Press, 1985). Allen and Hatfield (2004). Porter, Enid M., *The Folklore of East Anglia* (Batsford, 1974). Gerard (1597). Culpeper (1652). Salmon (1693). Allen and Hatfield (2004). Kemsey (1838). Chevallier (1996). Tongue, Ruth L., *Somerset Folklore*, ed. Briggs, K. M. (Folklore Society, 1965). Milliken, W. and Bridgewater, S., *Flora Celtica: Plants and People in Scotland* (Birlinn, 2004). Darwin (1996).

Fairweather, Barbara, *Highland Plant Lore* (Glencoe and North Lorn Folk Museum, *c*.1980). Jefferies, Richard, *Wild Life in a Southern County* (Nelson, n.d.). **WOOD SORREL** Watts, Donald C., *Elsevier's Dictionary of Plant Names and their Origins* (Elsevier, 2000). Pechey (1694). Grieve, Mrs M., *A Modern Herbal*, ed. Leyel, Mrs C. F. (Jonathan Cape, 1931). Fairweather, Barbara, *Highland Plant Lore* (Glencoe and North Lorn Folk Museum, *c*.1980). Allen and Hatfield (2004). Grieve, Mrs M. (1931). Gerard (1597). Culpeper (1652). Kemsey (1838). **WOODY NIGHTSHADE** Poem from Rigg, James, *Wild Flower Lyrics and other Poems* (Alexander Gardner, 1897). Culpeper (1652). Hodgson, William, Flora of Cumberland (Carlisle: W. Meals, 1898). Bown, Deni, *The Royal Horticultural Society Encyclopedia of Herbs and their Uses* (Dorling Kindersley, 1995). Salmon (1693). Allen and Hatfield (2004). Ranson, Florence, *British Herbs* (Penguin, 1949). Taylor, Dr Mark R., 'Magic, witchcraft, charm-cures and customs in East Anglia', data for a never-published book, collected largely by correspondence, while Regional Medical Officer in Norwich 1920–27 (Norfolk Record Office, MS 4322, 57X1). Allen and Hatfield (2004). Gerard (1597). Culpeper (1652). Pechey (1694). Salmon (1693). Kemsey (1838). Chevallier (1996). **WORMWOOD** Allen and Hatfield (2004). Allen, Andrew, *A Dictionary of Sussex Folk Medicine* (Countryside Books, 1995). Mr M. G. R—, Lakenheath, pers. com. collected by author (1990). Coffey, Timothy, *The History and Folklore of North American Wildflowers* (Facts on File, New York, 1993). Pechey (1694). Kemsey (1838). Chevallier (1996). Quelch (1941). Tongue, Ruth L., *Somerset Folklore*, ed. Briggs, K. M. (Folklore Society, 1965). Lafont, Ann-Marie, *Devon's Heritage: A Herbal Folklore* (Badger Books, 1984). Dyer, T. F. Thiselton, *The Folk-lore of Plants* (London, 1889); facsimile reprint (Llanerch Press, 1994). Chevallier (1996). Ernst, Edzard, ed., *Herbal Medicine: A Concise Overview for Professionals* (Butterworth-Heinemann, 2000). **WOUNDWORT** Johnson, C. Pierpoint, *The Useful Plants of Great Britain*, illus. Sowerby, John E. (Kent & Co., 1862). Gerard (1597). Allen and Hatfield (2004). Culpeper (1652). Pechey (1694). Wren, R. C., *Potter's New Cyclopaedia of Botanical Drugs and Preparations*, 8th edn (Health Science Press, 1975). Hoffmann, David, *The Holistic Herbal* (Findhorn Press, 1986). Wren, R. C., *Potter's New Cyclopaedia of Botanical Drugs and Preparations*, revised by Williamson, Elizabeth M. and Evans, Fred J. (C. W. Daniel Company, 1988). **YARROW** Porter, Enid M., *The Folklore of East Anglia* (Batsford, 1974). Milliken, W. and Bridgewater, S., *Flora Celtica: Plants and People in Scotland* (Birlinn, 2004). Mrs A. A—, Norfolk, pers. com. collected by author (1989). Allen and Hatfield (2004). Essex Age Concern Essay (1991). Milliken, W. and Bridgewater, S. (2004). Salmon (1693). Gerard (1597). Culpeper (1652). Gunton Household Book. Grieve, Mrs M., *A Modern Herbal*, ed. Leyel, Mrs C. F. (Jonathan Cape, 1931). Chevallier (1996). Newall, Carol A., Anderson, Linda A. and Phillipson, J. David, *Herbal Medicines: A Guide for Health Professionals* (Pharmaceutical Press, 1996). Halliwell, James Orchard, *Popular Rhymes and*

Nursery Tales (John Russell Smith, 1849). Watts, Donald C., *Elsevier's Dictionary of Plant Names and their Origins* (Elsevier, 2000). 'Tich', Tranmere, pers. com. collected by author (1985). **YELLOW FLAG IRIS** Darwin (1996). Pechey (1694). Vickery (1995). Milliken, W. and Bridgewater, S., *Flora Celtica: Plants and People in Scotland* (Birlinn, 2004). Allen and Hatfield (2004). Milliken, W. and Bridgewater, S. (2004). Allen and Hatfield (2004). Mr F. C. W—, Norwich, pers. com. collected by author (1989). Gerard (1597). Culpeper (1652). Johnson, C. Pierpoint, *The Useful Plants of Great Britain*, illus. Sowerby, John E. (Kent & Co., 1862). Kemsey (1838). Wren, R. C., *Potter's New Cyclopaedia of Botanical Drugs and Preparations*, 8th edn (Health Science Press, 1975). Chiej, Roberto, *The Macdonald Encyclopedia of Medicinal Plants* (Macdonald, 1984). **YELLOW LOOSESTRIFE** Poem by Collins, quoted in Nuttall, G. Clarke, *Wild Flowers as They Grow*, 5 vols (Waverley Book Company, c.1920). Culpeper (1652). Coates, Doris E., *Tuppeny Rice and Treacle: Cottage Housekeeping (1900–1920)* (Reader's Union, 1976). Vickery (1995). Culpeper (1652). Kemsey (1838). Gerard (1597). Pechey (1694). Gerard (1597). Chevallier (1996). **YELLOW TOADFLAX** Watts, Donald C., *Elsevier's Dictionary of Plant Names and their Origins* (Elsevier, 2000). Allen and Hatfield (2004). Fairweather, Barbara, *Highland Plant Lore* (Glencoe and North Lorn Folk Museum, c.1980). Ray, John, *Catalogus Plantarum* (1660),

quoted in Vickery (1995). Burgess, J. T., *Old English Wild Flowers* (Frederick Warne, 1868). Gerard (1597). Culpeper (1652). Pechey (1694). Chevallier (1996). Grieve, Mrs M., *A Modern Herbal*, ed. Leyel, Mrs C. F. (Jonathan Cape, 1931). **YEW** Vickery (1995). Darwin (1996). Vickery (1995). Rootsey, Samuel, 'Observations upon some of the medical plants mentioned by Shakespeare', *Transactions of the Royal Medico-botanical Society* 1832–33 (Royal Medico-botanical Society, London). Gerard (1597). Parkinson (1629). Taylor, Dr Mark R., 'Magic, witchcraft, charm-cures and customs in East Anglia', data for a never-published book, collected largely by correspondence, while Regional Medical Officer in Norwich 1920–27 (Norfolk Record Office, MS 4322, 57x1). Allen and Hatfield (2004). Kightly, Charles, *Country Voices: Life and Lore in Farm and Village* (Thames and Hudson, 1984). Dyer, T. F. Thiselton, *The Folk-lore of Plants* (London, 1889); facsimile reprint (Llanerch Press, 1994). Addy, S. O., *Household Tales, with Other Traditional Remains collected in the Counties of York, Lincoln, Derby and Nottingham* (1895), quoted in Radford, E. and Radford, M. A., *Encyclopaedia of Superstitions*, edited and revised by Hole, Christina (Hutchinson, 1974). Chevallier (1996). Johnson, A. T. and Smith, H. A., *Plant Names Simplified*, 2nd edn (Hamlyn, 1972). Step, Edward, *Wayside and Woodland Trees* (Frederick Warne, n.d.). Darwin (1996).

Further Reading

Allen, David E. and Gabrielle Hatfield, *Medicinal Plants in Folk Tradition: An Ethnobotany of Britain and Ireland* (Timber Press, 1999). This book brings together for the first time a large number of records of the folk usage (as opposed to the official usage employed by health professionals) of our native medicinal plants.

Bown, Deni, *The Royal Horticultural Society Encyclopedia of Herbs and Their Uses* (Dorling Kindersley, 1995). This is a meticulously researched and comprehensive account of herbal plants from all over the world, giving their uses as well as their cultivation requirements. The colour photographs, mostly taken by the author, make recognition easy.

Chevallier, Andrew, *The Encyclopedia of Medicinal Plants* (Dorling Kindersley, 1996). This is an authoritative account of the plants (some native to Britain, but also many non-native) used by medical herbalists, and written by the leading herbalist responsible for setting up the first degree course in medical herbalism in this country. It is beautifully illustrated.

Griggs, Barbara, *New Green Pharmacy: The Story of Western Herbal Medicine* (second edition; Vermilion, 1997). This is a thorough and unrivalled account of the history of official medical herbalism in this country and its inter-relations with North American herbalism.

Mabey, Richard, *Flora Britannica* (Sinclair Stevenson, 1996). Contains some wonderful pictures of our native wild flowers. There are numerous accounts of first-hand floral memories of contributors and some accounts, though relatively few, of the flowers' medicinal usage.

Milliken, William, and Bridgewater, Sam, *Flora Celtica: Plants and People in Scotland* (Birlinn, 2004). The authors' botanical careers have taken them all over the world. In this book they provide a wonderfully rich account of the inter-relations between mankind and plants in Scotland. There are a large number of recent original records as well as historical insights. The book is a delight for its illustrations too.

Vickery, Roy, *A Dictionary of Plant Lore* (Oxford University Press, 1995). Written by the Curator of Flowering Plants at the Natural History Museum, London, this is a fascinating collection of folklore, much of it gathered first-hand by the author and some collected from written accounts.

Index

Note: Page numbers in **bold** denote the main entry for each plant

PENGUIN NATURAL HISTORY

THE SECRET LIFE OF TREES
COLIN TUDGE

'A love-letter to trees' *Financial Times*

What is a tree? As this celebration of trees shows, they are our countryside; our ancestors descended from them; they give us air to breathe. Yet while the stories of trees are as plentiful as leaves in a forest, they are rarely told.

Here, Colin Tudge travels from his own back garden round the world to explore the beauty, variety and ingenuity of trees everywhere: from how they live so long to how they talk to each other and why they came to exist in the first place. Lyrical and evocative, this book will make everyone fall in love with the trees around them.

'One of those books you want everyone to have already read' *Sunday Telegraph*

'Everyone interested in the natural world will enjoy *The Secret Life of Trees*. I found myself reading out whole chunks to friends' *The Times*, Books of the Year

'Wondrous and important ... You'll discover how the maple leaf turns red in the fall, why koalas have such small brains, and the five other tree-products, after the wood of the white willow, that make up a cricket bat ... a holy botanical litany' *Guardian*

'Magnificent. Tudge wanders, trailing astonishing facts and lore behind him' *Oldie*

PENGUIN REFERENCE

THE LORE OF THE LAND
WESTWOOD AND SIMPSON

Where can you find the 'Devil's footprints'?

What happened at the 'hangman's stone'?

Did Sweeney Todd, the demon barber of Fleet Street, really exist?

Where was King Arthur laid to rest?

Bringing together tales of hauntings, highwaymen, family curses and lovers' leaps, this magnificent guide will take you on a magical journey through England's legendary past.

'A real treasury' Philip Pullman

'A treasure-house of extraordinary tales, rooted in the wildly various and haunted landscapes of England' *Sunday Times*

'A fascinating county-by county guidebook to headless horsemen, bottomless pools, immured adulteresses and talking animals' *London Review of Books*

'Wonderful . . . Contains almost every myth, legend and ghost story ever told in England' Simon Hoggart, *Guardian*

Penguin Travel/Architecture

ENGLAND'S THOUSAND BEST HOUSES
SIMON JENKINS

'The perfect guide to England's best houses' *Country Life*

'Buy, beg, borrow or steal a copy to keep in the car' *Daily Mail*

'This wonderful book will be in everyone's car pocket for decades …
It makes me want to take a year off … and plunge off into what Jenkins has
memorably described as "the theatre of our shared memory"'
Adam Nicolson, *Evening Standard*

England's houses are a treasure trove of riches and a unique, living record of
the nation's history. Simon Jenkins's lavishly illustrated guide selects the finest
homes throughout the land, from Cornwall to Cumbria, in a glorious
celebration of English life.

• Ranges from famous stately homes and palaces to humble cottages and huts

• Organized county-by-county for easy use

• Features a star ratings system for each house

• Highlights the very best 100 of all the properties in the country

'A heritage enthusiast's *Ode To Joy* … Any passably cultured inhabitant of the
British Isles should ask for, say, three or four copies of this book'
Max Hastings, *Sunday Telegraph*

'This is the perfect book to have beside your bed or on the back seat of your car
… Jenkins's zeal is infectious. He quite rightly sees England's greatest houses as
collectively nothing less than a wonder of the world' Geordie Greig,
Literary Review

'A great book … a feast, enlivened by the sort of tasty snippets that only a
master journalist can produce' Hugh Massingberd, *Daily Telegraph*

Penguin Travel/Architecture

ENGLAND'S THOUSAND BEST CHURCHES
SIMON JENKINS

'Think of Simon Jenkins's book as a hip flask and carry it always' *Daily Mail*

'Marvellous … this is a book to be kept by the bed or, better still, in the car. A constant excuse to leave the bold highway and let the imagination, body and soul, wander a little' Anna Ford, *Sunday Telegraph*

England's Thousand Best Churches is a celebration of our most glorious and lasting national monuments. Simon Jenkins has travelled England to select the finest churches of all periods and styles, revealing not only an unparalleled collection of English art, but the history of a people.

• With churches from all periods and denominations

• Organized county-by-county for easy use

• Features a star ratings system for each church

• Highlights the very best 100

'Every house in England should have a copy of this book' Auberon Waugh, *Literary Review* Book of the Century

'So excellent are Paul Barker's pictures … so mouthwatering are Jenkins's descriptions of the buildings he loves, that you want to visit the churches instantly' Andrew Lloyd Webber, *Daily Telegraph*

'In his journeys through the English counties, greater knowledge has deepened his sense that so many of our churches are celebrations in wood and stone of the spirit of the people of England, and they continue to be doors into mystery' Richard Chartres, *The Times*

He just wanted a decent book to read ...

Not too much to ask, is it? It was in 1935 when Allen Lane, Managing Director of Bodley Head Publishers, stood on a platform at Exeter railway station looking for something good to read on his journey back to London. His choice was limited to popular magazines and poor-quality paperbacks – the same choice faced every day by the vast majority of readers, few of whom could afford hardbacks. Lane's disappointment and subsequent anger at the range of books generally available led him to found a company – and change the world.

'We believed in the existence in this country of a vast reading public for intelligent books at a low price, and staked everything on it'
Sir Allen Lane, 1902–1970, founder of Penguin Books

The quality paperback had arrived – and not just in bookshops. Lane was adamant that his Penguins should appear in chain stores and tobacconists, and should cost no more than a packet of cigarettes.

Reading habits (and cigarette prices) have changed since 1935, but Penguin still believes in publishing the best books for everybody to enjoy. We still believe that good design costs no more than bad design, and we still believe that quality books published passionately and responsibly make the world a better place.

So wherever you see the little bird – whether it's on a piece of prize-winning literary fiction or a celebrity autobiography, political tour de force or historical masterpiece, a serial-killer thriller, reference book, world classic or a piece of pure escapism – you can bet that it represents the very best that the genre has to offer.

Whatever you like to read – trust Penguin.